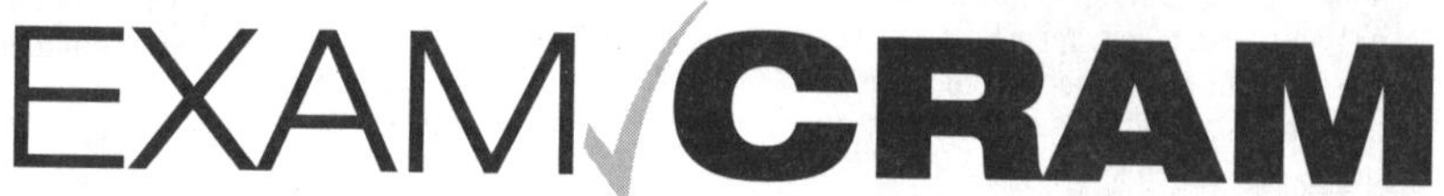

NCLEX-PN®

Practice Questions

Third Edition

Wilda Rinehart
Diann Sloan
Clara Hurd

800 East 96th Street, Indianapolis, Indiana 46240 USA

NCLEX-PN® Practice Questions, Third Edition

ISBN-13: 978-0-7897-4105-9
ISBN-10: 0-7897-4105-9

Library of Congress Cataloging-in-Publication Data

Rinehart, Wilda.
NCLEX-PN practice questions exam cram. -- 3rd ed. / Wilda Rinehart, Diann Sloan, Clara Hurd.
p. ; cm.
Includes index.
Rev. ed. of: NCLEX-PN exam prep / Wilda Rinehart, Diann Sloan, Clara Hurd. c2011.
ISBN-13: 978-0-7897-4105-9 (pbk. w/CD)
ISBN-10: 0-7897-4105-9 (pbk. w/CD)
I. Sloan, Diann. II. Hurd, Clara. III. Rinehart, Wilda. NCLEX-PN exam prep. IV. Title.
[DNLM: 1. Nursing, Practical--Examination Questions. WY 18.2]
LC classification not assigned
610.73076--dc23

2011032123

Printed in the United States on America
Fifth Printing: December 2012

Trademarks

All terms mentioned in this book that are known to be trademarks or service marks have been appropriately capitalized. Pearson cannot attest to the accuracy of this information. Use of a term in this book should not be regarded as affecting the validity of any trademark or service mark.

NCLEX® is a registered trademark of the National Council of State Boards of Nursing, Inc. (NCSBN), which does not sponsor or endorse this product.

Warning and Disclaimer

Every effort has been made to make this book as complete and as accurate as possible, but no warranty or fitness is implied. The information provided is on an "as is" basis. The author and the publisher shall have neither liability nor responsibility to any person or entity with respect to any loss or damages arising from the information contained in this book or from the use of the CD or programs accompanying it.

Bulk Sales

Que Publishing offers excellent discounts on this book when ordered in quantity for bulk purchases or special sales. For more information, please contact

U.S. Corporate and Government Sales
1-800-382-3419
corpsales@pearsontechgroup.com

For sales outside of the U.S., please contact

International Sales
international@pearsoned.com

Publisher
Paul Boger

Associate Publisher
David Dusthimer

Acquisitions Editor
Betsy Brown

Senior Development Editor
Christopher Cleveland

Managing Editor
Sandra Schroeder

Project Editor
Mandie Frank

Proofreader
Leslie Joseph

Technical Editor
Jacqueline Ruckel

Publishing Coordinator
Vanessa Evans

Multimedia Developer
Dan Scherf

Designer
Gary Adair

Page Layout
Studio Galou, LLC

Contents at a Glance

	Introduction	1
CHAPTER 1	Practice Exam 1 and Rationales	5
CHAPTER 2	Practice Exam 2 and Rationales	73
CHAPTER 3	Practice Exam 3 and Rationales	145
CHAPTER 4	Practice Exam 4 and Rationales	209
CHAPTER 5	Practice Exam 5 and Rationales	275
APPENDIX A	Things You Forgot	341
APPENDIX B	Need to Know More?	349
APPENDIX C	Alphabetical Listing of Nursing Boards in the United States and Protectorates	359

Table of Contents

Introduction 1

- Welcome to the NCLEX-PN® Practice Questions Exam Cram 1
- Taking the Computerized Adaptive Test 2
- The Cost of the Exam 2
- How to Prepare for the Exam 3
- What Will You Find in This Book? 3
- Hints for Using This Book 4
- Need Further Study? 4
- Contact the Authors 4

Chapter 1: Practice Exam 1 and Rationales 5

- Quick Check Answer Key 50
- Answers and Rationales 53

Chapter 2: Practice Exam 2 and Rationales 73

- Quick Check Answer Key 118
- Answers and Rationales 121

Chapter 3: Practice Exam 3 and Rationales 145

- Quick Check Answer Key 187
- Answers and Rationales 190

Chapter 4: Practice Exam 4 and Rationales 209

- Quick Check Answer Key 251
- Answers and Rationales 254

Chapter 5: Practice Exam 5 and Rationales 275

- Quick Check Answer Key 318
- Answers and Rationales 321

Appendix A: Things You Forgot 341

- Therapeutic Drug Levels 341

Vital Signs . . . 341
Intrapartal Normal Values . . . 342
Anticoagulant Therapy . . . 342
Standard Precautions . . . 343
Airborne Precautions . . . 343
Droplet Precautions . . . 344
Contact Precautions . . . 344
Revised Life Support Guidelines (American Heart Association) . . . 344
Defense Mechanisms . . . 345
Nutrition Notes . . . 345
Immunization Schedule . . . 347

Appendix B: Need to Know More? . . . 349
Pharmacology . . . 349
Care of the Client with Respiratory Disorders . . . 349
Care of the Client with Genitourinary Disorders . . . 350
Care of the Client with Hematological Disorders . . . 350
Care of the Client with Fluid and Electrolytes and Acid/Base Balance . . . 351
Care of the Client with Burns . . . 351
Care of the Client with Sensory Disorders . . . 352
Care of the Client with Neoplastic Disorders . . . 352
Care of the Client with Gastrointestinal Disorders . . . 353
Care of the Client with Musculoskeletal and Connective Tissue Disorder . . . 353
Care of the Client with Endocrine Disorders . . . 354
Care of the Client with Cardiac Disorders . . . 354
Care of the Client with Neurological Disorders . . . 355
Care of the Client with Psychiatric Disorders . . . 355
Care of the Client with Maternal-Newborn Care . . . 356
Care of the Pediatric Client . . . 356
Cultural Practices Influencing Nursing Care . . . 356
Legal Issues in Nursing Practice . . . 357

Appendix C: Alphabetical Listing of Nursing Boards in the United States and Protectorates . . . 359

About the Authors

Wilda Rinehart received an Associate Degree in Nursing from Northeast Mississippi Community College in Booneville, Mississippi. After working as a staff nurse and charge nurse, she became a public health nurse and served in that capacity for a number of years. In 1975, she received her nurse practitioner certification in the area of obstetrics-gynecology from the University of Mississippi Medical Center in Jackson, Mississippi. In 1979, she completed her Bachelor of Science degree in Nursing from Mississippi University for Women. In 1980, she completed her Master of Science degree in Nursing from the same university and accepted a faculty position at Northeast Mississippi Community College, where she taught medical-surgical nursing and maternal-newborn nursing. In 1982, she founded Rinehart and Associates Nursing Consultants. For the past 26 years, she and her associates have worked with nursing graduates and schools of nursing to assist graduates to pass the National Council Licensure Exam for Nursing. She has also worked as a curriculum consultant with faculty to improve test construction. Ms. Rinehart has served as a convention speaker throughout the southeastern United States and as a reviewer of medical-surgical and obstetric texts. She has co-authored materials used in seminars presented by Rinehart and Associates Nursing Review. As the president of Rinehart and Associates, she serves as the coordinator of a company dedicated to improving the quality of health through nursing education.

Dr. Diann Sloan received an Associate Degree in Nursing from Northeast Mississippi Community College, a Bachelor of Science degree in Nursing from the University of Mississippi, and a Master of Science degree in Nursing from Mississippi University for Women. In addition to her nursing degrees, she holds a Master of Science in Counseling Psychology from Georgia State University and a Doctor of Philosophy in Counselor Education, with minors in both Psychology and Educational Psychology, from Mississippi State University. She has completed additional graduate studies in healthcare administration at Western New England College and the University of Mississippi. Dr. Sloan has taught pediatric nursing, psychiatric mental health nursing, and medical surgical nursing in both associate degree and baccalaureate nursing programs. As a member of Rinehart and Associates Nursing Review, Dr. Sloan has conducted test construction workshops for faculty and nursing review seminars for both registered and practical nurse graduates. She has co-authored materials used in the item-writing workshops for nursing faculty and Rinehart and Associates Nursing Review. She is a member of Sigma Theta Tau nursing honor society.

Clara Hurd received an Associate Degree in Nursing from Northeast Mississippi Community College in Booneville, Mississippi (1975). Her experiences in nursing are clinically based, having served as a staff nurse in medical-surgical nursing. She has worked as an oncology, intensive care, orthopedic, neurological, and pediatric nurse. She received her Bachelor of Science degree in Nursing from the University of North Alabama in Florence, Alabama, and her Master of Science degree in Nursing from Mississippi University for Women in Columbus, Mississippi. Ms Hurd is a certified nurse educator. She currently serves as a nurse educator consultant and an independent contractor. Ms. Hurd has taught in both associate degree and baccalaureate degree nursing programs. She was a faculty member of Mississippi University for Women; Austin Peay State University in Clarksville, Tennessee; Tennessee State University inNashville, Tennessee; and Northeast Mississippi Community College. Ms. Hurd joined Rinehart and Associates in 1993. She has worked with students in preparing for the National Council Licensure Exam and with faculty as a consultant in writing test items. Ms. Hurd has also been a presenter at nursing conventions on various topics, including item-writing for nursing faculty. Her primary professional goal is to prepare the student and graduate for excellence in the delivery of healthcare.

Dedication

We would like to thank our families for tolerating our late nights and long hours. Also, thanks to Gene Sloan for his help without pay. Special thanks to all the graduates who have attended Rinehart and Associates Review Seminars. Thanks for allowing us to be a part of your success.

We are also delighted that Jessica Rinehart Wentz, RN, Whitney Hurd Miller, RN, and Brad Sloan, RN, chose nursing as their profession above so many other professions.

Acknowledgments

Our special thanks to our editors, support staff, and nurse reviewers for helping us to organize our thoughts and experiences into a text for students and practicing professionals. You made the task before us challenging and enjoyable.

We Want to Hear from You!

As the reader of this book, *you* are our most important critic and commentator. We value your opinion and want to know what we're doing right, what we could do better, what areas you'd like to see us publish in, and any other words of wisdom you're willing to pass our way.

As an associate publisher for Pearson, I welcome your comments. You can email or write me directly to let me know what you did or didn't like about this book—as well as what we can do to make our books better.

Please note that I cannot help you with technical problems related to the topic of this book. We do have a User Services group, however, where I will forward specific technical questions related to the book.

When you write, please be sure to include this book's title and author as well as your name, email address, and phone number. I will carefully review your comments and share them with the author and editors who worked on the book.

Email: feedback@pearsonitcertification.com

Mail: David Dusthimer
Associate Publisher
Pearson
800 East 96th Street
Indianapolis, IN 46240 USA

Reader Services

Visit our website and register this book at www.pearsonitcertification.com/register for convenient access to any updates, downloads, or errata that might be available for this book.

Introduction

Welcome to the NCLEX-PN® Practice Questions Exam Cram

This book helps you get ready to take and pass the Licensure Exam for Practical Nurses. This chapter discusses the NCLEX® exam in general and how the Exam Cram books can help you prepare for the test. It doesn't matter whether this is the first time you're going to take the exam or whether you have taken it previously; this book gives you the necessary information and techniques to obtain licensure.

The *NCLEX-PN® Practice Questions Exam Cram* helps you practice taking questions written in the NCLEX® format. Used with the Exam Cram review book *NCLEX-PN® Exam Cram*, it helps you understand and appreciate the subjects and materials you need to pass. The books are aimed at test preparation and review. They do not teach you everything you need to know about the subject of nursing. Instead, they present you with materials that you are likely to encounter on the exam. Using a simple approach, we help you understand the "need to know" information.

To pass the NCLEX®, you must understand how the exam is developed. The NCLEX-PN® consists of questions from the cognitive levels of knowledge, comprehension, application, and analysis. The majority of questions are written at the application and analysis level. Questions incorporate the five stages of the nursing process (assessment, diagnosis, planning, implementation, and evaluation) and the four categories of client needs. Client needs are divided into subcategories that define the content within each of the four major categories. These categories and subcategories are

- A. Safe, effective care environment:
    - Coordinated care: 13%-19%
    - Safety and infection control: 11%-17%
- B. Health promotion and maintenance: 7%–13%
- C. Psychosocial integrity: 7%-13%

- D. Physiological integrity:
    - Basic care and comfort: 9%-15%
    - Pharmacological and parenteral therapy: 11%-17%
    - Reduction of risk: 9%-15%
    - Physiological adaptation: 9%-15%

Taking the Computerized Adaptive Test

Computer-adaptive testing, commonly known as CAT, offers the candidate several advantages. First, the graduate can schedule the exam at a time that is convenient. It's also possible that you will not be tested on the entire 205-question set; if you answer the beginning questions correctly, the CAT might stop early in the session, with far fewer than the 205 questions you were expecting. When the engine has determined your ability level and it is satisfied that you are qualified to be a practical nurse, it will stop. The disadvantage of a CAT is that you cannot go back and change answers. When you make a decision and move on, that's it—no second guessing, like on a paper exam!

The Pearson Vue testing group is responsible for administering the exam. You can locate the center nearest you by visiting www.pearsonvue.com. If you are not familiar with the Pearson Vue testing centers, we recommend that you arrive at least 30 minutes early. If you are late, you will not be allowed to take the test. Bring two forms of identification with you, one of which must be a picture ID. Be sure that your form of identification matches your application. You will be photographed and fingerprinted upon entering the testing site, so don't let this increase your stress. The allotted time is 5 hours, and the candidate can receive results within approximately 7 days (in some states, even sooner). Remember, the exam is written at approximately the tenth-grade reading level, so keep a good dictionary handy during your studies.

The Cost of the Exam

A candidate wanting to write the licensure exam must fill out two applications: one to the National Council, and one to the state in which the candidate wants to be licensed. A separate fee must accompany each application. The fee required by the National Council is $200. State licensing fees vary. Licensure applications can be obtained on the National Council's website at www.ncsbn.org. Several states are members of the multistate licensure compact. This means that if you are issued a multistate license, you pay only one fee. This information also can be obtained by visiting the National Council's website.

How to Prepare for the Exam

Judicious use of this book, the *NCLEX® Exam Prep* book, and/or the *NCLEX-PN® Exam Cram* book, alone or with a review seminar such as that provided by Rinehart and Associates, can help you achieve your goal of becoming a licensed practical nurse. As you review for the NCLEX® exam, we suggest that you find a location where you can concentrate on the material each day. A minimum of 2 hours per day for at least 2 weeks is suggested. In *NCLEX-PN® Exam Cram*, we provide you with exam alerts, tips, notes, and sample questions, both multiple choice and alternate items. These questions will acquaint you with the type of questions that you will have during the exam. We have also formulated a mock exam with those difficult management and delegation questions that you can score to determine your readiness to test. Pay particular attention to the helpful hints and the Cram Sheet. Using these will help you gain and retain knowledge and will help reduce your stress as you prepare to test.

What Will You Find in This Book?

As seems obvious from the title, this book is all about practice questions! There are five full exams in this book, totaling 1,000 questions. Each chapter is set up with the questions and their possible answers first; the correct answers and rationales appear at the end of each chapter. In the margins next to each question, you will see a quick key to finding the location of its answer and rationales. Here's exactly what you will find in the chapters:

- **Practice Questions**—These are the numerous questions to help you learn, drill, and review.
- **Quick Check Answers**—When you finish answering the questions, you can quickly grade your exam from this section. Only correct answers are given here—no rationales are offered yet.
- **Answers and Rationales**—This section offers you the correct answers, as well as further explanation about the content posed in that question. Use this information to learn why an answer is correct and to reinforce the content in your mind for exam day.

You also will find a Cram Sheet at the beginning of this book specifically written for this exam. This is a very popular element that is also found in *NCLEX-PN® Exam Cram* (Que Publishing, ISBN 0-7897-3267-X). This item condenses all the necessary facts found in this exam into one easy-to-handle tearcard. The Cram Sheet is something you can carry with you to the exam location and use as a last-second study aid. Be aware that you can't take it into the exam room, though.

Hints for Using This Book

Because this book is a paper practice product, you might want to take advantage of the answer sheets in each chapter. These can be copied for multiple practice sessions. We suggest that you score your exam by subtracting the missed items from the total and then dividing the total answered correctly by the total number of questions. This gives you the percentage answered correctly. We also suggest that you achieve a score of at least 77% before you schedule your exam. If you do not, take the exam again until you do. The higher the score, the better your chance to do well on the NCLEX® exam!

You also will want to take advantage of the CD exam engine; it provides you with a computer-adaptive test very similar to the one you will experience during the NCLEX® exam. Every question in this book is on the CD, including the answer rationales.

Aside from being a test-preparation book, this book is useful if you are brushing up on your nursing knowledge. It is an excellent quick reference for the licensed nurse.

Need Further Study?

If you are having a hard time correctly answering questions, be sure to see this book's companion volume, the *NCLEX-PN® Exam Cram* (Que Publishing, ISBN 0-7897-3706-X). If you still need further study, you might want to take a class or look at one of the many other books available at your local bookstore.

Contact the Authors

The authors of this text are interested in you and want you to pass on the first attempt. If after reviewing with this text you would like to contact the authors, you may do so at Rinehart and Associates, PO Box 124, Booneville, MS 38829, or by visiting www.nclexreview.net.

CHAPTER ONE

Practice Exam 1 and Rationales

Quick Check

1. The nurse is caring for a client scheduled for removal of the pituitary gland. The nurse should be particularly alert for:

   - ❍ **A.** Nasal congestion
   - ❍ **B.** Abdominal tenderness
   - ❍ **C.** Muscle tetany
   - ❍ **D.** Oliguria

Quick Answers: **50**
Detailed Answer: **53**

2. A client with cancer is admitted to the oncology unit. Stat lab values reveal Hgb 12.6, WBC 6500, K+ 1.9, uric acid 7.0, Na+ 136, and platelets 178,000. The nurse evaluates that the client is experiencing which of the following?

   - ❍ **A.** Hypernatremia
   - ❍ **B.** Hypokalemia
   - ❍ **C.** Myelosuppression
   - ❍ **D.** Leukocytosis

Quick Answers: **50**
Detailed Answer: **53**

3. A 24-year-old female client is scheduled for surgery in the morning. Which of the following is the primary responsibility of the nurse?

   - ❍ **A.** Taking the vital signs
   - ❍ **B.** Obtaining the permit
   - ❍ **C.** Explaining the procedure
   - ❍ **D.** Checking the lab work

Quick Answers: **50**
Detailed Answer: **53**

Quick Check

4. The nurse is working in the emergency room when a client arrives with severe burns of the left arm, hands, face, and neck. Which action should receive priority?

Quick Answers: **50**
Detailed Answer: **53**

❍ **A.** Starting an IV
❍ **B.** Applying oxygen
❍ **C.** Obtaining blood gases
❍ **D.** Medicating the client for pain

5. The nurse is visiting a home health client with osteoporosis. The client has a new prescription for alendronate (Fosamax). Which instruction should be given to the client?

Quick Answers: **50**
Detailed Answer: **53**

❍ **A.** Rest in bed after taking the medication for at least 30 minutes
❍ **B.** Avoid rapid movements after taking the medication
❍ **C.** Take the medication with water only
❍ **D.** Allow at least 1 hour between taking the medicine and taking other medications

6. The nurse is making initial rounds on a client with a C5 fracture and crutchfield tongs. Which equipment should be kept at the bedside?

Quick Answers: **50**
Detailed Answer: **53**

❍ **A.** A pair of forceps
❍ **B.** A torque wrench
❍ **C.** A pair of wire cutters
❍ **D.** A screwdriver

7. An infant weighs 7 pounds at birth. The expected weight by 1 year should be:

Quick Answers: **50**
Detailed Answer: **53**

❍ **A.** 10 pounds
❍ **B.** 12 pounds
❍ **C.** 18 pounds
❍ **D.** 21 pounds

8. A client is admitted with a Ewing's sarcoma. Which symptoms would be expected due to this tumor's location?

Quick Answers: **50**
Detailed Answer: **53**

❍ **A.** Hemiplegia
❍ **B.** Aphasia
❍ **C.** Nausea
❍ **D.** Bone pain

Quick Check

9. The nurse is caring for a client with epilepsy who is being treated with carbamazepine (Tegretol). Which laboratory value might indicate a serious side effect of this drug?

 - ❍ **A.** Uric acid of 5mg/dL
 - ❍ **B.** Hematocrit of 33%
 - ❍ **C.** WBC 2,000 per cubic millimeter
 - ❍ **D.** Platelets 150,000 per cubic millimeter

Quick Answers: **50**
Detailed Answer: **53**

10. A 6-month-old client is admitted with possible intussuception. Which question during the nursing history is least helpful in obtaining information regarding this diagnosis?

 - ❍ **A.** "Tell me about his pain."
 - ❍ **B.** "What does his vomit look like?"
 - ❍ **C.** "Describe his usual diet."
 - ❍ **D.** "Have you noticed changes in his abdominal size?"

Quick Answers: **50**
Detailed Answer: **53**

11. The nurse is assisting a client with diverticulosis to select appropriate foods. Which food should be avoided?

 - ❍ **A.** Bran
 - ❍ **B.** Fresh peaches
 - ❍ **C.** Cucumber salad
 - ❍ **D.** Yeast rolls

Quick Answers: **50**
Detailed Answer: **53**

12. A client has rectal cancer and is scheduled for an abdominal perineal resection. What should be the priority nursing care during the post-op period?

 - ❍ **A.** Teaching how to irrigate the illeostomy
 - ❍ **B.** Stopping electrolyte loss in the incisional area
 - ❍ **C.** Encouraging a high-fiber diet
 - ❍ **D.** Facilitating perineal wound drainage

Quick Answers: **50**
Detailed Answer: **53**

13. The nurse is performing discharge teaching on a client with diverticulitis who has been placed on a low-roughage diet. Which food would have to be eliminated from this client's diet?

 - ❍ **A.** Roasted chicken
 - ❍ **B.** Noodles
 - ❍ **C.** Cooked broccoli
 - ❍ **D.** Custard

Quick Answers: **50**
Detailed Answer: **54**

Quick Check

14. The nurse is caring for a new mother. The mother asks why her baby has lost weight since he was born. The best explanation of the weight loss is:

Quick Answers: **50**
Detailed Answer: **54**

- ❍ **A.** The baby is dehydrated due to polyuria.
- ❍ **B.** The baby is hypoglycemic due to lack of glucose.
- ❍ **C.** The baby is allergic to the formula the mother is giving him.
- ❍ **D.** The baby can lose up to 10% of weight due to meconium stool, loss of extracellular fluid, and initiation of breast-feeding.

15. The nurse is caring for a client with laryngeal cancer. Which finding ascertained in the health history would not be common for this diagnosis?

Quick Answers: **50**
Detailed Answer: **54**

- ❍ **A.** Foul breath
- ❍ **B.** Dysphagia
- ❍ **C.** Diarrhea
- ❍ **D.** Chronic hiccups

16. A removal of the left lower lobe of the lung is performed on a client with lung cancer. Which post-operative measure would usually be included in the plan?

Quick Answers: **50**
Detailed Answer: **54**

- ❍ **A.** Closed chest drainage
- ❍ **B.** A tracheostomy
- ❍ **C.** A mediastenal tube
- ❍ **D.** Percussion vibration and drainage

17. Six hours after birth, the infant is found to have an area of swelling over the right parietal area that does not cross the suture line. The nurse should chart this finding as:

Quick Answers: **50**
Detailed Answer: **54**

- ❍ **A.** A cephalohematoma
- ❍ **B.** Molding
- ❍ **C.** Subdural hematoma
- ❍ **D.** Caput succedaneum

Quick Check

18. The nurse is assisting the RN with discharge instructions for a client with an implantable defibrillator. What discharge instruction is essential?

Quick Answers: **50**
Detailed Answer: **54**

- ❍ **A.** "You cannot eat food prepared in a microwave."
- ❍ **B.** "You should avoid moving the shoulder on the side of the pacemaker site for 6 weeks."
- ❍ **C.** "You should use your cellphone on your right side."
- ❍ **D.** "You will not be able to fly on a commercial airliner with the defibrillator in place."

19. A client in the cardiac step-down unit requires suctioning for excess mucous secretions. The nurse should be most careful to monitor the client for which dysrhythmia during this procedure?

Quick Answers: **50**
Detailed Answer: **54**

- ❍ **A.** Bradycardia
- ❍ **B.** Tachycardia
- ❍ **C.** Premature ventricular beats
- ❍ **D.** Heart block

20. The nurse is caring for a client scheduled for a surgical repair of a sacular abdominal aortic aneurysm. Which assessment is most crucial during the preoperative period?

Quick Answers: **50**
Detailed Answer: **54**

- ❍ **A.** Assessment of the client's level of anxiety
- ❍ **B.** Evaluation of the client's exercise tolerance
- ❍ **C.** Identification of peripheral pulses
- ❍ **D.** Assessment of bowel sounds and activity

21. A client with suspected renal disease is to undergo a renal biopsy. The nurse plans to include which statement in the teaching session?

Quick Answers: **50**
Detailed Answer: **54**

- ❍ **A.** "You will be sitting for the examination procedure."
- ❍ **B.** "Portions of the procedure will cause pain or discomfort."
- ❍ **C.** "You will be given some medication to anesthetize the area."
- ❍ **D.** "You will not be able to drink fluids for 24 hours before the study."

Quick Check

22. The nurse is performing an assessment on a client with possible pernicious anemia. Which data would support this diagnosis?

Quick Answers: **50**
Detailed Answer: **54**

❍ **A.** A weight loss of 10 pounds in 2 weeks

❍ **B.** Complaints of numbness and tingling in the extremities

❍ **C.** A red, beefy tongue

❍ **D.** A hemoglobin level of 12.0gm/dL

23. A client arrives in the emergency room with a possible fractured femur. The nurse should anticipate an order for:

Quick Answers: **50**
Detailed Answer: **55**

❍ **A.** Trendelenburg position

❍ **B.** Ice to the entire extremity

❍ **C.** Buck's traction

❍ **D.** An abduction pillow

24. A client with cancer is to undergo an intravenous pyelogram. The nurse should:

Quick Answers: **50**
Detailed Answer: **55**

❍ **A.** Force fluids 24 hours before the procedure

❍ **B.** Ask the client to void immediately before the study

❍ **C.** Hold medication that affects the central nervous system for 12 hours pre- and post-test

❍ **D.** Cover the client's reproductive organs with an x-ray shield

25. The nurse is caring for a client with a malignancy. The classification of the primary tumor is Tis. The nurse should plan care for a tumor:

Quick Answers: **50**
Detailed Answer: **55**

❍ **A.** That cannot be assessed

❍ **B.** That is in situ

❍ **C.** With increasing lymph node involvement

❍ **D.** With distant metastasis

26. A client is 2 days post-operative colon resection. After a coughing episode, the client's wound eviscerates. Which nursing action is most appropriate?

Quick Answers: **50**
Detailed Answer: **55**

❍ **A.** Reinsert the protruding organ and cover with 4×4s

❍ **B.** Cover the wound with a sterile 4×4 and ABD dressing

❍ **C.** Cover the wound with a sterile saline-soaked dressing

❍ **D.** Apply an abdominal binder and manual pressure to the wound

Quick Check

27. The nurse is preparing a client for surgery. Which item is most important to remove before sending the client to surgery?

Quick Answers: **50**
Detailed Answer: **55**

- ❍ **A.** Hearing aid
- ❍ **B.** Contact lenses
- ❍ **C.** Wedding ring
- ❍ **D.** Artificial eye

28. The nurse on the 3–11 shift is assessing the chart of a client with an abdominal aneurysm scheduled for surgery in the morning and finds that the consent form has been signed, but the client is unclear about the surgery and possible complications. Which is the most appropriate action?

Quick Answers: **50**
Detailed Answer: **55**

- ❍ **A.** Call the surgeon and ask him or her to see the client to clarify the information
- ❍ **B.** Explain the procedure and complications to the client
- ❍ **C.** Check in the physician's progress notes to see if understanding has been documented
- ❍ **D.** Check with the client's family to see if they understand the procedure fully

29. When assessing a client for risk of hyperphosphatemia, which piece of information is most important for the nurse to obtain?

Quick Answers: **50**
Detailed Answer: **55**

- ❍ **A.** A history of radiation treatment in the neck region
- ❍ **B.** A history of recent orthopedic surgery
- ❍ **C.** A history of minimal physical activity
- ❍ **D.** A history of the client's food intake

30. A client is admitted to the acute care unit. Initial laboratory values reveal serum sodium of 170meq/L. What behavior changes would be most common for this client?

Quick Answers: **50**
Detailed Answer: **55**

- ❍ **A.** Anger
- ❍ **B.** Mania
- ❍ **C.** Depression
- ❍ **D.** Psychosis

Quick Check

31. The nurse is obtaining a history of an 80-year-old client. Which statement made by the client might indicate a possible fluid and electrolyte imbalance?

Quick Answers: **50**
Detailed Answer: **55**

- ❍ **A.** "My skin is always so dry."
- ❍ **B.** "I often use a laxative for constipation."
- ❍ **C.** "I have always liked to drink a lot of ice tea."
- ❍ **D.** "I sometimes have a problem with dribbling urine."

32. A client visits the clinic after the death of a parent. Which statement made by the client's sister signifies abnormal grieving?

Quick Answers: **50**
Detailed Answer: **55**

- ❍ **A.** "My sister still has episodes of crying, and it's been 3 months since Daddy died."
- ❍ **B.** "Sally seems to have forgotten the bad things that Daddy did in his lifetime."
- ❍ **C.** "She really had a hard time after Daddy's funeral. She said that she had a sense of longing."
- ❍ **D.** "Sally has not been sad at all by Daddy's death. She acts like nothing has happened."

33. The nurse recognizes that which of the following would be most appropriate to wear when providing direct care to a client with a cough?

Quick Answers: **50**
Detailed Answer: **56**

- ❍ **A.** Mask
- ❍ **B.** Gown
- ❍ **C.** Gloves
- ❍ **D.** Shoe covers

34. The nurse is caring for a client with a diagnosis of hepatitis who is experiencing pruritis. Which would be the most appropriate nursing intervention?

Quick Answers: **50**
Detailed Answer: **56**

- ❍ **A.** Suggest that the client take warm showers B.I.D.
- ❍ **B.** Add baby oil to the client's bath water
- ❍ **C.** Apply powder to the client's skin
- ❍ **D.** Suggest a hot-water rinse after bathing

35. A client with pancreatitis has been transferred to the intensive care unit. Which order would the nurse anticipate?

Quick Answers: **50**
Detailed Answer: **56**

- ❍ **A.** Blood pressure every 15 minutes
- ❍ **B.** Insertion of a Levine tube
- ❍ **C.** Cardiac monitoring
- ❍ **D.** Dressing changes two times per day

Quick Check

36. The client is admitted to the unit after a cholescystectomy. Montgomery straps are utilized with this client. The nurse is aware that Montgomery straps are utilized on this client because:

❍ **A.** The client is at risk for evisceration.

❍ **B.** The client will require frequent dressing changes.

❍ **C.** The straps provide support for drains that are inserted in the incision.

❍ **D.** No sutures or clips are used to secure the incision.

Quick Answers: **50**
Detailed Answer: **56**

37. The physician has ordered that the client's medication be administered intrathecally. The nurse is aware that medications will be administered by which method?

❍ **A.** Intravenously

❍ **B.** Rectally

❍ **C.** Intramuscularly

❍ **D.** Into the cerebrospinal fluid

Quick Answers: **50**
Detailed Answer: **56**

38. Which client can best be assigned to the newly licensed practical nurse?

❍ **A.** The client receiving chemotherapy

❍ **B.** The client post–coronary bypass

❍ **C.** The client with a TURP

❍ **D.** The client with diverticulitis

Quick Answers: **50**
Detailed Answer: **56**

39. The nurse notes the patient care assistant looking through the personal items of the client with cancer. Which action should be taken by the registered nurse?

❍ **A.** Notify the police department as a robbery

❍ **B.** Report this behavior to the charge nurse

❍ **C.** Monitor the situation and note whether any items are missing

❍ **D.** Ignore the situation until items are reported missing

Quick Answers: **50**
Detailed Answer: **56**

40. The nurse overhears the patient care assistant speaking harshly to the client with dementia. The charge nurse should:

❍ **A.** Change the nursing assistant's assignment

❍ **B.** Explore the interaction with the nursing assistant

❍ **C.** Discuss the matter with the client's family

❍ **D.** Initiate a group session with the nursing assistant

Quick Answers: **50**
Detailed Answer: **56**

Quick Check

41. A home health nurse is planning for her daily visits. Which client should the home health nurse visit first?

Quick Answers: **50**
Detailed Answer: **57**

- ❍ **A.** A client with AIDS being treated with Foscarnet
- ❍ **B.** A client with a fractured femur in a long leg cast
- ❍ **C.** A client with laryngeal cancer with a laryngetomy
- ❍ **D.** A client with diabetic ulcers to the left foot

42. The nurse is assigned to care for an infant with physiologic jaundice. Which action by the nurse would facilitate elimination of the bilirubin?

Quick Answers: **50**
Detailed Answer: **57**

- ❍ **A.** Increasing the infant's fluid intake
- ❍ **B.** Maintaining the infant's body temperature at 98.6°F
- ❍ **C.** Minimizing tactile stimulation
- ❍ **D.** Decreasing caloric intake

43. The graduate licensed practical nurse is assigned to care for the client on ventilator support, pending organ donation. Which goal should receive priority?

Quick Answers: **50**
Detailed Answer: **57**

- ❍ **A.** Maintain the client's systolic blood pressure at 70mmHg or greater
- ❍ **B.** Maintain the client's urinary output greater than 300cc per hour
- ❍ **C.** Maintain the client's body temperature of greater than 33°F rectal
- ❍ **D.** Maintain the client's hematocrit less than 30%

44. Which action by the novice nurse indicates a need for further teaching?

Quick Answers: **50**
Detailed Answer: **57**

- ❍ **A.** The nurse fails to wear gloves to remove a dressing.
- ❍ **B.** The nurse applies an oxygen saturation monitor to the ear lobe.
- ❍ **C.** The nurse elevates the head of the bed to check the blood pressure.
- ❍ **D.** The nurse places the extremity in a dependent position to acquire a peripheral blood sample.

Quick Check

45. The nurse is preparing a client for mammography. To prepare the client for a mammogram, the nurse should tell the client:

Quick Answers: 50
Detailed Answer: 57

- ❍ **A.** To restrict her fat intake for 1 week before the test
- ❍ **B.** To omit creams, powders, or deodorants before the exam
- ❍ **C.** That mammography replaces the need for self-breast exams
- ❍ **D.** That mammography requires a higher dose of radiation than an x-ray

46. Which of the following roommates would be best for the client newly admitted with gastric resection?

Quick Answers: 50
Detailed Answer: 57

- ❍ **A.** A client with Crohn's disease
- ❍ **B.** A client with pneumonia
- ❍ **C.** A client with gastritis
- ❍ **D.** A client with phlebitis

47. The licensed practical nurse is working with a registered nurse and a patient care assistant. Which of the following clients should be cared for by the registered nurse?

Quick Answers: 50
Detailed Answer: 57

- ❍ **A.** A client 2 days post-appendectomy
- ❍ **B.** A client 1 week post-thyroidectomy
- ❍ **C.** A client 3 days post-splenectomy
- ❍ **D.** A client 2 days post-thoracotomy

48. The licensed practical nurse is observing a graduate nurse as she assesses the central venous pressure. Which observation would indicate that the graduate needs further teaching?

Quick Answers: 50
Detailed Answer: 57

- ❍ **A.** The graduate places the client in a supine position to read the manometer.
- ❍ **B.** The graduate turns the stop-cock to the off position from the IV fluid to the client.
- ❍ **C.** The graduate instructs the client to perform the Valsalva maneuver during the CVP reading.
- ❍ **D.** The graduate notes the level at the top of the meniscus.

Quick Check

49. Which of the following roommates would be most suitable for the client with myasthenia gravis?

Quick Answers: **50**
Detailed Answer: **57**

- ❍ **A.** A client with hypothyroidism
- ❍ **B.** A client with Crohn's disease
- ❍ **C.** A client with pylonephritis
- ❍ **D.** A client with bronchitis

50. The nurse employed in the emergency room is responsible for triage of four clients injured in a motor vehicle accident. Which of the following clients should receive priority in care?

Quick Answers: **50**
Detailed Answer: **57**

- ❍ **A.** A 10-year-old with lacerations of the face
- ❍ **B.** A 15-year-old with sternal bruises
- ❍ **C.** A 34-year-old with a fractured femur
- ❍ **D.** A 50-year-old with dislocation of the elbow

51. The client is receiving peritoneal dialysis. If the dialysate returns cloudy, the nurse should:

Quick Answers: **50**
Detailed Answer: **58**

- ❍ **A.** Document the finding
- ❍ **B.** Send a specimen to the lab
- ❍ **C.** Strain the urine
- ❍ **D.** Obtain a complete blood count

52. The client with cirrhosis of the liver is receiving Lactulose. The nurse is aware that the rationale for the order for Lactulose is:

Quick Answers: **50**
Detailed Answer: **58**

- ❍ **A.** To lower the blood glucose level
- ❍ **B.** To lower the uric acid level
- ❍ **C.** To lower the ammonia level
- ❍ **D.** To lower the creatinine level

53. The client with diabetes is preparing for discharge. During discharge teaching, the nurse assesses the client's ability to care for himself. Which statement made by the client would indicate a need for follow-up after discharge?

Quick Answers: **50**
Detailed Answer: **58**

- ❍ **A.** "I live by myself."
- ❍ **B.** "I have trouble seeing."
- ❍ **C.** "I have a cat in the house with me."
- ❍ **D.** "I usually drive myself to the doctor."

Quick Check

54. The client is receiving total parenteral nutrition (TPN). Which lab test should be evaluated while the client is receiving TPN?

Quick Answers: **50**
Detailed Answer: **58**

❍ **A.** Hemoglobin

❍ **B.** Creatinine

❍ **C.** Blood glucose

❍ **D.** White blood cell count

55. The client with a myocardial infarction comes to the nurse's station stating that he is ready to go home because there is nothing wrong with him. Which defense mechanism is the client using?

Quick Answers: **50**
Detailed Answer: **58**

❍ **A.** Rationalization

❍ **B.** Denial

❍ **C.** Projection

❍ **D.** Conversion reaction

56. Which laboratory test would be the least effective in making the diagnosis of a myocardial infarction?

Quick Answers: **50**
Detailed Answer: **58**

❍ **A.** AST

❍ **B.** Troponin

❍ **C.** CK-MB

❍ **D.** Myoglobin

57. The licensed practical nurse assigned to the post-partal unit is preparing to administer Rhogam to a postpartum client. Which woman is not a candidate for RhoGam?

Quick Answers: **50**
Detailed Answer: **58**

❍ **A.** A gravida IV para 3 that is Rh negative with an Rh-positive baby

❍ **B.** A gravida I para 1 that is Rh negative with an Rh-positive baby

❍ **C.** A gravida II para 0 that is Rh negative admitted after a stillbirth delivery

❍ **D.** A gravida IV para 2 that is Rh negative with an Rh-negative baby

58. The first exercise that should be performed by the client who had a mastectomy is:

Quick Answers: **50**
Detailed Answer: **58**

❍ **A.** Walking the hand up the wall

❍ **B.** Sweeping the floor

❍ **C.** Combing her hair

❍ **D.** Squeezing a ball

Quick Check

59. The client is scheduled for a Tensilon test to check for Myasthenia Gravis. Which medication should be kept available during the test?

Quick Answers: **50**
Detailed Answer: **58**

❍ **A.** Atropine sulfate

❍ **B.** Furosemide

❍ **C.** Prostigmin

❍ **D.** Promethazine

60. The client is scheduled for a pericentesis. Which instruction should be given to the client before the exam?

Quick Answers: **50**
Detailed Answer: **58**

❍ **A.** "You will need to lay flat during the exam."

❍ **B.** "You need to empty your bladder before the procedure."

❍ **C.** "You will be asleep during the procedure."

❍ **D.** "The doctor will inject a medication to treat your illness during the procedure."

61. To ensure safety while administering a nitroglycerine patch, the nurse should:

Quick Answers: **50**
Detailed Answer: **58**

❍ **A.** Wear gloves

❍ **B.** Shave the area where the patch will be applied

❍ **C.** Wash the area thoroughly with soap and rinse with hot water

❍ **D.** Apply the patch to the buttocks

62. A 25-year-old male is brought to the emergency room with a piece of metal in his eye. Which action by the nurse is correct?

Quick Answers: **50**
Detailed Answer: **59**

❍ **A.** Use a magnet to remove the object.

❍ **B.** Rinse the eye thoroughly with saline.

❍ **C.** Cover both eyes with paper cups.

❍ **D.** Patch the affected eye only.

63. The physician has ordered sodium warfarin (Coumadin) for the client with thrombophlebitis. The order should be entered to administer the medication at:

Quick Answers: **50**
Detailed Answer: **59**

❍ **A.** 0900

❍ **B.** 1200

❍ **C.** 1700

❍ **D.** 2100

Quick Check

64. The schizophrenic client has become disruptive and requires seclusion. Which staff member can institute seclusion?

Quick Answers: **50**
Detailed Answer: **59**

❍ **A.** The security guard

❍ **B.** The registered nurse

❍ **C.** The licensed practical nurse

❍ **D.** The nursing assistant

65. The client is admitted with chronic obstructive pulmonary disease. Blood gases reveal pH 7.36, CO_2 45, O_2 84, HCO3 28. The nurse would assess the client to be in:

Quick Answers: **50**
Detailed Answer: **59**

❍ **A.** Uncompensated acidosis

❍ **B.** Compensated alkalosis

❍ **C.** Compensated respiratory acidosis

❍ **D.** Uncompensated metabolic acidosis

66. The nurse is assessing the client recently returned from surgery. The nurse is aware that the best way to assess pain is to:

Quick Answers: **50**
Detailed Answer: **59**

❍ **A.** Take the blood pressure, pulse, and temperature

❍ **B.** Ask the client to rate his pain on a scale of 0–5

❍ **C.** Watch the client's facial expression

❍ **D.** Ask the client if he is in pain

67. The nursing is participating in discharge teaching for the post-partal client. The nurse is aware that an effective means of managing discomfort associated with an episiotomy after discharge is:

Quick Answers: **50**
Detailed Answer: **59**

❍ **A.** Promethazine

❍ **B.** Aspirin

❍ **C.** Sitz baths

❍ **D.** Ice packs

68. Which of the following post-operative diets is most appropriate for the client who has had a hemorroidectomy?

Quick Answers: **50**
Detailed Answer: **59**

❍ **A.** High-fiber

❍ **B.** Low-residue

❍ **C.** Bland

❍ **D.** Clear-liquid

Quick Check

69. The physician has ordered a culture for the client with suspected gonorrhea. The nurse should obtain which type of culture?

Quick Answers: **50**
Detailed Answer: **59**

❍ **A.** Blood

❍ **B.** Nasopharyngeal secretions

❍ **C.** Stool

❍ **D.** Genital secretions

70. The nurse is caring for a client with cerebral palsy. The nurse should provide frequent rest periods because:

Quick Answers: **50**
Detailed Answer: **59**

❍ **A.** Grimacing and writhing movements decrease with relaxation and rest.

❍ **B.** Hypoactive deep tendon reflexes become more active with rest.

❍ **C.** Stretch reflexes are increased with rest.

❍ **D.** Fine motor movements are improved.

71. The nurse is making assignments for the day. Which client should be assigned to the nursing assistant?

Quick Answers: **50**
Detailed Answer: **59**

❍ **A.** A client with Alzheimer's disease

❍ **B.** A client with pneumonia

❍ **C.** A client with appendicitis

❍ **D.** A client with thrombophebitis

72. A client with cancer develops xerostomia. The nurse can help alleviate the discomfort associated with xerostomia by:

Quick Answers: **50**
Detailed Answer: **59**

❍ **A.** Offering hard candy

❍ **B.** Administering analgesic medications

❍ **C.** Splinting swollen joints

❍ **D.** Providing saliva substitute

73. A home health nurse is making preparations for morning visits. Which one of the following clients should the nurse visit first?

Quick Answers: **50**
Detailed Answer: **60**

❍ **A.** A client with brain attack (stroke) with tube feedings

❍ **B.** A client with congestive heart failure complaining of nighttime dyspnea

❍ **C.** A client with a thoracotomy 6 months ago

❍ **D.** A client with Parkinson's disease

Quick Check

74. A client with glomerulonephritis is placed on a low-sodium diet. Which of the following snacks is suitable for the client with sodium restriction?

Quick Answers: **50**
Detailed Answer: **60**

❍ **A.** Peanut butter cookies

❍ **B.** Grilled cheese sandwich

❍ **C.** Cottage cheese and fruit

❍ **D.** Fresh peach

75. Due to a high census, it has been necessary for a number of clients to be transferred to other units within the hospital. Which client should be transferred to the postpartum unit?

Quick Answers: **50**
Detailed Answer: **60**

❍ **A.** A 66-year-old female with a gastroenteritis

❍ **B.** A 40-year-old female with a hysterectomy

❍ **C.** A 27-year-old male with severe depression

❍ **D.** A 28-year-old male with ulcerative colitis

76. During the change of shift, the oncoming nurse notes a discrepancy in the number of Percocet (Oxycodone) listed and the number present in the narcotic drawer. The nurse's first action should be to:

Quick Answers: **50**
Detailed Answer: **60**

❍ **A.** Notify the hospital pharmacist

❍ **B.** Notify the nursing supervisor

❍ **C.** Notify the Board of Nursing

❍ **D.** Notify the director of nursing

77. The nurse is assigning staff for the day. Which assignment should be given to the nursing assistant?

Quick Answers: **50**
Detailed Answer: **60**

❍ **A.** Taking the vital signs of the 5-month-old with bronchiolitis

❍ **B.** Taking the vital signs of the 10-year-old with a 2-day post-appendectomy

❍ **C.** Administering medication to the 2-year-old with periorbital cellulites

❍ **D.** Adjusting the traction of the 1-year-old with a fractured tibia

Quick Check

78. A new nursing graduate indicates in charting entries that he is a licensed practical nurse, although he has not yet received the results of the licensing exam. The graduate's action can result in what type of charge:

Quick Answers: **50**
Detailed Answer: **60**

❍ **A.** Fraud
❍ **B.** Tort
❍ **C.** Malpractice
❍ **D.** Negligence

79. A client with acute leukemia develops a low white blood cell count. In addition to the institution of isolation, the nurse should:

Quick Answers: **50**
Detailed Answer: **60**

❍ **A.** Request that foods be served with disposable utensils
❍ **B.** Ask the client to wear a mask when visitors are present
❍ **C.** Prep IV sites with mild soap and water and alcohol
❍ **D.** Provide foods in sealed single-serving packages

80. A 70-year-old male who is recovering from a stroke exhibits signs of unilateral neglect. Which behavior is suggestive of unilateral neglect?

Quick Answers: **50**
Detailed Answer: **60**

❍ **A.** The client is observed shaving only one side of his face.
❍ **B.** The client is unable to distinguish between two tactile stimuli presented simultaneously.
❍ **C.** The client is unable to complete a range of vision without turning his head side to side.
❍ **D.** The client is unable to carry out cognitive and motor activity at the same time.

81. The nurse is providing discharge teaching for a client taking disulfiram (Antabuse). The nurse should instruct the client to avoid eating:

Quick Answers: **50**
Detailed Answer: **60**

❍ **A.** Peanuts, dates, raisins
❍ **B.** Figs, chocolate, eggplant
❍ **C.** Pickles, salad with vinaigrette dressing, beef
❍ **D.** Milk, cottage cheese, ice cream

Quick Check

82. A client has been receiving cyanocobalamine (B12) injections for the past 6 weeks. Which laboratory finding indicates that the medication is having the desired effect?

Quick Answers: **50**
Detailed Answer: **60**

- ❍ **A.** Neutrophil count of 60%
- ❍ **B.** Basophil count of 0.5%
- ❍ **C.** Monocyte count of 2%
- ❍ **D.** Reticulocyte count of 1%

83. The nurse has just received a change-of-shift report. Which client should the nurse assess first?

Quick Answers: **50**
Detailed Answer: **60**

- ❍ **A.** A client 2 hours post-lobectomy with 150ccs drainage
- ❍ **B.** A client 2 days post-gastrectomy with scant drainage
- ❍ **C.** A client with pneumonia with an oral temperature of 102°F
- ❍ **D.** A client with a fractured hip in Buck's traction

84. Several clients are admitted to the emergency room following a three-car vehicle accident. Which clients can be assigned to share a room in the emergency department during the disaster?

Quick Answers: **50**
Detailed Answer: **61**

- ❍ **A.** The schizophrenic client having visual and auditory hallucinations and the client with ulcerative colitis
- ❍ **B.** The client who is 6 months pregnant with abdominal pain and the client with facial lacerations and a broken arm
- ❍ **C.** A child whose pupils are fixed and dilated and his parents, and the client with a frontal head injury
- ❍ **D.** The client who arrives with a large puncture wound to the abdomen and the client with chest pain

85. The home health nurse is planning for the day's visits. Which client should be seen first?

Quick Answers: **50**
Detailed Answer: **61**

- ❍ **A.** The 78-year-old who had a gastrectomy 3 weeks ago with a PEG tube
- ❍ **B.** The 5-month-old discharged 1 week ago with pneumonia who is being treated with amoxicillin liquid suspension
- ❍ **C.** The 50-year-old with MRSA being treated with Vancomycin via a PICC line
- ❍ **D.** The 30-year-old with an exacerbation of multiple sclerosis being treated with cortisone via a centrally placed venous catheter

Quick Check

86. The nurse is found to be guilty of charting blood glucose results without actually performing the procedure. After talking to the nurse, the charge nurse should:

Quick Answers: **50**
Detailed Answer: **61**

❍ **A.** Call the Board of Nursing

❍ **B.** File a formal reprimand

❍ **C.** Terminate the nurse

❍ **D.** Charge the nurse with a tort

87. Which information should be reported to the state Board of Nursing?

Quick Answers: **50**
Detailed Answer: **61**

❍ **A.** The facility fails to provide literature in both Spanish and English.

❍ **B.** The narcotic count has been incorrect on the unit for the past 3 days.

❍ **C.** The client fails to receive an itemized account of his bills and services received during his hospital stay.

❍ **D.** The nursing assistant assigned to the client with hepatitis fails to feed the client and give the bath.

88. Which nurse should be assigned to care for the postpartal client with preeclampsia?

Quick Answers: **51**
Detailed Answer: **61**

❍ **A.** The nurse with 2 weeks of experience on postpartum

❍ **B.** The nurse with 3 years of experience in labor and delivery

❍ **C.** The nurse with 10 years of experience in surgery

❍ **D.** The nurse with 1 year of experience in the neonatal intensive care unit

89. The client returns to the unit from surgery with a blood pressure of 90/50, pulse 132, respirations 30. Which action by the nurse should receive priority?

Quick Answers: **51**
Detailed Answer: **61**

❍ **A.** Continue to monitor the vital signs

❍ **B.** Contact the physician

❍ **C.** Ask the client how he feels

❍ **D.** Ask the LPN to continue the post-op care

Quick Check

90. Which assignment should not be performed by the licensed practical nurse?

Quick Answers: **51**
Detailed Answer: **61**

- ❍ **A.** Inserting a Foley catheter
- ❍ **B.** Discontinuing a nasogastric tube
- ❍ **C.** Obtaining a sputum specimen
- ❍ **D.** Initiating a blood transfusion

91. The nurse witnesses the nursing assistant hitting the client in the long-term care facility. The nursing assistant can be charged with:

Quick Answers: **51**
Detailed Answer: **61**

- ❍ **A.** Negligence
- ❍ **B.** Tort
- ❍ **C.** Assault
- ❍ **D.** Malpractice

92. The nurse is planning room assignments for the day. Which client should be assigned to a private room if only one is available?

Quick Answers: **51**
Detailed Answer: **61**

- ❍ **A.** The client with Cushing's disease
- ❍ **B.** The client with diabetes
- ❍ **C.** The client with acromegaly
- ❍ **D.** The client with myxedema

93. The nurse is making assignments for the day. Which client should be assigned to the pregnant nurse?

Quick Answers: **51**
Detailed Answer: **62**

- ❍ **A.** The client receiving linear accelerator radiation therapy for lung cancer
- ❍ **B.** The client with a radium implant for cervical cancer
- ❍ **C.** The client who has just been administered soluble brachytherapy for thyroid cancer
- ❍ **D.** The client who returned from placement of iridium seeds for prostate cancer

94. The client is receiving heparin for thrombophlebitis of the left lower extremity. Which of the following drugs reverses the effects of heparin?

Quick Answers: **51**
Detailed Answer: **62**

- ❍ **A.** Cyanocobalamine
- ❍ **B.** Protamine sulfate
- ❍ **C.** Streptokinase
- ❍ **D.** Sodium warfarin

Quick Check

95. The client is admitted with a BP of 210/120. Her doctor orders furosemide (Lasix) 40mg IV stat. How should the nurse administer the prescribed furosemide to this client?

Quick Answers: **51**
Detailed Answer: **62**

- ❍ **A.** By giving it over 1–2 minutes
- ❍ **B.** By hanging it IV piggyback
- ❍ **C.** With normal saline only
- ❍ **D.** By administering it through a venous access device

96. The physician prescribes captopril (Capoten) 25mg po tid for the client with hypertension. Which of the following adverse reactions can occur with administration of Capoten?

Quick Answers: **51**
Detailed Answer: **62**

- ❍ **A.** Tinnitus
- ❍ **B.** Persistent cough
- ❍ **C.** Muscle weakness
- ❍ **D.** Diarrhea

97. The doctor orders 2% nitroglycerin ointment in a 1-inch dose every 12 hours. Proper application of nitroglycerin ointment includes:

Quick Answers: **51**
Detailed Answer: **62**

- ❍ **A.** Rotating application sites
- ❍ **B.** Limiting applications to the chest
- ❍ **C.** Rubbing it into the skin
- ❍ **D.** Covering it with a gauze dressing

98. Lidocaine is a medication frequently ordered for the client experiencing:

Quick Answers: **51**
Detailed Answer: **62**

- ❍ **A.** Atrial tachycardia
- ❍ **B.** Ventricular tachycardia
- ❍ **C.** Heart block
- ❍ **D.** Ventricular brachycardia

99. The client is admitted to the emergency room with shortness of breath, anxiety, and tachycardia. His ECG reveals atrial fibrillation with a ventricular response rate of 130 beats per minute. The doctor orders quinidine sulfate. While he is receiving quinidine, the nurse should monitor his ECG for:

Quick Answers: **51**
Detailed Answer: **62**

- ❍ **A.** Peaked P wave
- ❍ **B.** Elevated ST segment
- ❍ **C.** Inverted T wave
- ❍ **D.** Prolonged QT interval

Quick Check

100. The physician has prescribed tranylcypromine sulfate (Parnate) 10mg bid. The nurse should teach the client to refrain from eating foods containing tyramine because it may cause:

Quick Answers: **51**
Detailed Answer: **62**

❍ **A.** Hypertension

❍ **B.** Hyperthermia

❍ **C.** Melanoma

❍ **D.** Urinary retention

101. The child with seizure disorder is being treated with Dilantin (phenytoin). Which of the following statements by the patient's mother indicates to the nurse that the patient is experiencing a side effect of Dilantin therapy?

Quick Answers: **51**
Detailed Answer: **63**

❍ **A.** "She is very irritable lately."

❍ **B.** "She sleeps quite a bit of the time."

❍ **C.** "Her gums look too big for her teeth."

❍ **D.** "She has gained about 10 pounds in the last 6 months."

102. A 5-year-old is admitted to the unit following a tonsillectomy. Which of the following would indicate a complication of the surgery?

Quick Answers: **51**
Detailed Answer: **63**

❍ **A.** Decreased appetite

❍ **B.** A low-grade fever

❍ **C.** Chest congestion

❍ **D.** Constant swallowing

103. A 6-year-old with cerebral palsy functions at the level of an 18-month-old. Which finding would support that assessment?

Quick Answers: **51**
Detailed Answer: **63**

❍ **A.** She dresses herself.

❍ **B.** She pulls a toy behind her.

❍ **C.** She can build a tower of eight blocks.

❍ **D.** She can copy a horizontal or vertical line.

104. Which information obtained from the mother of a child with cerebral palsy most likely correlates to the diagnosis?

Quick Answers: **51**
Detailed Answer: **63**

❍ **A.** She was born at 42 weeks gestation.

❍ **B.** She had meningitis when she was 6 months old.

❍ **C.** She had physiologic jaundice after delivery.

❍ **D.** She has frequent sore throats.

Quick Check

105. The 10-year-old is being treated for asthma. Before administering Theodur, the nurse should check the:

Quick Answers: **51**
Detailed Answer: **63**

- ❍ **A.** Urinary output
- ❍ **B.** Blood pressure
- ❍ **C.** Pulse
- ❍ **D.** Temperature

106. An elderly client is diagnosed with ovarian cancer. She has surgery followed by chemotherapy with a fluorouracil (Adrucil) IV. What should the nurse do if she notices crystals and cloudiness in the IV medication?

Quick Answers: **51**
Detailed Answer: **63**

- ❍ **A.** Discard the solution and order a new bag
- ❍ **B.** Warm the solution
- ❍ **C.** Continue the infusion and document the finding
- ❍ **D.** Discontinue the medication

107. The client is diagnosed with multiple myoloma. The doctor has ordered cyclophosphamide (Cytoxan). Which instruction should be given to the client?

Quick Answers: **51**
Detailed Answer: **63**

- ❍ **A.** "Walk about a mile a day to prevent calcium loss."
- ❍ **B.** "Increase the fiber in your diet."
- ❍ **C.** "Report nausea to the doctor immediately."
- ❍ **D.** "Drink at least eight large glasses of water a day."

108. The client is taking rifampin 600mg po daily to treat his tuberculosis. Which action by the nurse indicates understanding of the medication?

Quick Answers: **51**
Detailed Answer: **63**

- ❍ **A.** Telling the client that the medication will need to be taken with juice
- ❍ **B.** Telling the client that the medication will change the color of the urine
- ❍ **C.** Telling the client to take the medication before going to bed at night
- ❍ **D.** Telling the client to take the medication if night sweats occur

Quick Check

109. The client is taking prednisone 7.5mg po each morning to treat his systemic lupus errythymatosis. Which statement best explains the reason for taking the prednisone in the morning?

Quick Answers: **51**
Detailed Answer: **63**

- ❍ **A.** There is less chance of forgetting the medication if taken in the morning.
- ❍ **B.** There will be less fluid retention if taken in the morning.
- ❍ **C.** Prednisone is absorbed best with the breakfast meal.
- ❍ **D.** Morning administration mimics the body's natural secretion of corticosteroid.

110. A 20-year-old female has a prescription for tetracycline. While teaching the client how to take her medicine, the nurse learns that the client is also taking Ortho-Novum oral contraceptive pills. Which instructions should be included in the teaching plan?

Quick Answers: **51**
Detailed Answer: **63**

- ❍ **A.** The oral contraceptives will decrease the effectiveness of the tetracycline.
- ❍ **B.** Nausea often results from taking oral contraceptives and antibiotics.
- ❍ **C.** Toxicity can result when taking these two medications together.
- ❍ **D.** Antibiotics can decrease the effectiveness of oral contraceptives, so the client should use an alternate method of birth control.

111. A 60-year-old diabetic is taking glyburide (Diabeta) 1.25mg daily to treat Type II diabetes mellitus. Which statement indicates the need for further teaching?

Quick Answers: **51**
Detailed Answer: **63**

- ❍ **A.** "I will keep candy with me just in case my blood sugar drops."
- ❍ **B.** "I need to stay out of the sun as much as possible."
- ❍ **C.** "I often skip dinner because I don't feel hungry."
- ❍ **D.** "I always wear my medical identification."

112. The physician prescribes regular insulin, 5 units subcutaneous. Regular insulin begins to exert an effect:

Quick Answers: **51**
Detailed Answer: **63**

- ❍ **A.** In 5–10 minutes
- ❍ **B.** In 10–20 minutes
- ❍ **C.** In 30–60 minutes
- ❍ **D.** In 60–120 minutes

Quick Check

113. The client is admitted from the emergency room with multiple injuries sustained from an auto accident. His doctor prescribes a histamine blocker. The reason for this order is:

Quick Answers: **51**
Detailed Answer: **63**

- ❍ **A.** To treat general discomfort
- ❍ **B.** To correct electrolyte imbalances
- ❍ **C.** To prevent stress ulcers
- ❍ **D.** To treat nausea

114. The client with a recent liver transplant asks the nurse how long he will have to take cyclosporine (Sandimmune). Which response is correct?

Quick Answers: **51**
Detailed Answer: **64**

- ❍ **A.** 1 year
- ❍ **B.** 5 years
- ❍ **C.** 10 years
- ❍ **D.** The rest of his life

115. Shortly after the client was admitted to the postpartum unit, the nurse notes heavy lochia rubra with large clots. The nurse should anticipate an order for:

Quick Answers: **51**
Detailed Answer: **64**

- ❍ **A.** Methergine
- ❍ **B.** Stadol
- ❍ **C.** Magnesium sulfate
- ❍ **D.** Phenergan

116. The client is scheduled to have an intravenous cholangiogram. Before the procedure, the nurse should assess the patient for:

Quick Answers: **51**
Detailed Answer: **64**

- ❍ **A.** Shellfish allergies
- ❍ **B.** Reactions to blood transfusions
- ❍ **C.** Gallbladder disease
- ❍ **D.** Egg allergies

117. A new diabetic is learning to administer his insulin. He receives 10U of NPH and 12U of regular insulin each morning. Which of the following statements reflects understanding of the nurse's teaching?

Quick Answers: **51**
Detailed Answer: **64**

- ❍ **A.** "When drawing up my insulin, I should draw up the regular insulin first."
- ❍ **B.** "When drawing up my insulin, I should draw up the NPH insulin first."
- ❍ **C.** "It doesn't matter which insulin I draw up first."
- ❍ **D.** "I cannot mix the insulin, so I will need two shots."

Quick Check

118. A client with osteomylitis has an order for a trough level to be done because he is taking Gentamycin. When should the nurse call the lab to obtain the trough level?

Quick Answers: **51**
Detailed Answer: **64**

- ❍ **A.** Before the first dose
- ❍ **B.** 30 minutes before the fourth dose
- ❍ **C.** 30 minutes after the first dose
- ❍ **D.** 30 minutes after the fourth dose

119. A 4-year-old with cystic fibrosis has a prescription for Viokase pancreatic enzymes to prevent malabsorption. The correct time to give pancreatic enzyme is:

Quick Answers: **51**
Detailed Answer: **64**

- ❍ **A.** 1 hour before meals
- ❍ **B.** 2 hours after meals
- ❍ **C.** With each meal and snack
- ❍ **D.** On an empty stomach

120. Isoniazid (INH) has been prescribed for a family member exposed to tuberculosis. The nurse is aware that the length of time that the medication will be taken is:

Quick Answers: **51**
Detailed Answer: **64**

- ❍ **A.** 6 months
- ❍ **B.** 3 months
- ❍ **C.** 18 months
- ❍ **D.** 24 months

121. The client is admitted to the postpartum unit with an order to continue the infusion of Pitocin. Which finding indicates that the Pitocin is having the desired effect?

Quick Answers: **51**
Detailed Answer: **64**

- ❍ **A.** The fundus is deviated to the left.
- ❍ **B.** The fundus is firm and in the midline.
- ❍ **C.** The fundus is boggy.
- ❍ **D.** The fundus is two finger breadths below the umbilicus.

122. The nurse is teaching a group of new graduates about the safety needs of the client receiving chemotherapy. Before administering chemotherapy, the nurse should:

Quick Answers: **51**
Detailed Answer: **64**

- ❍ **A.** Administer a bolus of IV fluid
- ❍ **B.** Administer pain medication
- ❍ **C.** Administer an antiemetic
- ❍ **D.** Allow the patient a chance to eat

Quick Check

123. Before administering Methytrexate orally to the client with cancer, the nurse should check the:

Quick Answers: **51**
Detailed Answer: **64**

- ❍ **A.** IV site
- ❍ **B.** Electrolytes
- ❍ **C.** Blood gases
- ❍ **D.** Vital signs

124. Vitamin K (aquamephyton) is administered to a newborn shortly after birth for which of the following reasons?

Quick Answers: **51**
Detailed Answer: **64**

- ❍ **A.** To prevent dehydration
- ❍ **B.** To treat infection
- ❍ **C.** To replace electrolytes
- ❍ **D.** To facilitate clotting

125. The client with an ileostomy is being discharged. Which teaching should be included in the plan of care?

Quick Answers: **51**
Detailed Answer: **65**

- ❍ **A.** Use Karaya powder to seal the bag.
- ❍ **B.** Irrigate the ileostomy daily.
- ❍ **C.** Stomahesive is the best skin protector.
- ❍ **D.** Neosporin ointment can be used to protect the skin.

126. The client has an order for $FeSo_4$ liquid. Which method of administration would be best?

Quick Answers: **51**
Detailed Answer: **65**

- ❍ **A.** Administer the medication with milk
- ❍ **B.** Administer the medication with a meal
- ❍ **C.** Administer the medication with orange juice
- ❍ **D.** Administer the medication undiluted

127. The client arrives in the emergency room with a hyphema. Which action by the nurse would be best?

Quick Answers: **51**
Detailed Answer: **65**

- ❍ **A.** Elevate the head of the bed and apply ice to the eye
- ❍ **B.** Place the client in a supine position and apply heat to the knee
- ❍ **C.** Insert a Foley catheter and measure the intake and output
- ❍ **D.** Perform a vaginal exam and check for a discharge

Quick Check

128. The nurse is making assignments for the day. Which client should be assigned to the nursing assistant?

Quick Answers: **51**
Detailed Answer: **65**

❍ **A.** The 18-year-old with a fracture to two cervical vertebrae

❍ **B.** The infant with meningitis

❍ **C.** The elderly client with a thyroidectomy 4 days ago

❍ **D.** The client with a thoracotomy 2 days ago

129. The client arrives in the emergency room with a "bull's eye" rash. Which question would be most appropriate for the nurse to ask the client?

Quick Answers: **51**
Detailed Answer: **65**

❍ **A.** "Have you found any ticks on your body?"

❍ **B.** "Have you had any nausea in the last 24 hours?"

❍ **C.** "Have you been outside the country in the last 6 months?"

❍ **D.** "Have you had any fever for the past few days?"

130. Which of the following is the best indicator of the diagnosis of HIV?

Quick Answers: **51**
Detailed Answer: **65**

❍ **A.** White blood cell count

❍ **B.** ELISA

❍ **C.** Western Blot

❍ **D.** Complete blood count

131. The client has an order for gentamycin to be administered. Which lab results should be reported to the doctor before beginning the medication?

Quick Answers: **51**
Detailed Answer: **65**

❍ **A.** Hematocrit

❍ **B.** Creatinine

❍ **C.** White blood cell count

❍ **D.** Erythrocyte count

132. The nurse is caring for the client with a mastectomy. Which action would be contraindicated?

Quick Answers: **51**
Detailed Answer: **65**

❍ **A.** Taking the blood pressure in the side of the mastectomy

❍ **B.** Elevating the arm on the side of the mastectomy

❍ **C.** Positioning the client on the unaffected side

❍ **D.** Performing a dextrostix on the unaffected side

Quick Check

133. The charge nurse is making assignments for the day. After accepting the assignment to a client with leukemia, the nurse tells the charge nurse that her child has chickenpox. Which action should the charge nurse take?

Quick Answers: **51**
Detailed Answer: **65**

❍ **A.** Change the nurse's assignment to another client

❍ **B.** Explain to the nurse that there is no risk to the client

❍ **C.** Ask the nurse if the chickenpox have scabbed

❍ **D.** Ask the nurse if she has ever had the chickenpox

134. The client with brain cancer refuses to care for herself. Which action by the nurse would be best?

Quick Answers: **51**
Detailed Answer: **66**

❍ **A.** Alternate nurses caring for the client so that the staff will not get tired of caring for this client

❍ **B.** Talk to the client and explain the need for self-care

❍ **C.** Explore the reason for the lack of motivation seen in the client

❍ **D.** Talk to the doctor about the client's lack of motivation

135. The nurse is caring for the client who has been in a coma for 2 months. He has signed a donor card, but the wife is opposed to the idea of organ donation. How should the nurse handle the topic of organ donation with the wife?

Quick Answers: **51**
Detailed Answer: **66**

❍ **A.** Contact organ retrieval to come talk to the wife

❍ **B.** Tell her that because her husband signed a donor card, the hospital has the right to take the organs upon the death of her husband

❍ **C.** Drop the subject until a later time

❍ **D.** Refrain from talking about the subject until after the death of her husband

136. The nurse is assessing the abdomen. The nurse knows the best sequence to perform the assessment is:

Quick Answers: **51**
Detailed Answer: **66**

❍ **A.** Inspection, auscultation, palpation

❍ **B.** Auscultation, palpation, inspection

❍ **C.** Palpation, inspection, auscultation

❍ **D.** Inspection, palpation, auscultation

Quick Check

137. The nurse is assisting in the assessment of the patient admitted with abdominal pain. Why should the nurse ask about medications that the client is taking?

Quick Answers: **51**
Detailed Answer: **66**

❍ **A.** Interactions between medications can be identified.

❍ **B.** Various medications taken by mouth can affect the alimentary tract.

❍ **C.** This will provide an opportunity to educate the patient regarding the medications used.

❍ **D.** The types of medications might be attributable to an abdominal pathology not already identified.

138. The nurse is asked by the nurse aide, "Are peptic ulcers really caused by stress?" The nurse would be correct in replying with which of the following:

Quick Answers: **51**
Detailed Answer: **66**

❍ **A.** "Peptic ulcers result from overeating fatty foods."

❍ **B.** "Peptic ulcers are always caused from exposure to continual stress."

❍ **C.** "Peptic ulcers are like all other ulcers, which all result from stress."

❍ **D.** "Peptic ulcers are associated with *H. pylori*, although there are other ulcers that are associated with stress."

139. The client is newly diagnosed with juvenile onset diabetes. Which of the following nursing diagnoses is a priority?

Quick Answers: **51**
Detailed Answer: **66**

❍ **A.** Anxiety

❍ **B.** Pain

❍ **C.** Knowledge deficit

❍ **D.** Altered thought process

140. The nurse understands that the diagnosis of oral cancer is confirmed with:

Quick Answers: **51**
Detailed Answer: **66**

❍ **A.** Biopsy

❍ **B.** Gram Stain

❍ **C.** Scrape cytology

❍ **D.** Oral washings for cytology

Quick Check

141. The nurse is assisting in the care of a patient who is 2 days post-operative from a hemorroidectomy. The nurse would be correct in instructing the patient to:

Quick Answers: **51**
Detailed Answer: **66**

❍ **A.** Avoid a high-fiber diet because this can hasten the healing time

❍ **B.** Continue to use ice packs until discharge and then when at home

❍ **C.** Take 200mg of Colace bid to prevent constipation

❍ **D.** Use a sitz bath after each bowel movement to promote cleanliness and comfort

142. The nurse is caring for a patient with a colostomy. The patient asks, "Will I ever be able to swim again?" The nurse's best response would be:

Quick Answers: **51**
Detailed Answer: **66**

❍ **A.** "Yes, you should be able to swim again, even with the colostomy."

❍ **B.** "You should avoid immersing the colostomy in water."

❍ **C.** "No, you should avoid getting the colostomy wet."

❍ **D.** "Don't worry about that. You will be able to live just like you did before."

143. Which is true regarding the administration of antacids?

Quick Answers: **51**
Detailed Answer: **66**

❍ **A.** Antacids should be administered without regard to mealtimes.

❍ **B.** Antacids should be administered with each meal and snack of the day.

❍ **C.** Antacids should be administered within 1–2 hours of all other medications.

❍ **D.** Antacids should be administered with all other medications, for maximal absorption.

144. The nurse is preparing to administer a feeding via a nasogastric tube. The nurse would perform which of the following before initiating the feeding?

Quick Answers: **51**
Detailed Answer: **66**

❍ **A.** Assess for tube placement by aspirating stomach content

❍ **B.** Place the patient in a left-lying position

❍ **C.** Administer feeding with 50% H_20 concentration

❍ **D.** Ensure that the feeding solution has been warmed in a microwave for 2 minutes

Quick Check

145. The patient is prescribed metronidazole (Flagyl) for adjunct treatment for a duodenal ulcer. When teaching about this medication, the nurse would say:

Quick Answers: **51**
Detailed Answer: **67**

- ❍ **A.** "This medication should be taken only until you begin to feel better."
- ❍ **B.** "This medication should be taken on an empty stomach to increase absorption."
- ❍ **C.** "While taking this medication, you do not have to be concerned about being in the sun."
- ❍ **D.** "While taking this medication, alcoholic beverages and products containing alcohol should be avoided."

146. In planning care for the patient with ulcerative colitis, the nurse identifies which nursing diagnoses as a priority?

Quick Answers: **51**
Detailed Answer: **67**

- ❍ **A.** Anxiety
- ❍ **B.** Impaired skin integrity
- ❍ **C.** Fluid volume deficit
- ❍ **D.** Nutrition altered, less than body requirements

147. The nurse is teaching about irritable bowel syndrome (IBS). Which of the following would be most important?

Quick Answers: **51**
Detailed Answer: **67**

- ❍ **A.** Reinforcing the need for a balanced diet
- ❍ **B.** Encouraging the client to drink 16 ounces of fluid with each meal
- ❍ **C.** Telling the client to eat a diet low in fiber
- ❍ **D.** Instructing the client to limit his intake of fruits and vegetables

148. The nurse is planning care for the patient with celiac disease. In teaching about the diet, the nurse should instruct the patient to avoid which of the following for breakfast?

Quick Answers: **51**
Detailed Answer: **67**

- ❍ **A.** Cream of wheat
- ❍ **B.** Banana
- ❍ **C.** Puffed rice
- ❍ **D.** Cornflakes

Quick Check

149. The nurse is caring for a patient with suspected diverticulitis. The nurse would be most prudent in questioning which of the following diagnostic tests ordered?

❍ **A.** Colonoscopy

❍ **B.** Barium enema

❍ **C.** Complete blood count

❍ **D.** Computed tomography (CT) scan

Quick Answers: **51**
Detailed Answer: **67**

150. When the nurse is gathering information for the assessment, the patient states, "My stomach hurts about 2 hours after I eat." Based upon this information, the nurse knows the patient likely has a:

❍ **A.** Gastric ulcer

❍ **B.** Duodenal ulcer

❍ **C.** Peptic ulcer

❍ **D.** Curling's ulcer

Quick Answers: **51**
Detailed Answer: **67**

151. The registered nurse is conducting an in-service for colleagues about peptic ulcers. The nurse would be correct in identifying which of the following as a causative factor?

❍ **A.** *N. gonorrhea*

❍ **B.** *H. influenza*

❍ **C.** *H. pylori*

❍ **D.** *E. coli*

Quick Answers: **51**
Detailed Answer: **67**

152. The nurse is caring for the patient's post-surgical removal of a 6mm oral cancerous lesion. The priority nursing measure would be to:

❍ **A.** Maintain a patent airway

❍ **B.** Perform meticulous oral care every 2 hours

❍ **C.** Ensure that the incisional area is kept as dry as possible

❍ **D.** Assess the client frequently for pain using the visual analogue scale

Quick Answers: **51**
Detailed Answer: **67**

Quick Check

153. The nurse is assisting in the care of a patient with diverticulosis. Which of the following assessment findings would necessitate a report to the doctor?

Quick Answers: 51
Detailed Answer: 67

- ❍ **A.** Bowel sounds of 5–20 seconds
- ❍ **B.** Intermittent left lower-quadrant pain
- ❍ **C.** Constipation alternating with diarrhea
- ❍ **D.** Hemoglobin 26% and hematocrit 32

154. The nurse is assessing the client admitted for possible oral cancer. The nurse identifies which of the following as a late-occurring symptom of oral cancer?

Quick Answers: 51
Detailed Answer: 67

- ❍ **A.** Warmth
- ❍ **B.** Odor
- ❍ **C.** Pain
- ❍ **D.** Ulcer with flat edges

155. An obstetrical client decides to have an epidural anesthetic to relieve pain during labor. Following administration of the anesthesia, the nurse should:

Quick Answers: 51
Detailed Answer: 67

- ❍ **A.** Monitor the client for seizures
- ❍ **B.** Monitor the client for orthostatic hypotension
- ❍ **C.** Monitor the client for respiratory depression
- ❍ **D.** Monitor the client for hematuria

156. The nurse is performing an assessment of an elderly client with a total hip repair. Based on this assessment, the nurse decides to medicate the client with an analgesic. Which finding most likely prompted the nurse to decide to administer the analgesic?

Quick Answers: 51
Detailed Answer: 68

- ❍ **A.** The client's blood pressure is 130/86.
- ❍ **B.** The client is unable to concentrate.
- ❍ **C.** The client's pupils are dilated.
- ❍ **D.** The client grimaces during care.

Quick Check

157. A client who has chosen to breastfeed complains to the nurse that her nipples became very sore while she was breastfeeding her older child. Which measure will help her to avoid soreness of the nipples?

Quick Answers: **51**
Detailed Answer: **68**

- ❍ **A.** Feeding the baby during the first 48 hours after delivery
- ❍ **B.** Breaking suction by placing a finger between the baby's mouth and the breast when she terminates the feeding
- ❍ **C.** Applying warm, moist soaks to the breast several times per day
- ❍ **D.** Wearing a support bra

158. The nurse asked the client if he has an advance directive. The reason for asking the client this question is:

Quick Answers: **51**
Detailed Answer: **68**

- ❍ **A.** She is curious about his plans regarding funeral arrangements.
- ❍ **B.** Much confusion can occur with the client's family if he does not have an advanced directive.
- ❍ **C.** An advanced directive allows the medical personnel to make all decisions for the client.
- ❍ **D.** An advanced directive allows active euthanasia.

159. The doctor has ordered a Transcutaneous Electrical Nerve Stimulation (TENS) unit for the client with chronic back pain. The nurse teaching the client with a TENS unit should tell the client:

Quick Answers: **51**
Detailed Answer: **68**

- ❍ **A.** "You may be electrocuted if you use water with this unit."
- ❍ **B.** "Please report skin irritation to the doctor."
- ❍ **C.** "The unit may be used anywhere on the body without fear of adverse reactions."
- ❍ **D.** "A cream should be applied to the skin before applying the unit."

Quick Check

160. The doctor has ordered a patient-controlled analgesia (PCA) pump for the client with chronic pain. The client asks the nurse if he can become overdosed with pain medication using this machine. The nurse demonstrates understanding of the PCA if she states:

Quick Answers: **51**
Detailed Answer: **68**

❍ **A.** "The machine will administer only the amount that you need to control your pain without your taking any action."

❍ **B.** "The machine has a locking device that prevents over-dosing to occur."

❍ **C.** "The machine will administer one large dose every 4 hours to relieve your pain."

❍ **D.** "The machine is set to deliver medication only if you need it."

161. The 84-year-old male has returned from the recovery room following a total hip repair. He complains of pain and is medicated by morphine sulfate and promethazine. Which medication should be kept available for the client being treated with opoid analgesics?

Quick Answers: **51**
Detailed Answer: **68**

❍ **A.** Nalozone (Narcan)

❍ **B.** Ketorolac (Toradol)

❍ **C.** Acetylsalicylic acid (aspirin)

❍ **D.** Atropine sulfate (Atropine)

162. The nurse is taking the vital signs of the client admitted with cancer of the pancreas. The nurse is aware that the fifth vital sign is:

Quick Answers: **51**
Detailed Answer: **68**

❍ **A.** Anorexia

❍ **B.** Pain

❍ **C.** Insomnia

❍ **D.** Fatigue

163. The client with AIDS tells the nurse that he has been using acupuncture to help with his pain. The nurse should question the client regarding this treatment because acupuncture:

Quick Answers: **51**
Detailed Answer: **68**

❍ **A.** Uses pressure from the fingers and hands to stimulate the energy points in the body

❍ **B.** Uses oils extracted from plants and herbs

❍ **C.** Uses needles to stimulate certain points on the body to treat pain

❍ **D.** Uses manipulation of the skeletal muscles to relieve stress and pain

Quick Check

164. The client has an order for heparin to prevent post-surgical thrombi. Immediately following a heparin injection, the nurse should:

Quick Answers: **51**
Detailed Answer: **68**

❍ **A.** Aspirate for blood

❍ **B.** Check the pulse rate

❍ **C.** Massage the site

❍ **D.** Check the site for bleeding

165. Which of the following lab studies should be done periodically if the client is taking sodium warfarin (Coumadin)?

Quick Answers: **51**
Detailed Answer: **69**

❍ **A.** Stool specimen for occult blood

❍ **B.** White blood cell count

❍ **C.** Blood glucose

❍ **D.** Erthyrocyte count

166. The doctor has ordered 80mg of furosemide (Lasix) two times per day. The nurse notes the patient's potassium level to be 2.5meq/L. The nurse should:

Quick Answers: **51**
Detailed Answer: **69**

❍ **A.** Administer the Lasix as ordered

❍ **B.** Administer half the dose

❍ **C.** Offer the patient a potassium-rich food

❍ **D.** Withhold the drug and call the doctor

167. The doctor is preparing to remove chest tubes from the client's left chest. In preparation for the removal, the nurse should instruct the client to:

Quick Answers: **51**
Detailed Answer: **69**

❍ **A.** Breathe normally

❍ **B.** Hold his breath and bear down

❍ **C.** Take a deep breath

❍ **D.** Sneeze on command

168. The nurse identifies ventricular tachycardia on the heart monitor. Which action should the nurse prepare to take?

Quick Answers: **51**
Detailed Answer: **69**

❍ **A.** Administer atropine sulfate

❍ **B.** Check the potassium level

❍ **C.** Administer an antiarrythmic medication such as Lidocaine

❍ **D.** Defibrillate at 360 joules

Quick Check

169. A client is being monitored using a central venous pressure monitor. If the pressure is 2cm of water, the nurse should:

Quick Answers: 51
Detailed Answer: 69

- A. Call the doctor immediately
- B. Slow the intravenous infusion
- C. Listen to the lungs for rales
- D. Administer a diuretic

170. The nurse is evaluating the client's pulmonary artery pressure. The nurse is aware that this test will evaluate:

Quick Answers: 51
Detailed Answer: 69

- A. Pressure in the left ventricle
- B. The systolic, diastolic, and mean pressure of the pulmonary artery
- C. The pressure in the pulmonary veins
- D. The pressure in the right ventricle

171. The physician has ordered atropine sulfate 0.4mg IM before surgery. The medication is supplied in 0.8mg per milliliter. The nurse should administer how many milliliters of the medication?

Quick Answers: 51
Detailed Answer: 69

- A. 0.25mL
- B. 0.5mL
- C. 1mL
- D. 1.25mL

172. If the nurse is unable to illicit the deep tendon reflexes of the patella, the nurse should ask the client to:

Quick Answers: 51
Detailed Answer: 69

- A. Pull against the palms
- B. Grimace the facial muscles
- C. Cross the legs at the ankles
- D. Perform Valsalva maneuver

173. A client with an abdominal aortic aneurysm is admitted in preparation for surgery. Which of the following should be reported to the doctor?

Quick Answers: 51
Detailed Answer: 69

- A. An elevated white blood cell count
- B. An abdominal bruit
- C. A negative Babinski reflex
- D. Pupils that are equal and reactive to light

Quick Check

174. A 4-year-old male is admitted to the unit with nephotic syndrome. He is extremely edematous. To decrease the discomfort associated with scrotal edema, the nurse should:

Quick Answers: **51**
Detailed Answer: **69**

- ❍ **A.** Apply ice to the scrotum
- ❍ **B.** Elevate the scrotum on a small pillow
- ❍ **C.** Apply heat to the abdominal area
- ❍ **D.** Administer a diuretic

175. The nurse is taking the blood pressure of an obese client. If the blood pressure cuff is too small, the results will be:

Quick Answers: **51**
Detailed Answer: **69**

- ❍ **A.** A false elevation
- ❍ **B.** A false low reading
- ❍ **C.** A blood pressure reading that is correct
- ❍ **D.** A subnormal finding

176. The client is admitted with thrombophlebitis and an order for heparin. The medication should be administered using:

Quick Answers: **51**
Detailed Answer: **70**

- ❍ **A.** Buretrol
- ❍ **B.** A tuberculin syringe
- ❍ **C.** Intravenous controller
- ❍ **D.** Three-way stop-cock

177. The client is admitted to the hospital in chronic renal failure. A diet low in protein is ordered. The rationale for alow-protein diet is:

Quick Answers: **51**
Detailed Answer: **70**

- ❍ **A.** Protein breaks down into blood urea nitrogen and metabolic waste.
- ❍ **B.** High protein increases the sodium and potassium levels.
- ❍ **C.** A high-protein diet decreases albumin production.
- ❍ **D.** A high-protein diet depletes calcium and phosphorous.

178. The client is admitted to the unit after a motor vehicle accident with a temperature of 102°F rectally. The nurse is aware that the most likely explanation for the elevated temperature is:

Quick Answers: **51**
Detailed Answer: **70**

- ❍ **A.** There was damage to the hypothalamus.
- ❍ **B.** He has an infection from the abrasions to the head and face.
- ❍ **C.** He will require a cooling blanket to decrease the temperature.
- ❍ **D.** There was damage to the frontal lobe of the brain.

Quick Check

179. The nurse is caring for the client following a cerebral vascular accident. Which portion of the brain is responsible for taste, smell, and hearing?

Quick Answers: **51**
Detailed Answer: **70**

❍ **A.** Occipital

❍ **B.** Frontal

❍ **C.** Temporal

❍ **D.** Parietal

180. A 20-year-old is admitted to the rehabilitation unit following a motorcycle accident. Which would be the appropriate method for measuring the client for crutches?

Quick Answers: **51**
Detailed Answer: **70**

❍ **A.** Measuring five finger breaths under the axilla

❍ **B.** Measuring 3 inches under the axilla

❍ **C.** Measuring the client with the elbows flexed 10°

❍ **D.** Measuring the client with the crutches 20 inches from the side of the foot

181. The nurse is doing bowel and bladder retraining for the client with paraplegia. Which of the following is not a factor for the nurse to consider?

Quick Answers: **51**
Detailed Answer: **70**

❍ **A.** Dietary patterns

❍ **B.** Mobility

❍ **C.** Fluid intake

❍ **D.** Sexual function

182. The client returns to the recovery room following repair of an intrathoracic aneurysm. Which finding would require further investigation?

Quick Answers: **51**
Detailed Answer: **70**

❍ **A.** Pedal pulses bounding and regular

❍ **B.** Urinary output 20mL in the past hour

❍ **C.** Blood pressure 108/50

❍ **D.** Oxygen saturation 97%

183. The nurse is teaching the client regarding use of sodium warfarin. Which statement made by the client would require further teaching?

Quick Answers: **51**
Detailed Answer: **70**

❍ **A.** "I will have blood drawn every month."

❍ **B.** "I will assess my skin for a rash."

❍ **C.** "I take aspirin for a headache."

❍ **D.** "I will use an electric razor to shave."

Quick Check

184. A client with a femoral popliteal bypass graft is assigned to a semiprivate room. The most suitable roommate for this client is the client with:

❍ **A.** Hypothyroidism

❍ **B.** Diabetic ulcers

❍ **C.** Ulcerative colitis

❍ **D.** Pneumonia

Quick Answers: **52**
Detailed Answer: **70**

185. The nurse has just received shift report and is preparing to make rounds. Which client should be seen first?

❍ **A.** The client who has a history of a cerebral aneurysm with an oxygen saturation rate of 99%

❍ **B.** The client who is three days post–coronary artery bypass graft with a temperature of 100.2°F

❍ **C.** The client who was admitted 1 hour ago with shortness of breath

❍ **D.** The client who is being prepared for discharge following a femoral popliteal bypass graft

Quick Answers: **52**
Detailed Answer: **70**

186. The doctor has ordered antithrombolic stockings to be applied to the legs of the client with peripheral vascular disease. The nurse knows that the proper method of applying the stockings is:

❍ **A.** Before rising in the morning

❍ **B.** With the client in a standing position

❍ **C.** After bathing and applying powder

❍ **D.** Before retiring in the evening

Quick Answers: **52**
Detailed Answer: **71**

187. The nurse is preparing a client with an axillo-popliteal bypass graft for discharge. The client should be taught to avoid:

❍ **A.** Using a recliner to rest

❍ **B.** Resting in supine position

❍ **C.** Sitting in a straight chair

❍ **D.** Sleeping in right Sim's position

Quick Answers: **52**
Detailed Answer: **71**

188. While caring for a client with hypertension, the nurse notes the following vital signs: BP of 140/20, pulse 120, respirations 36, temperature 100.8°F. The nurse's initial action should be to:

❍ **A.** Call the doctor

❍ **B.** Recheck the vital signs

❍ **C.** Obtain arterial blood gases

❍ **D.** Obtain an ECG

Quick Answers: **52**
Detailed Answer: **71**

Quick Check

189. The nurse is caring for a client with peripheral vascular disease. To correctly assess the oxygen saturation level, the monitor may be placed on the:

- ❍ **A.** Abdomen
- ❍ **B.** Ankle
- ❍ **C.** Earlobe
- ❍ **D.** Chin

Quick Answers: **52**
Detailed Answer: **71**

190. Dalteparin (Fragmin) has been ordered for a client with pulmonary embolis. Which statement made by the graduate nurse indicates inadequate understanding of the medication?

- ❍ **A.** "I will administer the medication before meals."
- ❍ **B.** "I will administer the medication in the abdomen."
- ❍ **C.** "I will check the PTT before administering the medication."
- ❍ **D.** "I will not need to aspirate when I give Dalteparin."

Quick Answers: **52**
Detailed Answer: **71**

191. The client has a prescription for a calcium carbonate compound to neutralize stomach acid. The nurse should assess the client for:

- ❍ **A.** Constipation
- ❍ **B.** Hyperphosphatemia
- ❍ **C.** Hypomagnesemia
- ❍ **D.** Diarrhea

Quick Answers: **52**
Detailed Answer: **71**

192. A client who has been receiving urokinase has a large bloody bowel movement. What nursing action would be best for the nurse to take immediately?

- ❍ **A.** Administer vitamin K IM
- ❍ **B.** Discontinue the urokinase
- ❍ **C.** Reduce the urokinase and administer heparin
- ❍ **D.** Stop the urokinase, notify the physician, and prepare to administer amicar

Quick Answers: **52**
Detailed Answer: **71**

193. Which of the following best describes the language of a 24-month-old?

- ❍ **A.** Doesn't understand yes and no
- ❍ **B.** Understands the meaning of words
- ❍ **C.** Able to verbalize needs
- ❍ **D.** Continually asks "Why?" to most topics

Quick Answers: **52**
Detailed Answer: **71**

Quick Check

194. In terms of cognitive development, a 2-year-old would be expected to:

Quick Answers: **52**
Detailed Answer: **71**

❍ **A.** Think abstractly

❍ **B.** Use magical thinking

❍ **C.** Understand conservation of matter

❍ **D.** See things from the perspective of others

195. The nurse is ready to begin an exam on a 9-month-old infant. The child is sitting in his mother's lap. What should the nurse do first?

Quick Answers: **52**
Detailed Answer: **72**

❍ **A.** Check the Babinski reflex

❍ **B.** Listen to the heart and lung sounds

❍ **C.** Palpate the abdomen

❍ **D.** Check tympanic membranes

196. Which of the following examples represents parallel play?

Quick Answers: **52**
Detailed Answer: **72**

❍ **A.** Jenny and Tommy share their toys.

❍ **B.** Jimmy plays with his car beside Mary, who is playing with her doll.

❍ **C.** Kevin plays a game of Scrabble with Kathy and Sue.

❍ **D.** Mary plays with a handheld game while sitting in her mother's lap.

197. Assuming that all have achieved normal cognitive and emotional development, which of the following children is at greatest risk for accidental poisoning?

Quick Answers: **52**
Detailed Answer: **72**

❍ **A.** A 6-month-old

❍ **B.** A 4-year-old

❍ **C.** A 10-year-old

❍ **D.** A 13-year-old

198. An important intervention in monitoring the dietary compliance of a client with bulimia is:

Quick Answers: **52**
Detailed Answer: **72**

❍ **A.** Allowing the client privacy during mealtimes

❍ **B.** Praising her for eating all her meals

❍ **C.** Observing her for 1–2 hours after meals

❍ **D.** Encouraging her to choose foods she likes and to eat in moderation

Quick Check

199. The client is admitted for evaluation of aggressive behavior and diagnosed with antisocial personality disorder. A key part of the care of such a client is:

- ❍ **A.** Setting realistic limits
- ❍ **B.** Encouraging the client to express remorse for behavior
- ❍ **C.** Minimizing interactions with other clients
- ❍ **D.** Encouraging the client to act out feelings of rage

Quick Answers: **52**
Detailed Answer: **72**

200. A client with a diagnosis of passive-aggressive personality disorder is seen at the local mental health clinic. A common characteristic of persons with passive-aggressive personality disorder is:

- ❍ **A.** Superior intelligence
- ❍ **B.** Underlying hostility
- ❍ **C.** Dependence on others
- ❍ **D.** Ability to share feelings

Quick Answers: **52**
Detailed Answer: **72**

Quick Check Answer Key

1. A
2. B
3. A
4. B
5. C
6. B
7. D
8. D
9. C
10. C
11. C
12. D
13. C
14. D
15. C
16. A
17. A
18. C
19. A
20. C
21. B
22. C
23. C
24. B
25. B
26. C
27. B
28. A
29. A
30. B
31. B
32. D
33. A
34. B
35. B
36. B
37. D
38. D
39. B
40. B
41. C
42. A
43. A
44. A
45. B
46. D
47. D
48. C
49. A
50. B
51. B
52. C
53. B
54. C
55. B
56. A
57. D
58. D
59. A
60. B
61. A
62. C
63. C
64. B
65. C
66. B
67. C
68. D
69. D
70. A
71. A
72. D
73. B
74. D
75. B
76. B
77. B
78. A
79. D
80. A
81. C
82. D
83. A
84. B
85. D
86. B
87. B

88. B
89. B
90. D
91. C
92. A
93. A
94. B
95. A
96. B
97. A
98. B
99. D
100. A
101. C
102. D
103. B
104. B
105. C
106. A
107. D
108. B
109. D
110. D
111. C
112. C
113. C
114. D
115. A
116. A
117. A
118. B
119. C
120. A
121. B
122. C
123. D
124. D
125. C
126. C
127. A
128. C
129. A
130. C
131. B
132. A
133. D
134. C
135. A
136. A
137. B
138. D
139. C
140. A
141. D
142. A
143. C
144. A
145. D
146. C
147. A
148. A
149. B
150. B
151. C
152. A
153. D
154. C
155. C
156. D
157. B
158. B
159. B
160. B
161. A
162. B
163. C
164. D
165. A
166. D
167. B
168. C
169. A
170. B
171. B
172. A
173. A
174. B
175. A
176. B
177. A
178. A
179. C
180. B
181. D
182. B
183. C

184. A

185. C

186. A

187. C

188. A

189. C

190. C

191. A

192. D

193. C

194. B

195. B

196. B

197. B

198. C

199. A

200. B

Answers and Rationales

1. **Answer A is correct.** Removal of the pituitary gland is usually done by a transsphenoidal approach, through the nose. Nasal congestion further interferes with the airway. Answers B, C, and D are not correct because they are not directly associated with the pituitary gland.

2. **Answer B is correct.** Hypokalemia is evident from the lab values listed. The other laboratory findings are within normal limits, making answers A, C, and D incorrect.

3. **Answer A is correct.** The primary responsibility of the nurse is to take the vital signs before any surgery. The actions in answers B, C, and D are the responsibility of the doctor and, therefore, are incorrect for this question.

4. **Answer B is correct.** The client with burns to the neck needs airway assessment and supplemental oxygen, so applying oxygen is the priority. The next action should be to start an IV and medicate for pain, making answers A and C incorrect. Answer D, obtaining blood gases, is ordered by the doctor.

5. **Answer C is correct.** Fosamax should be taken with water only. The client should also remain upright for at least 30 minutes after taking the medication. Answers A, B, and D are not applicable to taking Fosamax and, thus, are incorrect.

6. **Answer B is correct.** A torque wrench is kept at the bedside to tighten and loosen the screws of crutchfield tongs. This wrench controls the amount of pressure that is placed on the screws. A pair of forceps, wire cutters, and a screwdriver, in answers A, C, and D, would not be used and, thus, are incorrect.

7. **Answer D is correct.** A birth weight of 7 pounds would indicate 21 pounds in 1 year, or triple his birth weight. Answers A, B, and C therefore are incorrect.

8. **Answer D is correct.** Sarcoma is a type of bone cancer; therefore, bone pain would be expected. Answers A, B, and C are not specific to this type of cancer and are incorrect.

9. **Answer C is correct.** Tegretol can suppress the bone marrow and decrease the white blood cell count; thus, a lab value of WBC 2,000 per cubic millimeter indicates side effects of the drug. Answers A and D are within normal limits, and answer B is a lower limit of normal; therefore answers A, B, and D are incorrect.

10. **Answer C is correct.** The least-helpful questions are those describing his usual diet. A, B, and D are useful in determining the extent of disease process and, thus, are incorrect.

11. **Answer C is correct.** The client with diverticulitis should avoid foods with seeds. The foods in answers A, B, and D are allowed; in fact, bran cereal and fruit will help prevent constipation.

12. **Answer D is correct.** The client with a perineal resection will have a perineal incision. Drains will be used to facilitate wound drainage. This will help prevent infection of the surgical site. The client will not have an illeostomy, as in answer A; he will have some electrolyte loss, but treatment is not focused on preventing the loss, so answer B is incorrect. A high-fiber diet, in answer C, is not ordered at this time.

13. **Answer C is correct.** The client with diverticulitis should avoid eating foods that are gas forming and that increase abdominal discomfort, such as cooked broccoli. Foods such as those listed in answers A, B, and D are allowed.

14. **Answer D is correct.** After birth, meconium stool, loss of extracellular fluid, and initiation of breastfeeding cause the infant to lose body mass. There is no evidence to indicate dehydration, hypoglycemia, or allergy to the infant formula; thus, answers A, B, and C are incorrect.

15. **Answer C is correct.** Diarrhea is not common in clients with mouth and throat cancer. All the findings in answers A, B, and D are expected findings.

16. **Answer A is correct.** The client with a lung resection will have chest tubes and a drainage-collection device. He probably will not have a tracheostomy or medicastenal tube, and he will not have an order for percussion, vibration, or drainage. Therefore, answers B, C, and D are incorrect.

17. **Answer A is correct.** A swelling over the right parietal area is a cephalohematoma, an area of bleeding outside the cranium. This type of hematoma does not cross the suture line because it is outside the cranium but beneath the periosteum. Answer B, molding, is overlapping of the bones of the cranium and, thus, incorrect. In answer C, a subdural hematoma, or intracranial bleeding, is ominous and can be seen only on a CAT scan or x-ray. A caput succedaneum, in answer D, crosses the suture line and is edema.

18. **Answer C is correct.** The client with an internal defibrillator should learn to use any battery-operated machinery on the opposite side. He should also take his pulse rate and report dizziness or fainting. Answers A, B, and D are incorrect because the client can eat food prepared in the microwave, move his shoulder on the affected side, and fly in an airplane.

19. **Answer A is correct.** Suctioning can cause a vagal response and bradycardia. Answer B is unlikely and, therefore, not most important, although it can occur. Answers C and D can occur as well, but they are less likely.

20. **Answer C is correct.** The assessment that is most crucial to the client is the identification of peripheral pulses because the aorta is clamped during surgery. This decreases blood circulation to the kidneys and lower extremities. The nurse must also assess for the return of circulation to the lower extremities. Answer A is of lesser concern, answer B is not advised at this time, and answer D is of lesser concern than answer A.

21. **Answer B is correct.** Portions of the exam are painful, especially when the sample is being withdrawn, so this should be included in the session with the client. Answer A is incorrect because the client will be positioned prone, not in a sitting position, for the exam. Anesthesia is not commonly given before this test, making answer C incorrect. Answer D is incorrect because the client can eat and drink following the test.

22. **Answer C is correct.** A red, beefy tongue is characteristic of the client with pernicious anemia. Answer A, a weight loss of 10 pounds in 2 weeks, is abnormal but is not seen in pernicious anemia. Numbness and tingling, in answer B, can be associated with anemia but are not particular to pernicious anemia. This is more likely associated with peripheral vascular diseases involving vasculature. In answer D, the hemoglobin is low normal.

23. **Answer C is correct.** The client with a fractured femur will be placed in Buck's traction to realign the leg and to decrease spasms and pain. The Trendelenburg position is the wrong position for this client, so answer A is incorrect. Ice might be ordered after repair, but not for the entire extremity, so answer B is incorrect. An abduction pillow is ordered after a total hip replacement, not for a fractured femur; therefore, answer D is incorrect.

24. **Answer B is correct.** The client having an intravenous pyelogram will have orders for laxatives or enemas, so asking the client to void before the test is in order. A full bladder or bowel can obscure the visualization of the kidney ureters and urethra. In answers A, C, and D, there is no need to force fluids before the procedure, to withhold medications, or to cover the reproductive organs.

25. **Answer B is correct.** Cancer in situ means that the cancer is still localized to the primary site. Cancer is graded in terms of tumor, grade, node involvement, and mestatasis. Answer A is incorrect because it is an untrue statement. Answer C is incorrect because *T* indicates tumor, not node involvement. Answer D is incorrect because a tumor that is in situ is not metastasized.

26. **Answer C is correct.** If the client eviscerates, the abdominal content should be covered with a sterile saline-soaked dressing. Reinserting the content should not be the action and will require that the client return to surgery; thus, answer A is incorrect. Answers B and D are incorrect because they are not appropriate to this case.

27. **Answer B is correct.** It is most important to remove the contact lenses because leaving them in can lead to corneal drying, particularly with contact lenses that are not extended-wear lenses. Leaving in the hearing aid or artificial eye will not harm the client. Leaving the wedding ring on is also allowed; usually, the ring is covered with tape. Therefore, answers A, C, and D are incorrect.

28. **Answer A is correct.** It is the responsibility of the physician to explain and clarify the procedure to the client. Answers B, C, and D are incorrect because they are not within the nurse's purview.

29. **Answer A is correct.** Previous radiation to the neck might have damaged the parathyroid glands, which are located on the thyroid gland, and interfered with calcium and phosphorus regulation. Answer B has no significance to this case; answers C and D are more related to calcium only, not to phosphorus regulation.

30. **Answer B is correct.** The client with serum sodium of 170meq/L has hypernatremia and might exhibit manic behavior. Answers A, C, and D are not associated with hypernatremia and are, therefore, incorrect.

31. **Answer B is correct.** Frequent use of laxatives can lead to diarrhea and electrolyte loss. Answers A, C, and D are not of particular significance in this case and, therefore, are incorrect.

32. **Answer D is correct.** Abnormal grieving is exhibited by a lack of feeling sad; if the client's sister appears not to grieve, it might be abnormal grieving. This family member might be suppressing feelings of grief. Answers A, B, and C are all normal expressions of grief and, therefore, incorrect.

33. **Answer A is correct.** If the nurse is exposed to the client with a cough, the best item to wear is a mask. If the answer had included a mask, gloves, and a gown, all would be appropriate, but in this case, only one item is listed; therefore, answers B and C are incorrect. Shoe covers are not necessary, so answer D is incorrect.

34. **Answer B is correct.** Oils can be applied to help with the dry skin and to decrease itching, so adding baby oil to bath water is soothing to the skin. Answer A is incorrect because bathing twice a day is too frequent and can cause more dryness. Answer C is incorrect because powder is also drying. Rinsing with hot water, as stated in answer D, dries out the skin as well.

35. **Answer B is correct.** The client with pancreatitis frequently has nausea and vomiting. Lavage is often used to decompress the stomach and rest the bowel, so the insertion of a Levine tube should be anticipated. Answers A and C are incorrect because blood pressures are not required every 15 minutes, and cardiac monitoring might be needed, but this is individualized to the client. Answer D is incorrect because there are no dressings to change on this client.

36. **Answer B is correct.** Montgomery straps are used to secure dressings that require frequent dressing changes because the client with a cholecystectomy usually has a large amount of drainage on the dressing. Montgomery straps are also used for clients who are allergic to several types of tape. This client is not at higher risk of evisceration than other clients, so answer A is incorrect. Montgomery straps are not used to secure the drains, so answer C is incorrect. Sutures or clips are used to secure the wound of the client who has had gallbladder surgery, so answer D is incorrect.

37. **Answer D is correct.** Intrathecal medications are administered into the cerebrospinal fluid. This method of administering medications is reserved for the client with metastases, the client with chronic pain, or the client with cerebrospinal infections. Answers A, B, and C are incorrect because intravenous, rectal, and intramuscular injections are entirely different procedures.

38. **Answer D is correct.** The best client to assign to the newly licensed nurse is the most stable client; in this case, it is the client with diverticulitis. The client receiving chemotherapy and the client with a coronary bypass both need nurses experienced in these areas, so answers A and B are incorrect. Answer D is incorrect because the client with a transurethral prostatectomy might bleed, so this client should be assigned to a nurse who knows how much bleeding is within normal limits.

39. **Answer B is correct.** The best action at this time is to report the incident to the charge nurse. Further action might be needed, but it should be determined by the charge nurse. Answers A, C, and D are incorrect because notifying the police is overreacting at this time, and monitoring or ignoring the situation is an inadequate response.

40. **Answer B is correct.** The best action for the nurse to take is to explore the interaction with the nursing assistant. This will allow for clarification of the situation. Changing the assignment in answer A might need to be done, but talking to the nursing assistant is the first step. Answer C is incorrect because discussing the incident with the family is not necessary at this time; it might cause more problems. Answer C is not a first step, even though initiating a group session might be a plan for the future.

41. **Answer C is correct.** The client with laryngeal cancer has a potential airway alteration and should be seen first. The clients in answers A, B, and D are not in immediate danger and can be seen later in the day.

42. **Answer A is correct.** Bilirubin is excreted through the kidneys, thus the need for increased fluids. Maintaining the body temperature is important but will not assist in eliminating bilirubin; therefore, answer B is incorrect. Answers C and D are incorrect because they do not relate to the question.

43. **Answer A is correct.** When the cadaver client is being prepared to donate an organ, the systolic blood pressure should be maintained at 70mmHg or greater to ensure a blood supply to the donor organ. Answers B, C, and D are incorrect because they are unnecssary actions for organ donation.

44. **Answer A is correct.** The nurse who fails to wear gloves to remove a contaminated dressing needs further instruction. Answers B, C, and D are incorrect because they indicate an understanding of the correct method of completing these tasks.

45. **Answer B is correct.** The client having a mammogram should be instructed to omit deodorants or powders beforehand because powders and deodorants can be interpreted as abnormal. Answer A is incorrect because there is no need for dietary restrictions before a mammogram. Answer C is incorrect because the mammogram does not replace the need for self-breast exams. Answer D is incorrect because a mammogram does not require higher doses of radiation than an x-ray.

46. **Answer D is correct.** The most suitable roommate for the client with gastric resection is the client with phlebitis because phlebitis is an inflammation of the blood vessel and is not infectious. Crohn's disease clients, in answer A, have frequent stools that might spread infections to the surgical client. The client in answer B with pneumonia is coughing and will disturb the gastric client. The client with gastritis, in answer C, is vomiting and has diarrhea, which also will disturb the gastric client.

47. **Answer D is correct.** The most critical client should be assigned to the registered nurse; in this case, that is the client 2 days post-thoracotomy. The clients in answers A and B are ready for discharge, and the client in answer C who had a splenectomy 3 days ago is stable enough to be assigned to an LPN.

48. **Answer C is correct.** The client should breathe normally during a central venous pressure monitor reading. Answer A indicates understanding because the client should be placed supine if he can tolerate being in that position. Answers B and D indicate understanding because the stop-cock should be turned off to the IV fluid, and the reading should be done at the top of the meniscus.

49. **Answer A is correct.** The most suitable roommate for the client with myasthenia gravis is the client with hypothyroidism because he is quiet. The client with Crohn's disease in answer B will be up to the bathroom frequently; the client with pylonephritis in answer C has a kidney infection and will be up to urinate frequently. The client in answer D with bronchitis will be coughing and will disturb any roommate.

50. **Answer B is correct.** The teenager with sternal bruising might be experiencing airway and oxygenation problems and, thus, should be seen first. In answer A, the 10-year-old with lacerations might look bad but is not in distress. The client in answer C with a

fractured femur should be immobilized but can be seen after the client with sternal bruising. The client in answer D with the dislocated elbow can be seen later as well.

51. **Answer B is correct.** If the dialysate returns cloudy, infection might be present and must be evaluated. Documenting the finding, as stated in answer A, as not enough; straining the urine, in answer C, is incorrect; and dialysate, in answer D, is not urine at all. However, the physician might order a white blood cell count.

52. **Answer C is correct.** Lactulose is administered to the client with cirrhosis to lower ammonia levels. Answers A, B, and D are incorrect because this does not have an effect on the other lab values.

53. **Answer B is correct.** A client with diabetes who has trouble seeing would require follow-up after discharge. The lack of visual acuity for the client preparing and injecting insulin might require help. Answers A, C, and D will not prevent the client from being able to care for himself and, thus, are incorrect.

54. **Answer C is correct.** When the client is receiving TPN, the blood glucose level should be drawn. TPN is a solution that contains large amounts of glucose. Answers A, B, and D are not directly related to the question and are incorrect.

55. **Answer B is correct.** The client who says he has nothing wrong is in denial about his myocardial infarction. Rationalization is making excuses for what happened, projection is projecting feeling or thoughts onto others, and conversion reaction is converting a psychological trauma into a physical illness; thus, answers A, C, and D are incorrect.

56. **Answer A is correct.** Answer A, AST, is not specific for myocardial infarction. Troponin, CK-MB, and myoglobin, in answers B, C, and D, are more specific, although myoglobin is also elevated in burns and trauma to muscles.

57. **Answer D is correct.** The mothers in answers A, B, and C all require RhoGam and, thus, are incorrect. The mother in answer D is the only one who does not require a RhoGam injection.

58. **Answer D is correct.** The first exercise that should be done by the client with a mastectomy is squeezing the ball. Answers A, B, and C are incorrect as the first step; they are implemented later.

59. **Answer A is correct.** Atropine sulfate is the antidote for Tensilon and is given to treat cholenergic crises. Furosemide (answer B) is a diuretic, Prostigmin (answer C) is the treatment for myasthenia gravis, and Promethazine (answer D) is an antiemetic, antianxiety medication. Thus, answers B, C, and D are incorrect.

60. **Answer B is correct.** The client scheduled for a pericentesis should be told to empty the bladder, to prevent the risk of puncturing the bladder when the needle is inserted. A pericentesis is done to remove fluid from the peritoneal cavity. The client will be positioned sitting up or leaning over a table, making answer A incorrect. The client is usually awake during the procedure, and medications are not commonly inserted into the peritoneal cavity during this procedure; thus, answers C and D are incorrect (although this could depend on the circumstances).

61. **Answer A is correct.** To protect herself, the nurse should wear gloves when applying a nitroglycerine patch or cream. Answer B is incorrect because shaving the shin might abrade the area. Answer C is incorrect because washing with hot water will vasodilate

and increase absorption. The patches should be applied to areas above the waist, making answer D incorrect.

62. **Answer C is correct.** Covering both eyes prevents consensual movement of the affected eye. The nurse should not attempt to remove the object from the eye because this might cause trauma, as stated in answer A. Rinsing the eye, as stated in answer B, might be ordered by the doctor, but this is not the first step for the nurse. Answer D is not correct because often when one eye moves, the other also does.

63. **Answer C is correct.** Sodium warfarin is administered in the late afternoon, at approximately 1700 hours. This allows for accurate bleeding times to be drawn in the morning. Therefore, answers A, B, and D are incorrect.

64. **Answer B is correct.** The registered nurse is the only one of these who can legally put the client in seclusion. The only other healthcare worker who is allowed to initiate seclusion is the doctor; therefore, answers A, C, and D are incorrect.

65. **Answer C is correct.** The client is experiencing compensated metabolic acidosis. The pH is within the normal range but is lower than 7.40, so it is on the acidic side. The CO_2 level is elevated, the oxygen level is below normal, and the bicarb level is slightly elevated. In respiratory disorders, the pH will be the inverse of the CO_2 and bicarb levels. This means that if the pH is low, the CO_2 and bicarb levels will be elevated. Answers A, B, and D are incorrect because they do not fall into the range of symptoms.

66. **Answer B is correct.** The best way to evaluate pain levels is to ask the client to rate his pain on a scale. In answer A, the blood pressure, pulse, and temperature can alter for other reasons than pain. Answers C and D are not as effective in determining pain levels.

67. **Answer C is correct.** A sitz bath will help with swelling and improve healing. Ice packs, in answer D, can be used immediately after delivery. Answers A and B are not used in this instance.

68. **Answer D is correct.** After surgery, the client will be placed on a clear-liquid diet and progressed to a regular diet. Stool softeners will be included in the plan of care, to avoid constipation. Later, a high-fiber diet, in answer A, is encouraged, but this is not the first diet after surgery. Answers B and C are not diets for this type of surgery.

69. **Answer D is correct.** A culture for gonorrhea is taken from the genital secretions. The culture is placed in a warm environment, where it can grow nisseria gonorrhea. Answers A, B, and C are incorrect because these cultures do not test for gonorrhea.

70. **Answer A is correct.** Frequent rest periods help to relax tense muscles and preserve energy. Answers B, C, and D are incorrect because they are untrue statements.

71. **Answer A is correct.** The client with Alzheimer's disease is the most stable of these clients and can be assigned to the nursing assistant, who can perform duties such as feeding and assisting the client with activities of daily living. The clients in answers B, C, and D are less stable and should be attended by a registered nurse.

72. **Answer D is correct.** Xerostomia is dry mouth, and offering the client a saliva substitute will help the most. Eating hard candy in answer A can further irritate the mucosa and cut the tongue and lips. Administering an analgesic might not be necessary; thus,

answer B is incorrect. Splinting swollen joints, in answer C, is not associated with xerostomia.

73. **Answer B is correct.** The client with congestive heart failure who is complaining of nighttime dyspnea should be seen first because airway is no. 1 in nursing care. In answers A, C, and D, the clients are more stable.

74. **Answer D is correct.** The fresh peach is the lowest in sodium of these choices. Answers A, B, and C have much higher amounts of sodium.

75. **Answer B is correct.** The best client to transport to the postpartum unit is the 40-year-old female with a hysterectomy. The nurses on the postpartum unit will be aware of normal amounts of bleeding and will be equipped to care for this client. The clients in answers A and D will be best cared for on a medical-surgical unit. The client with depression in answer C should be transported to the psychiatric unit.

76. **Answer B is correct.** The first action the nurse should take is to report the finding to the nurse supervisor and follow the chain of command. If it is found that the pharmacy is in error, it should be notified, as stated in answer A. Answers C and D, notifying the director of nursing and the Board of Nursing, might be necessary if theft is found, but not as a first step; thus, these are incorrect answers.

77. **Answer B is correct.** The client with the appendectomy is the most stable of these clients and can be assigned to a nursing assistant. The client with bronchiolitis has an alteration in the airway, the client with periorbital cellulitis has an infection, and the client with a fracture might be an abused child. Therefore, answers A, C, and D are incorrect.

78. **Answer A is correct.** Identifying oneself as a nurse without a license defrauds the public and can be prosecuted. A tort is a wrongful act; malpractice is failing to act appropriately as a nurse or acting in a way that harm comes to the client; and negligence is failing to perform care. Therefore, answers B, C, and D are incorrect.

79. **Answer D is correct.** Because the client is immune-suppressed, foods should be served in sealed containers, to avoid food contaminants. Answer B is incorrect because of possible infection from visitors. Answer A is not necessary, but the utensils should be cleaned thoroughly and rinsed in hot water. Answer C might be a good idea, but alcohol can be drying and can cause the skin to break down.

80. **Answer A is correct.** The client with unilateral neglect will neglect one side of the body. Answers B, C, and D are not associated with unilateral neglect.

81. **Answer C is correct.** The client taking antabuse should not eat or drink anything containing alcohol or vinegar. The other foods in answers A, B, and D are allowed.

82. **Answer D is correct.** Cyanocolamine is a B12 medication that is used for pernicious anemia, and a reticulocyte count of 1% indicates that it is having the desired effect. Answers A, B, and C are white blood cells and have nothing to do with this medication.

83. **Answer A is correct.** The first client to be seen is the one who recently returned from surgery. The other clients in answers B, C, and D are more stable and can be seen later.

84. **Answer B is correct.** Out of all of these clients, it is best to hold the pregnant client and the client with a broken arm and facial lacerations in the same room. The clients in answer A need to be placed in separate rooms because these clients are disruptive or have infections. In the case of answer C, the child is terminal and should be in a private room with his parents.

85. **Answer D is correct.** The priority client is the one with multiple sclerosis who is being treated with cortisone via the central line. This client is at highest risk for complications. MRSA, in answer C, is methicillin-resistant staphylococcus aureas. Vancomycin is the drug of choice and can be administered later, but its use must be scheduled at specific times of the day to maintain a therapeutic level. Answers A and B are incorrect because these clients are more stable.

86. **Answer B is correct.** The action after discussing the problem with the nurse is to document the incident and file a formal reprimand. If the behavior continues or if harm has resulted to the client, the nurse may be terminated and reported to the Board of Nursing, but this is not the first step. A tort is a wrongful act committed against a client or his belongings. Answers A, C, and D are incorrect.

87. **Answer B is correct.** The Joint Commission on Accreditation of Hospitals will probably be interested in the problems in answers A and C. The failure of the nursing assistant to assist the client with hepatitis should be reported to the charge nurse. If the behavior continues, termination may result. Answer D is incorrect because failure to feed and bathe the client should be reported to the superior, not the Board of Nursing.

88. **Answer B is correct.** The nurse in answer B has the most experience with possible complications involved with preeclampsia. The nurse in answer A is a new nurse to this unit and should not be assigned to this client; the nurses in answers C and D have no experience with the postpartal client and also should not be assigned to this client.

89. **Answer B is correct.** The vital signs are abnormal and should be reported to the doctor immediately. Answer A, continuing to monitor the vital signs, can result in deterioration of the client's condition. Answer C, asking the client how he feels, would supply only subjective data. Involving the LPN, in answer D, is not the best solution to help this client because he is unstable.

90. **Answer D is correct.** A licensed practical nurse should not be assigned to initiate a blood transfusion. The LPN can assist with the transfusion and check ID numbers for the RN. The licensed practical nurse can be assigned to insert Foley and French urinary catheters, discontinue Levine and Gavage gastric tubes, and obtain all types of specimens, so answers A, B, and C are incorrect.

91. **Answer C is correct.** Assault is defined as striking or touching the client inappropriately, so a nurse assistant striking a client could be charged with assault. Answer A, negligence, is failing to perform care for the client. Answer B, a tort, is a wrongful act committed on the client or their belongings. Answer D, malpractice, is failure to perform an act that the nursing assistant knows should be done, or the act of doing something wrong that results in harm to the client.

92. **Answer A is correct.** The client with Cushing's disease has adrenocortical hypersecretion. This increase in the level of cortisone causes the client to be immune suppressed. In answer B, the client with diabetes poses no risk to other clients. The client

in answer C has an increase in growth hormone and poses no risk to himself or others. The client in answer D has hyperthyroidism or myxedema, and poses no risk to others or himself.

93. **Answer A is correct.** The pregnant nurse should not be assigned to any client with radioactivity present. Therefore, the client receiving linear accelerator therapy is correct because this client travels to the radium department for therapy, and the radiation stays in the department; the client is not radioactive. The client in answer B does pose a risk to the pregnant client. The client in answer C is radioactive in very small doses. For approximately 72 hours, the client should dispose of urine and feces in special containers and use plastic spoons and forks. The client in answer D is also radioactive in small amounts, especially upon return from the procedure.

94. **Answer B is correct.** The antidote for heparin is protamine sulfate. Cyanocobalamine is B12, Streptokinase is a thrombolytic, and sodium warfarin is an anticoagulant. Therefore, answers A, C, and D are incorrect.

95. **Answer A is correct.** Lasix should be given approximately 1mL per minute to prevent hypotension. Answers B, C, and D are incorrect because it is not necessary to be given in an IV piggyback, with saline, or through a venous access device (VAD).

96. **Answer B is correct.** A persistent cough might be related to an adverse reaction to Captoten. Answers A and D are incorrect because tinnitus and diarrhea are not associated with the medication. Muscle weakness might occur when beginning the treatment but is not an adverse effect; thus, answer C is incorrect.

97. **Answer A is correct.** Sites for the application of nitroglycerin should be rotated, to prevent skin irritation. It can be applied to the back and upper arms, not to the lower extremities, making answer B incorrect. Answer C is contraindicated to the question, and answer D is incorrect because the medication should be covered with a prepared dressing made of a thin paper substance, not gauze.

98. **Answer B is correct.** Lidocaine is used to treat ventricular tachycardia. This medication slowly exerts an antiarrhythmic effect by increasing the electric stimulation threshold of the ventricles without depressing the force of ventricular contractions. It is not used for atrial arrhythmias; thus, answer A is incorrect. Answers C and D are incorrect because it slows the heart rate, so it is not used for heart block or brachycardia.

99. **Answer D is correct.** Quinidine can cause widened Q-T intervals and heart block. Other signs of myocardial toxicity are notched P waves and widened QRS complexes. The most common side effects are diarrhea, nausea, and vomiting. The client might experience tinnitus, vertigo, headache, visual disturbances, and confusion. Answers A, B, and C are not related to the use of quinidine.

100. **Answer A is correct.** If the client eats foods high in tyramine, he might experience malignant hypertension. Tyramine is found in cheese, sour cream, Chianti wine, sherry, beer, pickled herring, liver, canned figs, raisins, bananas, avocados, chocolate, soy sauce, fava beans, and yeast. These episodes are treated with Regitine, an alpha-adrenergic blocking agent. Answers B, C, and D are not related to the question.

101. **Answer C is correct.** Hyperplasia of the gums is associated with Dilantin therapy. Answer A is not related to the therapy; answer B is a side effect, and answer D is not related to the question.

102. **Answer D is correct.** A complication of a tonsillectomy is bleeding, and constant swallowing may indicate bleeding. Decreased appetite is expected after a tonsillectomy, as is a low-grade temperature; thus, answers A and B are incorrect. In answer C, chest congestion is not normal but is not associated with the tonsillectomy.

103. **Answer B is correct.** Children at 18 months of age like push-pull toys. Children at approximately 3 years of age begin to dress themselves and build a tower of eight blocks. At age four, children can copy a horizontal or vertical line. Therefore, answers A, C, and D are incorrect.

104. **Answer B is correct.** The diagnosis of meningitis at age 6 months correlates to a diagnosis of cerebral palsy. Cerebral palsy, a neurological disorder, is often associated with birth trauma or infections of the brain or spinal column. Answers A, C and D are not related to the question.

105. **Answer C is correct.** Theodur is a bronchodilator, and a side effect of bronchodilators is tachycardia, so checking the pulse is important. Extreme tachycardia should be reported to the doctor. Answers A, B, and D are not necessary.

106. **Answer A is correct.** Crystals in the solution are not normal and should not be administered to the client. Discard the bad solution immediately. Answer B is incorrect because warming the solution will not help. Answer C is incorrect, and answer D requires a doctor's order.

107. **Answer D is correct.** Cytoxan can cause hemorrhagic cystitis, so the client should drink at least eight glasses of water a day. Answers A and B are not necessary and, so, are incorrect. Nausea often occurs with chemotherapy, so answer C is incorrect.

108. **Answer B is correct.** Rifampin can change the color of the urine and body fluid. Teaching the client about these changes is best because he might think this is a complication. Answer A is not necessary, answer C is not true, and answer D is not true because this medication should be taken regularly during the course of the treatment.

109. **Answer D is correct.** Taking corticosteroids in the morning mimics the body's natural release of cortisol. Answers A is not necessarily true, and answers B and C are not true.

110. **Answer D is correct.** Taking antibiotics and oral contraceptives together decreases the effectiveness of the oral contraceptives. Answers A, B, and C are not necessarily true.

111. **Answer C is correct.** The client should be taught to eat his meals even if he is not hungry, to prevent a hypoglycemic reaction. Answers A, B, and D are incorrect because they indicate an understanding of the nurse's teaching.

112. **Answer C is correct.** The time of onset for regular insulin is 30–60 minutes; therefore, answers A, B, and D are incorrect.

113. **Answer C is correct.** Histamine blockers are frequently ordered for clients who are hospitalized for prolonged periods and who are in a stressful situation. They are not

used to treat discomfort, correct electrolytes, or treat nausea; therefore, answers A, B, and D are incorrect.

114. **Answer D is correct.** Cyclosporin is an immunosuppressant, and the client with a liver transplant will be on immunosuppressants for the rest of his life. Answers A, B, and C, therefore, are incorrect.

115. **Answer A is correct.** Methergine is a drug that causes uterine contractions. It is used for postpartal bleeding that is not controlled by Pitocin. Answers B, C, and D are incorrect: Stadol is an analgesic; magnesium sulfate is used for preeclampsia; and phenergan is an antiemetic.

116. **Answer A is correct.** Clients having dye procedures should be assessed for allergies to iodine or shellfish. Answers B and D are incorrect because there is no need for the client to be assessed for reactions to blood or eggs. Because an IV cholangiogram is done to detect gallbladder disease, there is no need to ask about answer C.

117. **Answer A is correct.** Regular insulin should be drawn up before the NPH. They can be given together, so there is no need for two injections, making answer D incorrect. Answer B is obviously incorrect, and answer C is incorrect because it does matter which is drawn first: Contamination of NPH into regular insulin will result in a hypoglycemic reaction at unexpected times.

118. **Answer B is correct.** Trough levels are the lowest blood levels and should be done 30 minutes before the third IV dose or 30 minutes before the fourth IM dose. Answers A, C, and D are incorrect.

119. **Answer C is correct.** Viokase is a pancreatic enzyme that is used to facilitate digestion. It should be given with meals and snacks, and it works well in foods such as applesauce. Answers A, B, and D are incorrect times to administer this medication.

120. **Answer A is correct.** The expected time for contact to tuberculosis is 1 year. Therefore, answers B, C, and D are incorrect.

121. **Answer B is correct.** Pitocin is used to cause the uterus to contract and decrease bleeding. A uterus deviated to the left, as stated in answer A, indicates a full bladder. It is not desirable to have a boggy uterus, making answer C incorrect. This lack of muscle tone will increase bleeding. Answer D is incorrect because the position of the uterus is not related to the use of Pitocin.

122. **Answer C is correct.** Before chemotherapy, an antiemetic should be given because most chemotherapy agents cause nausea. It is not necessary to give a bolus of IV fluids, medicate for pain, or allow the client to eat; therefore, answers A, B, and D are incorrect.

123. **Answer D is correct.** The vital signs should be taken before any chemotherapy agent. If it is an IV infusion of chemotherapy, the nurse should check the IV site as well. Answers B and C are incorrect because it is not necessary to check the electrolytes or blood gasses.

124. **Answer D is correct.** Vitamin K is given after delivery because the newborn's intestinal tract is sterile and lacks vitamin K needed for clotting. Answer A is incorrect because vitamin K is not directly given to prevent dehydration, but will facilitate clotting.

Answers B and C are incorrect because vitamin K does not prevent infection or replace electrolytes.

125. Answer C is correct. The best protector for the client with an ileostomy to use is stomahesive. Answer A is not correct because the bag will not seal if the client uses Karaya powder. Answer B is incorrect because there is no need to irrigate an ileostomy. Neosporin, answer D, is not used to protect the skin because it is an antibiotic.

126. Answer C is correct. $FeSO_4$ or iron should be given with ascorbic acid (vitamin C). This helps with the absorption. It should not be given with meals or milk because this decreases the absorption; thus, answers A and B are incorrect. Giving it undiluted, as stated in answer D, is not good because it tastes bad.

127. Answer A is correct. Hyphema is blood in the anterior chamber of the eye and around the eye. The client should have the head of the bed elevated and ice applied. Answers B, C, and D are incorrect and do not treat the problem.

128. Answer C is correct. The most stable client is the client with the thyroidectomy 4 days ago. Answers A, B, and D are incorrect because the other clients are less stable and require a registered nurse.

129. Answer A is correct. The "bull's eye" rash is indicative of Lyme's disease, a disease spread by ticks. The signs and symptoms include elevated temp-erature, headache, nausea, and the rash. Although answers B and D are important, the question asks which would be *best*. Answer C has no significance.

130. Answer C is correct. The most definitive diagnostic tool for HIV is the Western Blot. The white blood cell count, as stated in answer A, is not the best indicator, but a white blood cell count of less than 3,500 requires investigation. The ELISA test, answer B, is a screening exam. Answer D is not specific enough.

131. Answer B is correct. Gentamycin is a drug from the aminoglycocide classification. These drugs are toxic to the auditory nerve and the kidneys. The hematocrit is not of significant consideration in this client; therefore, answer A is incorrect. Answer C is incorrect because we would expect the white blood cell count to be elevated in this client because gentamycin is an antibiotic. Answer D is incorrect because the erythrocyte count is also particularly significant to check.

132. Answer A is correct. The nurse should not take the blood pressure on the affected side. Also, venopunctures and IVs should not be used in the affected area. Answers B, C, and D are all indicated for caring for the client. The arm should be elevated to decrease edema. It is best to position the client on the unaffected side and perform a dextrostix on the unaffected side.

133. Answer D is correct. The nurse who has had the chickenpox has immunity to the illness. Answer A is incorrect because more information is needed to determine whether a change in assignment is necessary. Answer B is incorrect because there could be a risk to the immune-suppressed client. Answer C is incorrect because the client who is immune-suppressed could still be at risk from the nurse's exposure to the chickenpox, even if scabs are present.

134. **Answer C is correct.** The nurse should explore the cause for the lack of motivation. The client might be anemic and lack energy, might be in pain, or might be depressed. Alternating staff, as stated in answer A, will prevent a bond from being formed with the nurse. Answer B is not enough, and answer D is not necessary.

135. **Answer A is correct.** Contacting organ retrieval to talk to the family member is the best choice because a trained specialist has the knowledge to assist the wife with making the decision to donate or not to donate the client's organs. The hospital will certainly honor the wishes of family members even if the patient has signed a donor card. Answer B is incorrect; answer C might be done, but there might not be time; and answer D is not good nursing etiquette and, therefore, is incorrect.

136. **Answer A is correct.** The nurse should inspect first, then auscultate, and finally palpate. If the nurse palpates first the assessment might be unreliable. Therefore, answers B, C, and D are incorrect.

137. **Answer B is correct.** Many medications can irritate the stomach and contribute to abdominal pain. For answer A, the primary reason for asking about medications is not to identify interactions between medication. Although this might provide an opportunity for teaching, this is not the best time to teach. Therefore, answers C and D are incorrect.

138. **Answer D is correct.** *H. pylori* bacteria and stress are directly related to peptic ulcers. Answers A and B are incorrect because peptic ulcers are not caused by overeating or always caused by continued stress. Answer C is incorrect because peptic ulcers are related to but not directly caused by stress.

139. **Answer C is correct.** The new diabetic has a knowledge deficit. Answers A, B, and D are not supported within the stem and so are incorrect.

140. **Answer A is correct.** The best diagnostic tool for cancer is the biopsy. Other assessment includes checking the lymph nodes. Answers B, C, and D will not confirm a diagnosis of oral cancer.

141. **Answer D is correct.** The use of a sitz bath will help with the pain and swelling associated with a hemorroidectomy. The client should eat foods high in fiber, so answer A is incorrect. Ice packs, as stated in answer B, are ordered immediately after surgery only. Answer C, a stool softener, can be ordered, but only by the doctor.

142. **Answer A is correct.** The client with a colostomy can swim and carry on activities as before the colostomy; therefore, answers B and C are incorrect. Answer D shows a lack of empathy.

143. **Answer C is correct.** Antacids should be administered within 1–2 hours of other medications. If antacids are taken with many medications, they render the other medications inactive. All other answers are incorrect.

144. **Answer A is correct.** Before beginning feedings, an x-ray is often obtained to check for placement. Aspirating stomach content and checking the pH for acidity is the best method of checking for placement. Other methods include placing the end in water and checking for bubbling, and injecting air and listening over the epigastric area. Answers B and C are not correct. Answer D is incorrect because warming in the microwave is contraindicated.

145. **Answer D is correct.** Alcohol will cause extreme nausea if consumed with Flagyl. Answer A is incorrect because the full course of treatment should be taken. The medication should be taken with a full 8oz. of water, with meals, and the client should avoid direct sunlight because he will most likely be photosensitive; therefore, answers A, B, and C are incorrect.

146. **Answer C is correct.** Fluid volume deficit can lead to metabolic acidosis and electrolyte loss. The other nursing diagnoses in answers A, B, and D might be applicable but are of lesser priority.

147. **Answer A is correct.** The nurse should reinforce the need for a diet balanced in all nutrients and fiber. Foods that often cause diarrhea and bloating associated with irritable bowel syndrome include fried foods, caffeinated beverages, alcohol, and spicy foods. Therefore, answers B, C, and D are incorrect.

148. **Answer A is correct.** Clients with celiac disease should refrain from eating foods containing gluten. Foods with gluten include wheat barley, oats, and rye. The other foods are allowed.

149. **Answer B is correct.** A barium enema is contraindicated in the client with diverticulitis because it can cause bowel perforation. Answers A, C, and D are appropriate diagnostic studies for the client with diverticulitis.

150. **Answer B is correct.** Individuals with ulcers within the duodenum typically complain of pain occurring 2–3 hours after a meal, as well as at night. The pain is usually relieved by eating. The pain associated with gastric ulcers, answer A, occurs 30 minutes after eating. Answer C is too vague and does not distinguish the type of ulcer. Answer D is associated with stress.

151. **Answer C is correct.** *H. pylori* bacteria has been linked to peptic ulcers. Answers A, B, and D are not typically cultured within the stomach, duodenum, or esophagus, and are not related to the development of peptic ulcers.

152. **Answer A is correct.** Maintaining a patient's airway is paramount in the post-operative period. This is the priority of nursing care. Answers B, C, and D are applicable but are not the priority. The nurse should instruct the client to perform mouth care using a soft sponge toothette or irrigate the mouth with normal saline. The incision should be kept as dry as possible, and pain should be treated. Pain medications should be administered PRN.

153. **Answer D is correct.** Low hemoglobin and hematocrit might indicate intestinal bleeding. Answers A, B, and C are normal lab values.

154. **Answer C is correct.** Pain is a late sign of oral cancer. Answers A, B, and D are incorrect because a feeling of warmth, odor, and a flat ulcer in the mouth are all early occurrences of oral cancer.

155. **Answer C is correct.** Epidural anesthesia involves injecting an anesthetic into the epidural space. If the anesthetic rises above the respiratory center, the client will have impaired breathing; thus, monitoring for respiratory depression is necessary. Answer A, seizure activity, is not likely after an epidural. Answer B, orthostatic hypotension, occurs when the client stands up but is not a monitoring action. The client with an epidural anesthesia must remain flat on her back and should not stand up for 24 hours. Answer D, hematuria, is not related to epidural anesthesia.

176. **Answer B is correct.** To safely administer heparin, the nurse should obtain an infusion controller. Too rapid infusion of heparin can result in hemorrhage. Answers A, C, and D are incorrect. It is not necessary to have a buretrol, an infusion filter, or a three-way stop-cock.

177. **Answer A is correct.** A low-protein diet is required because protein breaks down into nitrogenous waste and causes an increased workload on the kidneys. Answers B, C, and D are incorrect.

178. **Answer A is correct.** Damage to the hypothalamus can result in an elevated temperature because this portion of the brain helps to regulate body temperature. Answers B, C, and D are incorrect because there is no data to support the possibility of an infection, a cooling blanket might not be required, and the frontal lobe is not responsible for regulation of the body temperature.

179. **Answer C is correct.** The temporal lobe is responsible for taste, smell, and hearing. The occipital lobe is responsible for vision. The frontal lobe is responsible for judgment, foresight, and behavior. The parietal lobe is responsible for ideation, sensory functions, and language. Therefore, answers A, B, and D are incorrect.

180. **Answer B is correct.** To correctly measure the client for crutches, the nurse should measure approximately 3 inches under the axilla. Answer A allows for too much distance under the arm. The elbows should be flexed approximately 35°, not 10°, as stated in answer C. The crutches should be approximately 6 inches from the side of the foot, not 20 inches, as stated in answer D.

181. **Answer D is correct.** When assisting the client with bowel and bladder training, the least helpful factor is the sexual function. Dietary history, mobility, and fluid intake are important factors; these must be taken into consideration because they relate to constipation, urinary function, and the ability to use the urinal or bedpan. Therefore, answers A, B, and C are incorrect.

182. **Answer B is correct.** Because the aorta is clamped during surgery, the blood supply to the kidneys is impaired. This can result in renal damage. A urinary output of 20mL is oliguria. In answer A, the pedal pulses that are thready and regular are within normal limits. For answer C, it is desirable for the client's blood pressure to be slightly low after surgical repair of an aneurysm. The oxygen saturation of 97% in answer D is within normal limits and, therefore, incorrect.

183. **Answer C is correct.** The client taking an anticoagulant should not take aspirin because it will further thin the blood. He should return to have a Protime drawn for bleeding time, report a rash, and use an electric razor. Therefore, answers A, B, and D are incorrect.

184. **Answer A is correct.** The best roommate for the post-surgical client is the client with hypothyroidism. This client is sleepy and has no infectious process. Answers B, C, and D are incorrect because the client with a diabetic ulcer, ulcerative colitis, or pneumonia can transmit infection to the post-surgical client.

185. **Answer C is correct.** The client admitted 1 hour ago with shortness of breath should be seen first because this client might require oxygen therapy. The client in answer A with a low-grade temperature can be assessed after the client with shortness of breath. The client in answer B can also be seen later. This client will have some

inflammatory process after surgery, so a temperature of 100.2°F is not unusual. The low-grade temperature should be re-evaluated in 1 hour. The client in answer D can be reserved for later.

186. Answer A is correct. The best time to apply antithrombolytic stockings is in the morning before rising. If the doctor orders them later in the day, the client should return to bed, wait 30 minutes, and apply the stockings. Answers B, C, and D are incorrect because there is likely to be more peripheral edema if the client is standing or has just taken a bath; before retiring in the evening is wrong because, late in the evening, more peripheral edema will be present.

187. Answer C is correct. The client with a femoral popliteal bypass graft should avoid activities that can occlude the femoral artery graft. Sitting in the straight chair and wearing tight clothes are prohibited for this reason. Resting in a supine position, resting in a recliner, or sleeping in right Sim's are allowed, as stated in answers A, B, and D.

188. Answer A is correct. The client is exhibiting a widened pulse pressure, tachycardia, and tachypnea. The next action after obtaining these vital signs is to notify the doctor for additional orders. Rechecking the vitals signs, as in answer B, is wasting time. It is the doctor's call to order arterial blood gases and an ECG.

189. Answer C is correct. If the finger cannot be used, the next best place to apply the oxygen monitor is to the earlobe. It can also be placed on the forehead, but the choices in answers A, B, and D are incorrect.

190. Answer C is correct. It is necessary to check the PTT *as well* as administer in the abdomen, as stated in answer C. It is not necessary to administer this medication before meals; thus, answer A is incorrect. Answer D is incorrect because the nurse should not aspirate after the injection.

191. Answer A is correct. The client taking calcium preparations will frequently develop constipation so the client should be assessed for any problems related to bowel elimination. Answers B, C, and D are not problems related to the use of calcium carbonate.

192. Answer D is correct. Urokinase is a thrombolytic used to destroy a clot following a myocardial infraction. If the client exhibits overt signs of bleeding, the nurse should stop the medication, call the doctor immediately, and prepare the antidote, which is Amicar. Answer B is not correct because simply stopping the urokinase is not enough. In answer A, vitamin K is not the antidote for urokinase, and reducing the urokinase, as stated in answer B, is not enough.

193. Answer C is correct. Children at age 2 can reach for objects that they desire and use simple words such as *cookie* to express what they want. They already understand "yes" and "no," so answer A is incorrect. Simple language patterns begin to develop after this age, even though children at this age might understand some words; therefore, answer B is not a good choice. Later, at about age 3 or 4, they begin to ask "Why?," making answer D incorrect.

194. Answer B is correct. A 2-year-old is expected only to use magical thinking, such as believing that a toy bear is a real bear. Answers A, C, and D are not expected until the child is much older. Abstract thinking, conservation of matter, and the ability to look at things from the perspective of others are not skills for small children.

195. Answer B is correct. The first action that the nurse should take when beginning to examine the infant is to listen to the heart and lungs. If the nurse elicits the Babinski reflex, palpates the abdomen, or looks in the child's ear first, the child will begin to cry and it will be difficult to obtain an objective finding while listening to the heart and lungs. Therefore, answers A, C, and D are incorrect.

196. Answer B is correct. Parallel play is play that is demonstrated by two children playing side by side but not together. The play in answers A and C is participative play because the children are playing together. The play in answer D is solitary play because the mother is not playing with Mary.

197. Answer B is correct. The 4-year-old is more prone to accidental poisoning because children at this age are much more mobile and this makes them more likely to ingest poisons than the other children. Answers A, C, and D are incorrect because the 6-month-old is still too small to be extremely mobile, the 10-year-old has begun to understand risk, and the 13-year-old is also aware of the risks of poisoning and is less likely to ingest poisons than the 4-year-old.

198. Answer C is correct. To prevent the client from inducing vomiting after eating, the client should be observed for 1–2 hours after meals. Allowing privacy as stated in answer A will only give the client time to vomit. Praising the client for eating all of a meal does not correct the psychological aspects of the disease; thus, answer B is incorrect. Encouraging the client to choose favorite foods might increase stress and the chance of choosing foods that are low in calories and fats.

199. Answer A is correct. Clients with antisocial personality disorder must have limits set on their behavior because they are artful in manipulating others. Answer B is not correct because they do express feelings and remorse. Answers C and D are incorrect because it is unnecessary to minimize interactions with others or encourage them to act out rage more than they already do.

200. Answer B is correct. The client with passive-aggressive personality disorder often has underlying hostility that is exhibited as acting-out behavior. Answers A, C, and D are incorrect. Although these individuals might have a high IQ, it cannot be said that they have superior intelligence. They also do not necessarily have dependence on others or an inability to share feelings.

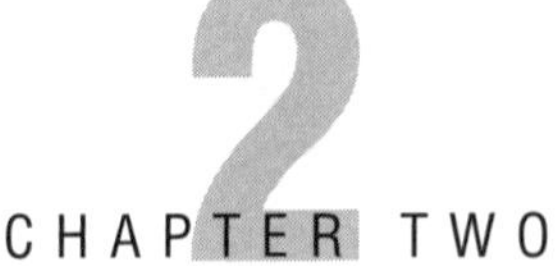

Practice Exam 2 and Rationales

Quick Check

1. A papular lesion is noted on the perineum of the laboring client. Which initial action is most appropriate?

Quick Answers: **118**
Detailed Answer: **121**

- ❍ **A.** Document the finding
- ❍ **B.** Report the finding to the doctor
- ❍ **C.** Prepare the client for a C-section
- ❍ **D.** Continue primary care as prescribed

2. A client with a diagnosis of human papillomavirus (HPV) is at risk for which of the following?

Quick Answers: **118**
Detailed Answer: **121**

- ❍ **A.** Lymphoma
- ❍ **B.** Vaginal cancer
- ❍ **C.** Leukemia
- ❍ **D.** Systemic lupus

3. The client seen in the family planning clinic tells the nurse that she has a painful lesion on the perineum. The nurse is aware that the most likely source of the lesion is:

Quick Answers: **118**
Detailed Answer: **121**

- ❍ **A.** Syphilis
- ❍ **B.** Herpes
- ❍ **C.** Candidiasis
- ❍ **D.** Condylomata

4. A client visiting a family planning clinic is suspected of having an STI. The most diagnostic test for treponema pallidum is:

Quick Answers: **118**
Detailed Answer: **121**

- ❍ **A.** Venereal Disease Research Lab (VDRL)
- ❍ **B.** Rapid plasma reagin (RPR)
- ❍ **C.** Florescent treponemal antibody (FTA)
- ❍ **D.** Thayer-Martin culture (TMC)

Quick Check

5. Which laboratory finding is associated with HELLP syndrome in the obstetric client?

Quick Answers: **118**
Detailed Answer: **121**

❍ **A.** Elevated blood glucose
❍ **B.** Elevated platelet count
❍ **C.** Elevated creatinine clearance
❍ **D.** Elevated hepatic enzymes

6. The nurse is assessing the deep tendon reflexes of the client with hypomagnesemia. Which method is used to elicit the biceps reflex?

Quick Answers: **118**
Detailed Answer: **121**

❍ **A.** The nurse places her thumb on the muscle inset in the antecubital space and taps the thumb briskly with the reflex hammer.
❍ **B.** The nurse loosely suspends the client's arm in an open hand while tapping the back of the client's elbow.
❍ **C.** The nurse instructs the client to dangle her legs as the nurse strikes the area below the patella with the blunt side of the reflex hammer.
❍ **D.** The nurse instructs the client to place her arms loosely at her side as the nurse strikes the muscle insert just above the wrist.

7. Which medication should be used with caution in the obstetric client with diabetes?

Quick Answers: **118**
Detailed Answer: **121**

❍ **A.** Magnesium sulfate
❍ **B.** Brethine
❍ **C.** Stadol
❍ **D.** Ancef

8. A multigravida is scheduled for an amniocentesis at 32 weeks gestation to determine the L/S ratio and phosphatidyl glycerol level. The L/S ratio is 1:1. The nurse's assessment of this data is:

Quick Answers: **118**
Detailed Answer: **121**

❍ **A.** The infant is at low risk for congenital anomalies.
❍ **B.** The infant is at high risk for intrauterine growth retardation.
❍ **C.** The infant is at high risk for respiratory distress syndrome.
❍ **D.** The infant is at high risk for birth trauma.

Quick Check

9. Which observation in the newborn of a mother who is alcohol dependent would require immediate nursing intervention?

Quick Answers: **118**
Detailed Answer: **121**

❍ **A.** Crying
❍ **B.** Wakefulness
❍ **C.** Jitteriness
❍ **D.** Yawning

10. The nurse caring for a client receiving magnesium sulfate must closely observe for side effects associated with drug therapy. An expected side effect of magnesium sulfate is:

Quick Answers: **118**
Detailed Answer: **121**

❍ **A.** Decreased urinary output
❍ **B.** Hypersomnolence
❍ **C.** Absence of knee jerk reflex
❍ **D.** Decreased respiratory rate

11. The 57-year-old male client has elected to have epidural anesthesia as the anesthetic during a hernia repair. If the client experiences hypotension, the nurse would:

Quick Answers: **118**
Detailed Answer: **122**

❍ **A.** Place him in the Trendelenburg position
❍ **B.** Obtain an order for Benedryl
❍ **C.** Administer oxygen per nasal cannula
❍ **D.** Speed the IV infusion of normal saline

12. A client has cancer of the pancreas. The nurse should be most concerned with which nursing diagnosis?

Quick Answers: **118**
Detailed Answer: **122**

❍ **A.** Alteration in nutrition
❍ **B.** Alteration in bowel elimination
❍ **C.** Alteration in skin integrity
❍ **D.** Ineffective individual coping

13. The nurse is caring for a client with ascites. Which is the best method to use for determining early ascites?

Quick Answers: **118**
Detailed Answer: **122**

❍ **A.** Inspection of the abdomen for enlargement
❍ **B.** Bimanual palpation for hepatomegaly
❍ **C.** Daily measurement of abdominal girth
❍ **D.** Assessment for a fluid wave

Quick Check

14. The client arrives in the emergency department after a motor vehicle accident. Nursing assessment findings include BP 80/34, pulse rate 120, and respirations 20. Which is the client's most appropriate priority nursing diagnosis?

❍ **A.** Alteration in cerebral tissue perfusion
❍ **B.** Fluid volume deficit
❍ **C.** Ineffective airway clearance
❍ **D.** Alteration in sensory perception

Quick Answers: **118**
Detailed Answer: **122**

15. Which information obtained from the visit to a client with hemophilia would cause the most concern? The client:

❍ **A.** Likes to play football
❍ **B.** Drinks several carbonated drinks per day
❍ **C.** Has two sisters with sickle cell tract
❍ **D.** Is taking acetaminophen to control pain

Quick Answers: **118**
Detailed Answer: **122**

16. The nurse on oncology is caring for a client with a white blood count of 800, a platelet count of 150,000, and a red blood cell count of 250,000. During evening visitation, a visitor is noted to be coughing and sneezing. What action should the nurse take?

❍ **A.** Ask the visitor to wash his hands
❍ **B.** Document the visitor's condition in the chart
❍ **C.** Ask the visitor to leave and not return until the client's white blood cell count is 1,000
❍ **D.** Provide the visitor with a mask and gown

Quick Answers: **118**
Detailed Answer: **122**

17. The nurse is caring for the client admitted after trauma to the neck in an automobile accident. The client suddenly becomes unresponsive and pale, with a BP of 60 systolic. The initial nurse's action should be to:

❍ **A.** Place the client in Trendelenburg position
❍ **B.** Increase the infusion of normal saline
❍ **C.** Administer atropine IM
❍ **D.** Obtain a crash cart

Quick Answers: **118**
Detailed Answer: **122**

18. Immediately following the removal of a chest tube, the nurse would:

❍ **A.** Order a chest x-ray
❍ **B.** Take the blood pressure
❍ **C.** Cover the insertion site with a Vaseline gauze
❍ **D.** Ask the client to perform the Valsalva maneuver

Quick Answers: **118**
Detailed Answer: **122**

Quick Check

19. A client being treated with sodium warfarin has an INR of 9.0. Which intervention would be most important to include in the nursing care plan?

Quick Answers: **118**
Detailed Answer: **123**

❍ **A.** Assess for signs of abnormal bleeding
❍ **B.** Anticipate an increase in the dosage
❍ **C.** Instruct the client regarding the drug therapy
❍ **D.** Increase the frequency of neurological assessments

20. Which snack selection by a client with osteoporosis indicates that the client understands the dietary management of the disease?

Quick Answers: **118**
Detailed Answer: **123**

❍ **A.** A glass of orange juice
❍ **B.** A blueberry muffin
❍ **C.** A cup of yogurt
❍ **D.** A banana

21. The elderly client with hypomagnesemia is admitted to the unit with an order for magnesium sulfate. Which action by the nurse indicates understanding of magnesium sulfate?

Quick Answers: **118**
Detailed Answer: **123**

❍ **A.** The nurse places a sign over the bed not to check blood pressures in the left arm.
❍ **B.** The nurse places a padded tongue blade at the bedside.
❍ **C.** The nurse measures the urinary output hourly.
❍ **D.** The nurse darkens the room.

22. The nurse is caring for a 10-year-old client scheduled for surgery. The client's mother tells the nurse that her religion forbids blood transfusions. What nursing action is most appropriate?

Quick Answers: **118**
Detailed Answer: **123**

❍ **A.** Document the mother's statement in the chart
❍ **B.** Encourage the mother to reconsider
❍ **C.** Explain the consequences of no treatment
❍ **D.** Notify the physician of the mother's refusal

23. A client is admitted to the unit 3 hours after an injury with second-degree burns to the face, neck, and head. The nurse would be most concerned with the client developing which of the following?

Quick Answers: **118**
Detailed Answer: **123**

❍ **A.** Hypovolemia
❍ **B.** Laryngeal edema
❍ **C.** Hypernatremia
❍ **D.** Hyperkalemia

Quick Check

24. The nurse is evaluating nutritional outcomes for an elderly client with anorexia. Which data best indicates that the plan of care is effective?

Quick Answers: **118**
Detailed Answer: **123**

❍ **A.** The client selects a balanced diet from the menu.

❍ **B.** The client's hematocrit improves.

❍ **C.** The client's tissue turgor improves.

❍ **D.** The client gains weight.

25. The client is admitted following repair of a fractured femur with cast application. Which nursing assessment should be reported to the doctor?

Quick Answers: **118**
Detailed Answer: **123**

❍ **A.** Pain

❍ **B.** Warm toes

❍ **C.** Pedal pulses rapid

❍ **D.** Paresthesia of the toes

26. Which would be an expected finding during injection of dye with a cardiac catheterization?

Quick Answers: **118**
Detailed Answer: **123**

❍ **A.** Cold extremity distant to the injection site

❍ **B.** Warmth in the extremity

❍ **C.** Extreme chest pain

❍ **D.** Itching in the extremities

27. Which action by the healthcare worker indicates a need for further teaching?

Quick Answers: **118**
Detailed Answer: **124**

❍ **A.** The nursing assistant wears gloves while giving the client a bath.

❍ **B.** The nurse wears goggles while drawing blood from the client.

❍ **C.** The doctor washes his hands before examining the client.

❍ **D.** The nurse wears gloves to take the client's vital signs.

28. The client is having electroconvulsive therapy for treatment of severe depression. Which of the following indicates that the client's ECT has been effective?

Quick Answers: **118**
Detailed Answer: **124**

❍ **A.** The client loses consciousness.

❍ **B.** The client vomits.

❍ **C.** The client's ECG indicates tachycardia.

❍ **D.** The client has a grand mal seizure.

Quick Check

29. The 5-year-old is being tested for pinworms. To collect a specimen for assessment of pinworms, the nurse should teach the mother to:

Quick Answers: **118**
Detailed Answer: **124**

❍ **A.** Examine the perianal area with a flashlight 2–3 hours after the child is asleep and to collect any eggs on a clear tape

❍ **B.** Scrape the skin with a piece of cardboard and bring it to the clinic

❍ **C.** Obtain a stool specimen in the afternoon

❍ **D.** Bring a hair sample to the clinic for evaluation

30. Which instruction should be given regarding the medication used to treat enterobiasis (pinworms)?

Quick Answers: **118**
Detailed Answer: **124**

❍ **A.** Treatment is not recommended for children less than 10 years of age.

❍ **B.** The entire family should be treated.

❍ **C.** Medication therapy will continue for 1 year.

❍ **D.** Intravenous antibiotic therapy will be ordered.

31. Which client should be assigned to the pregnant licensed practical nurse?

Quick Answers: **118**
Detailed Answer: **124**

❍ **A.** The client who just returned after receiving linear accelerator radiation therapy for lung cancer

❍ **B.** The client with a radium implant for cervical cancer

❍ **C.** The client who has just been administered soluble brachytherapy for thyroid cancer

❍ **D.** The client who has returned from placement of iridium seeds for prostate cancer

32. Which client should be assigned to a private room if only one is available?

Quick Answers: **118**
Detailed Answer: **124**

❍ **A.** The client with Cushing's syndrome

❍ **B.** The client with diabetes

❍ **C.** The client with acromegaly

❍ **D.** The client with myxedema

Quick Check

33. The nurse caring for a client on the pediatric unit administers adult-strength Digitalis to the 3-pound infant. As a result of her actions, the baby suffers permanent heart and brain damage. The nurse can be charged with:

❍ **A.** Negligence
❍ **B.** Tort
❍ **C.** Assault
❍ **D.** Malpractice

Quick Answers: **118**
Detailed Answer: **124**

34. Which assignment should not be performed by the licensed practical nurse?

❍ **A.** Inserting a Foley catheter
❍ **B.** Discontinuing a nasogastric tube
❍ **C.** Obtaining a sputum specimen
❍ **D.** Initiating a blood transfusion

Quick Answers: **118**
Detailed Answer: **125**

35. The client returns to the unit from surgery with a blood pressure of 90/50, pulse 132, and respirations 30. Which action by the nurse should receive priority?

❍ **A.** Continuing to monitor the vital signs
❍ **B.** Contacting the physician
❍ **C.** Asking the client how he feels
❍ **D.** Asking the LPN to continue the post-op care

Quick Answers: **118**
Detailed Answer: **125**

36. Which nurse should be assigned to care for the postpartal client with preeclampsia? The nurse with:

❍ **A.** 2 weeks of experience in postpartum
❍ **B.** 3 years of experience in labor and delivery
❍ **C.** 10 years of experience in surgery
❍ **D.** 1 year of experience in the neonatal intensive care unit

Quick Answers: **118**
Detailed Answer: **125**

37. Which information should be reported to the state Board of Nursing?

❍ **A.** The facility fails to provide literature in both Spanish and English.
❍ **B.** The narcotic count has been incorrect on the unit for the past 3 days.
❍ **C.** The client fails to receive an itemized account of his bills and services received during his hospital stay.
❍ **D.** The nursing assistant assigned to the client with hepatitis fails to feed the client and give the bath.

Quick Answers: **118**
Detailed Answer: **125**

Quick Check

38. The nurse is suspected of charting the administration of a medication that he did not give. After talking to the nurse, the charge nurse should:

Quick Answers: 118
Detailed Answer: 125

- ❍ **A.** Call the Board of Nursing
- ❍ **B.** File a formal reprimand
- ❍ **C.** Terminate the nurse
- ❍ **D.** Charge the nurse with a tort

39. The nurse is making rounds. Which client should be seen first?

Quick Answers: 118
Detailed Answer: 125

- ❍ **A.** The 78-year-old who had a gastrectomy 3 weeks ago and has a PEG tube
- ❍ **B.** The 5-month-old discharged 1 week ago with pneumonia who is being treated with amoxicillin liquid suspension
- ❍ **C.** The 50-year-old with MRSA (methcillin-resistant staphylococcus aurea)
- ❍ **D.** The 30-year-old with an exacerbation of multiple sclerosis being treated with cortisone intravenously

40. The emergency room is flooded with clients injured in a tornado. Which clients can be assigned to share a room in the emergency department during the disaster?

Quick Answers: 118
Detailed Answer: 125

- ❍ **A.** A schizophrenic client having visual and auditory hallucinations and the client with ulcerative colitis
- ❍ **B.** The client who is 6 months pregnant with abdominal pain and the client with facial lacerations and a broken arm
- ❍ **C.** A child whose pupils are fixed and dilated and his parents, and a client with a frontal head injury
- ❍ **D.** The client who arrives with a large puncture wound to the abdomen and the client with chest pain

41. The nurse is caring for a 6-year-old client admitted with the diagnosis of conjunctivitis. Before administering eyedrops, the nurse should recognize that it is essential to consider which of the following?

Quick Answers: 118
Detailed Answer: 125

- ❍ **A.** The eye should be cleansed with warm water, removing any exudate, before instilling the eyedrops.
- ❍ **B.** The child should be allowed to instill his own eyedrops.
- ❍ **C.** The mother should be allowed to instill the eyedrops.
- ❍ **D.** If the eye is clear of any redness or edema, the eyedrops should be held.

Quick Check

42. The nurse is discussing meal planning with the mother of a 2-year-old toddler. Which of the following statements, if made by the mother, would require a need for further instruction?

Quick Answers: **118**
Detailed Answer: **126**

- ❍ **A.** "It is okay to give my child white grape juice for breakfast."
- ❍ **B.** "My child can have a grilled cheese sandwich for lunch."
- ❍ **C.** "We are going on a trip, and I have bought hot dogs to grill for his lunch."
- ❍ **D.** "For a snack, my child can have ice cream."

43. A 2-year-old toddler is seen in the pediatrician's office. During physical assessment, the nurse would anticipate the need for which intervention?

Quick Answers: **118**
Detailed Answer: **126**

- ❍ **A.** Ask the parent/guardian to leave the room when assessments are being performed
- ❍ **B.** Ask the parent/guardian to remove the child's toys during examination
- ❍ **C.** Ask the parent/guardian to stay with the child during the examination
- ❍ **D.** If the child is screaming, tell him this is inappropriate behavior

44. Which instruction should be given to the client who is fitted for a behind-the-ear hearing aid?

Quick Answers: **118**
Detailed Answer: **126**

- ❍ **A.** Remove the mold and clean every week
- ❍ **B.** Store the hearing aid in a cool place
- ❍ **C.** Clean the lint from the hearing aide with a toothpick
- ❍ **D.** Change the batteries weekly

45. A priority nursing diagnosis for a child being admitted from surgery following a tonsillectomy is:

Quick Answers: **118**
Detailed Answer: **126**

- ❍ **A.** Body image disturbance
- ❍ **B.** Impaired verbal communication
- ❍ **C.** Risk for aspiration
- ❍ **D.** Pain

Quick Check

46. A client with bacterial pneumonia is admitted to the pediatric unit. What would the nurse expect the admitting assessment to reveal?

Quick Answers: **118**
Detailed Answer: **126**

❍ **A.** High fever
❍ **B.** Nonproductive cough
❍ **C.** Rhinitis
❍ **D.** Vomiting and diarrhea

47. The nurse is caring for a client admitted with acute laryngotracheobronchitis (LTB). Because of the possibility of complete obstruction of the airway, which of the following should the nurse have available?

Quick Answers: **118**
Detailed Answer: **126**

❍ **A.** Intravenous access supplies
❍ **B.** Emergency intubation equipment
❍ **C.** Intravenous fluid administration pump
❍ **D.** Supplemental oxygen

48. The 45-year-old client is seen in the clinic with hyperthyroidism. What would the nurse expect the admitting assessment to reveal?

Quick Answers: **118**
Detailed Answer: **126**

❍ **A.** Bradycardia
❍ **B.** Decreased appetite
❍ **C.** Exophthalmos
❍ **D.** Weight gain

49. The nurse is providing dietary instructions to the mother of an 8-year-old child diagnosed with celiac disease. Which of the following foods, if selected by the mother, would indicate her understanding of the dietary instructions?

Quick Answers: **118**
Detailed Answer: **126**

❍ **A.** Whole-wheat bread
❍ **B.** Spaghetti and meatballs
❍ **C.** Hamburger on white bread with ketchup
❍ **D.** Cheese omelet

50. The nurse is caring for a 9-year-old child admitted with asthma. During the morning rounds, the nurse finds an O_2 sat of 78%. Which of the following actions should the nurse take first?

Quick Answers: **118**
Detailed Answer: **126**

❍ **A.** Check the arterial blood gases
❍ **B.** Do nothing; this is a normal O_2 sat for this client
❍ **C.** Apply oxygen
❍ **D.** Assess the child's pulse

Quick Check

51. A gravida II para 0 is admitted to the labor and delivery unit. The doctor performs an amniotomy. Which observation would the nurse expect to make after the amniotomy?

Quick Answers: **118**
Detailed Answer: **127**

- ❍ **A.** Fetal heart tones 160bpm
- ❍ **B.** A moderate amount of straw-colored fluid
- ❍ **C.** A small amount of greenish fluid
- ❍ **D.** A small segment of the umbilical cord

52. The client is admitted to the unit. Vaginal exam reveals that she is 3cm dilated. Which of the following statements would the nurse expect her to make?

Quick Answers: **118**
Detailed Answer: **127**

- ❍ **A.** "I can't decide what to name the baby."
- ❍ **B.** "It feels good to push with each contraction."
- ❍ **C.** "Don't touch me. I'm trying to concentrate."
- ❍ **D.** "When can I get my epidural?"

53. The client is having fetal heart rates of 100–110bpm during the contractions. The first action the nurse should take is:

Quick Answers: **118**
Detailed Answer: **127**

- ❍ **A.** Reassess the fetal heart tones in 15 minutes
- ❍ **B.** Turn the client to her left side
- ❍ **C.** Get the client up and walk her in the hall
- ❍ **D.** Move the client to the delivery room

54. The nurse is monitoring the client admitted for induction of labor. The nurse knows that Pitocin has been effective when:

Quick Answers: **118**
Detailed Answer: **127**

- ❍ **A.** The client has a rapid, painless delivery.
- ❍ **B.** The client's cervix is effaced.
- ❍ **C.** The client has infrequent contractions.
- ❍ **D.** The client has progressive cervical dilation.

55. A vaginal exam reveals a breech presentation. The nurse should take which of the following actions at this time?

Quick Answers: **118**
Detailed Answer: **127**

- ❍ **A.** Prepare the client for a Caesarean section
- ❍ **B.** Apply the fetal heart monitor
- ❍ **C.** Place the client in Trendelenburg position
- ❍ **D.** Perform an ultrasound exam

Quick Check

56. The nurse is caring for a gravida 1 admitted in labor. Which finding would suggest the need for an internal fetal monitor?

Quick Answers: **118**
Detailed Answer: **127**

- ❍ **A.** The cervix is dilated 5cm.
- ❍ **B.** The fetal heart tones are difficult to assess using the external toco monitor.
- ❍ **C.** The fetus is at station 0.
- ❍ **D.** Contractions are every 3 minutes.

57. Which nursing diagnoses is most appropriate for the client as she completes the latent phase of labor?

Quick Answers: **118**
Detailed Answer: **127**

- ❍ **A.** Impaired gas exchange related to hyperventilation
- ❍ **B.** Alteration in oxygen perfusion related to maternal position
- ❍ **C.** Impaired physical mobility related to fetal-monitoring equipment
- ❍ **D.** Potential fluid volume deficit related to decreased fluid intake

58. As the client reaches 8cm dilation, the nurse notes a pattern on the fetal monitor that shows a drop in the fetal heart rate of 30bpm beginning at the peak of the contraction and ending at the end of the contraction. The FHR baseline is 165–175bpm with variability of 0–2bpm. What is the most likely explanation of this pattern?

Quick Answers: **118**
Detailed Answer: **127**

- ❍ **A.** The baby is asleep.
- ❍ **B.** The umbilical cord is compressed.
- ❍ **C.** There is a vagal response.
- ❍ **D.** There is uteroplacental insufficiency.

59. The nurse notes variable decelerations on the fetal monitor strip. The most appropriate initial action would be to:

Quick Answers: **118**
Detailed Answer: **128**

- ❍ **A.** Notify her doctor
- ❍ **B.** Document the finding
- ❍ **C.** Reposition the client
- ❍ **D.** Readjust the monitor

Quick Check

60. Which of the following is a characteristic of a reassuring fetal heart rate pattern?

Quick Answers: **118**
Detailed Answer: **128**

- ❍ **A.** A fetal heart rate of 170–180bpm
- ❍ **B.** A baseline variability of 25–35bpm
- ❍ **C.** Ominous periodic changes
- ❍ **D.** Acceleration of FHR with fetal movements

61. The nurse asks the client with an epidural anesthesia to void every hour during the labor. The rationale for this intervention is:

Quick Answers: **118**
Detailed Answer: **128**

- ❍ **A.** The bladder fills more rapidly because of the medication used for the epidural.
- ❍ **B.** Her level of consciousness is such that she is in a trancelike state.
- ❍ **C.** The sensation of the bladder filling is diminished or lost.
- ❍ **D.** She is embarrassed to ask for the bedpan that frequently.

62. A client in the family planning clinic asks the nurse about the most likely time for her to conceive. The nurse explains that conception is most likely to occur when:

Quick Answers: **118**
Detailed Answer: **128**

- ❍ **A.** Estrogen levels are low.
- ❍ **B.** Lutenizing hormone is high.
- ❍ **C.** The endometrial lining is thin.
- ❍ **D.** The progesterone level is low.

63. A client tells the nurse that she plans to use the rhythm method of birth control. The nurse is aware that the success of the rhythm method depends on the:

Quick Answers: **118**
Detailed Answer: **128**

- ❍ **A.** Age of the client
- ❍ **B.** Frequency of intercourse
- ❍ **C.** Regularity of the menses
- ❍ **D.** Range of the client's temperature

64. A client with diabetes asks the nurse for advice regarding methods of birth control. Which method of birth control is most suitable for the client with diabetes?

Quick Answers: **118**
Detailed Answer: **128**

- ❍ **A.** Intrauterine device
- ❍ **B.** Oral contraceptives
- ❍ **C.** Diaphragm
- ❍ **D.** Contraceptive sponge

Quick Check

65. The doctor suspects that the client has an ectopic pregnancy. Which symptom is consistent with a diagnosis of ectopic pregnancy?

Quick Answers: 118
Detailed Answer: 128

- ❍ **A.** Painless vaginal bleeding
- ❍ **B.** Abdominal cramping
- ❍ **C.** Throbbing pain in the upper quadrant
- ❍ **D.** Sudden, stabbing pain in the lower quadrant

66. The nurse is teaching a pregnant client about nutritional needs during pregnancy. Which menu selection will best meet the nutritional needs of the pregnant client?

Quick Answers: 118
Detailed Answer: 128

- ❍ **A.** Hamburger pattie, green beans, French fries, and iced tea
- ❍ **B.** Roast beef sandwich, potato chips, baked beans, and cola
- ❍ **C.** Baked chicken, fruit cup, potato salad, coleslaw, yogurt, and iced tea
- ❍ **D.** Fish sandwich, gelatin with fruit, and coffee

67. The client with hyperemesis gravidarum is at risk for developing:

Quick Answers: 118
Detailed Answer: 129

- ❍ **A.** Respiratory alkalosis without dehydration
- ❍ **B.** Metabolic acidosis with dehydration
- ❍ **C.** Respiratory acidosis without dehydration
- ❍ **D.** Metabolic alkalosis with dehydration

68. A client tells the doctor that she is about 20 weeks pregnant. The most definitive sign of pregnancy is:

Quick Answers: 118
Detailed Answer: 129

- ❍ **A.** Elevated human chorionic gonadatropin
- ❍ **B.** The presence of fetal heart tones
- ❍ **C.** Uterine enlargement
- ❍ **D.** Breast enlargement and tenderness

69. The nurse is caring for a neonate whose mother is diabetic. The nurse will expect the neonate to be:

Quick Answers: 118
Detailed Answer: 129

- ❍ **A.** Hypoglycemic, small for gestational age
- ❍ **B.** Hyperglycemic, large for gestational age
- ❍ **C.** Hypoglycemic, large for gestational age
- ❍ **D.** Hyperglycemic, small for gestational age

Quick Check

70. Which of the following instructions should be included in the nurse's teaching regarding oral contraceptives?

Quick Answers: **118**
Detailed Answer: **129**

- ❍ **A.** Weight gain should be reported to the physician.
- ❍ **B.** An alternate method of birth control is needed when taking antibiotics.
- ❍ **C.** If the client misses one or more pills, two pills should be taken per day for 1 week.
- ❍ **D.** Changes in the menstrual flow should be reported to the physician.

71. The nurse is discussing breastfeeding with a postpartum client. Breastfeeding is contraindicated in the postpartum client with:

Quick Answers: **118**
Detailed Answer: **129**

- ❍ **A.** Diabetes
- ❍ **B.** Positive HIV
- ❍ **C.** Hypertension
- ❍ **D.** Thyroid disease

72. A client is admitted to the labor and delivery unit complaining of vaginal bleeding with very little discomfort. The nurse's first action should be to:

Quick Answers: **118**
Detailed Answer: **129**

- ❍ **A.** Assess the fetal heart tones
- ❍ **B.** Check for cervical dilation
- ❍ **C.** Check for firmness of the uterus
- ❍ **D.** Obtain a detailed history

73. A client telephones the emergency room stating that she thinks that she is in labor. The nurse should tell the client that labor has probably begun when:

Quick Answers: **118**
Detailed Answer: **129**

- ❍ **A.** Her contractions are 2 minutes apart.
- ❍ **B.** She has back pain and a bloody discharge.
- ❍ **C.** She experiences abdominal pain and frequent urination.
- ❍ **D.** Her contractions are 5 minutes apart.

Quick Check

74. The nurse is teaching a group of prenatal clients about the effects of cigarette smoke on fetal development. Which characteristic is associated with babies born to mothers who smoked during pregnancy?

Quick Answers: **118**
Detailed Answer: **129**

- ❍ **A.** Low birth weight
- ❍ **B.** Large for gestational age
- ❍ **C.** Preterm birth, but appropriate size for gestation
- ❍ **D.** Growth retardation in weight and length

75. The physician has ordered an injection of RhoGam for the postpartum client whose blood type is A negative but whose baby is O positive. To provide postpartum prophylaxis, RhoGam should be administered:

Quick Answers: **118**
Detailed Answer: **130**

- ❍ **A.** Within 72 hours of delivery
- ❍ **B.** Within 1 week of delivery
- ❍ **C.** Within 2 weeks of delivery
- ❍ **D.** Within 1 month of delivery

76. After the physician performs an amniotomy, the nurse's first action should be to assess the:

Quick Answers: **118**
Detailed Answer: **130**

- ❍ **A.** Degree of cervical dilation
- ❍ **B.** Fetal heart tones
- ❍ **C.** Client's vital signs
- ❍ **D.** Client's level of discomfort

77. A client is admitted to the labor and delivery unit. The nurse performs a vaginal exam and determines that the client's cervix is 5cm dilated with 75% effacement. Based on the nurse's assessment, the client is in which phase of labor?

Quick Answers: **118**
Detailed Answer: **130**

- ❍ **A.** Active
- ❍ **B.** Latent
- ❍ **C.** Transition
- ❍ **D.** Early

78. A newborn with narcotic abstinence syndrome is admitted to the nursery. Nursing care of the newborn should include:

Quick Answers: **118**
Detailed Answer: **130**

- ❍ **A.** Teaching the mother to provide tactile stimulation
- ❍ **B.** Wrapping the newborn snugly in a blanket
- ❍ **C.** Placing the newborn in the infant seat
- ❍ **D.** Initiating an early infant-stimulation program

Quick Check

79. A client elects to have epidural anesthesia to relieve the discomfort of labor. Following the initiation of epidural anesthesia, the nurse should give priority to:

Quick Answers: **118**
Detailed Answer: **130**

- ❍ **A.** Checking for cervical dilation
- ❍ **B.** Placing the client in a supine position
- ❍ **C.** Checking the client's blood pressure
- ❍ **D.** Obtaining a fetal heart rate

80. The nurse is aware that the best way to prevent post-operative wound infection in the surgical client is to:

Quick Answers: **118**
Detailed Answer: **130**

- ❍ **A.** Administer a prescribed antibiotic
- ❍ **B.** Wash her hands for 2 minutes before care
- ❍ **C.** Wear a mask when providing care
- ❍ **D.** Ask the client to cover her mouth when she coughs

81. The elderly client is admitted to the emergency room. Which symptom is the client with a fractured hip most likely to exhibit?

Quick Answers: **118**
Detailed Answer: **130**

- ❍ **A.** Pain
- ❍ **B.** Disalignment
- ❍ **C.** Cool extremity
- ❍ **D.** Absence of pedal pulses

82. The nurse knows that the 60-year-old female client's susceptibility to osteoporosis is most likely related to:

Quick Answers: **118**
Detailed Answer: **130**

- ❍ **A.** Lack of exercise
- ❍ **B.** Hormonal disturbances
- ❍ **C.** Lack of calcium
- ❍ **D.** Genetic predisposition

83. A 2-year-old is admitted for repair of a fractured femur and is placed in Bryant's traction. Which finding by the nurse indicates that the traction is working properly?

Quick Answers: **118**
Detailed Answer: **131**

- ❍ **A.** The infant no longer complains of pain.
- ❍ **B.** The buttocks are 15° off the bed.
- ❍ **C.** The legs are suspended in the traction.
- ❍ **D.** The pins are secured within the pulley.

Quick Check

84. A client with a fractured hip has been placed in traction. Which statement is true regarding balanced skeletal traction? Balanced skeletal traction:

Quick Answers: **118**
Detailed Answer: **131**

- ❍ **A.** Utilizes a pin through bones
- ❍ **B.** Requires that both legs be secured
- ❍ **C.** Utilizes Kirschner wires
- ❍ **D.** Is used primarily to heal the fractured hips

85. The client is admitted for an open reduction internal fixation of a fractured hip. Immediately following surgery, the nurse should give priority to assessing the client for:

Quick Answers: **118**
Detailed Answer: **131**

- ❍ **A.** Hypovolemia
- ❍ **B.** Pain
- ❍ **C.** Nutritional status
- ❍ **D.** Immobilizer

86. Which statement made by the family member caring for the client with a percutaneous gastrotomy tube indicates understanding of the nurse's teaching?

Quick Answers: **118**
Detailed Answer: **131**

- ❍ **A.** "I must flush the tube with water after feedings and clamp the tube."
- ❍ **B.** "I must check placement four times per day."
- ❍ **C.** "I will report to the doctor any signs of indigestion."
- ❍ **D.** "If my father is unable to swallow, I will discontinue the feeding and call the clinic."

87. The nurse is assessing the client with a total knee replacement 2 hours post-operative. Which information requires notification of the doctor?

Quick Answers: **118**
Detailed Answer: **131**

- ❍ **A.** Bleeding on the dressing is 2cm in diameter.
- ❍ **B.** The client has a low-grade temperature.
- ❍ **C.** The client's hemoglobin is 6g/dL.
- ❍ **D.** The client voids after surgery.

Quick Check

88. The nurse is caring for the client with a 5-year-old diagnosed with plumbism. Which information in the health history is most likely related to the development of plumbism?

Quick Answers: **119**
Detailed Answer: **131**

- ❍ **A.** The client has traveled out of the country in the last 6 months.
- ❍ **B.** The client's parents are skilled stained-glass artists.
- ❍ **C.** The client lives in a house built in 1990.
- ❍ **D.** The client has several brothers and sisters.

89. A client with a total hip replacement requires special equipment. Which equipment would assist the client with a total hip replacement with prevention of dislocation of the prosthesis?

Quick Answers: **119**
Detailed Answer: **131**

- ❍ **A.** An abduction pillow
- ❍ **B.** A straight chair
- ❍ **C.** A pair of crutches
- ❍ **D.** A soft mattress

90. The client with a joint replacement is scheduled to receive Lovenox (enoxaparin). Which lab value should be reported to the doctor?

Quick Answers: **119**
Detailed Answer: **132**

- ❍ **A.** PT of 20 seconds
- ❍ **B.** PTT of 300 seconds
- ❍ **C.** Protime of 30 seconds
- ❍ **D.** INR 3

91. An elderly client with abdominal surgery is admitted to the unit following surgery. In anticipation of complications of anesthesia and narcotic administration, the nurse should:

Quick Answers: **119**
Detailed Answer: **132**

- ❍ **A.** Administer oxygen via nasal cannula
- ❍ **B.** Have Narcan (naloxane) available
- ❍ **C.** Prepare to administer blood products
- ❍ **D.** Prepare to do cardioresuscitation

92. Which roommate would be most suitable for the 6-year-old male with a fractured femur in Russell's traction?

Quick Answers: **119**
Detailed Answer: **132**

- ❍ **A.** 16-year-old female with scoliosis
- ❍ **B.** 12-year-old male with a fractured femur
- ❍ **C.** 10-year-old male with sarcoma
- ❍ **D.** 6-year-old male with osteomylitis

Quick Check

93. A client with rheumatoid arthritis has a prescription for hydroxychloroquine (Plaquenil). Which instruction should be included in the discharge teaching?

Quick Answers: **119**
Detailed Answer: **132**

- ❍ **A.** Take the medication with milk
- ❍ **B.** Report joint pain
- ❍ **C.** Allow 6 weeks for optimal effects
- ❍ **D.** Have eye exams every six months

94. A client with a fractured tibia has a plaster-of-Paris cast applied to immobilize the fracture. Which action by the nurse indicates understanding of a plaster-of-Paris cast? The nurse:

Quick Answers: **119**
Detailed Answer: **132**

- ❍ **A.** Handles the cast with the fingertips
- ❍ **B.** Bivalves the cast
- ❍ **C.** Dries the cast with a hair dryer
- ❍ **D.** Allows 24 hours before bearing weight

95. The teenager with a fiberglass cast asks the nurse if it will be okay to allow his friends to autograph his cast. Which response would be best?

Quick Answers: **119**
Detailed Answer: **132**

- ❍ **A.** "It will be alright for your friends to autograph the cast."
- ❍ **B.** "Because the cast is made of plaster, autographing can weaken the cast."
- ❍ **C.** "If they don't use chalk to autograph, it is okay."
- ❍ **D.** "Autographing or writing on the cast in any form will harm the cast."

96. The nurse is assigned to care for the client with a Steinmen pin. During pin care, she notes that the LPN uses sterile gloves and Q-tips to clean the pin. Which action should the nurse take at this time?

Quick Answers: **119**
Detailed Answer: **132**

- ❍ **A.** Assist the LPN with opening sterile packages and peroxide
- ❍ **B.** Tell the LPN that clean gloves are allowed
- ❍ **C.** Tell the LPN that the registered nurse should perform pin care
- ❍ **D.** Ask the LPN to clean the weights and pulleys with peroxide

Quick Check

97. A child with scoliosis has a spica cast applied. Which action specific to the spica cast should be taken?

Quick Answers: **119**
Detailed Answer: **132**

- ❍ **A.** Checking the bowel sounds
- ❍ **B.** Assessing the blood pressure
- ❍ **C.** Offering pain medication
- ❍ **D.** Checking for swelling

98. The client with a cervical fracture is placed in traction. Which type of traction will be utilized at the time of discharge?

Quick Answers: **119**
Detailed Answer: **132**

- ❍ **A.** Russell's traction
- ❍ **B.** Buck's traction
- ❍ **C.** Halo traction
- ❍ **D.** Crutchfield tong traction

99. A client with a total knee replacement has a CPM applied during the post-operative period. Which statement made by the nurse indicates understanding of the CPM machine?

Quick Answers: **119**
Detailed Answer: **132**

- ❍ **A.** "Use of the CPM will permit the client to ambulate during the therapy."
- ❍ **B.** "The CPM machine controls should be positioned distal to the site."
- ❍ **C.** "If the client complains of pain during the therapy, I will turn off the machine and call the doctor."
- ❍ **D.** "Use of the CPM machine will alleviate the need for physical therapy after the client is discharged."

100. A client with a fractured hip is being taught correct use of the walker. The nurse is aware that the correct use of the walker is achieved if the:

Quick Answers: **119**
Detailed Answer: **133**

- ❍ **A.** Palms rest lightly on the handles
- ❍ **B.** Elbows are flexed 0°
- ❍ **C.** Client walks to the front of the walker
- ❍ **D.** Client carries the walker

101. When assessing a laboring client, the nurse finds a prolapsed cord. The nurse should:

Quick Answers: **119**
Detailed Answer: **133**

- ❍ **A.** Attempt to replace the cord
- ❍ **B.** Place the client on her left side
- ❍ **C.** Elevate the client's hips
- ❍ **D.** Cover the cord with a dry, sterile gauze

Quick Check

102. The nurse is caring for a 30-year-old male admitted with a stab wound. While in the emergency room, a chest tube is inserted. Which of the following explains the primary rationale for insertion of chest tubes?

Quick Answers: **119**
Detailed Answer: **133**

❍ **A.** The tube will allow for equalization of the lung expansion.

❍ **B.** Chest tubes serve as a method of draining blood and serous fluid, and assist in reinflating the lungs.

❍ **C.** Chest tubes relieve pain associated with a collapsed lung.

❍ **D.** Chest tubes assist with cardiac function by stabilizing lung expansion.

103. A client who delivered this morning tells the nurse that she plans to breastfeed her baby. The nurse is aware that successful breastfeeding is most dependent on the:

Quick Answers: **119**
Detailed Answer: **133**

❍ A Mother's educational level

❍ **B.** Infant's birth weight

❍ **C.** Size of the mother's breast

❍ **D.** Mother's desire to breastfeed

104. The nurse is monitoring the progress of a client in labor. Which finding should be reported to the physician immediately?

Quick Answers: **119**
Detailed Answer: **133**

❍ **A.** The presence of scant bloody discharge

❍ **B.** Frequent urination

❍ **C.** The presence of green-tinged amniotic fluid

❍ **D.** Moderate uterine contractions

105. The nurse is measuring the duration of the client's contractions. Which statement is true regarding the measurement of the duration of contractions?

Quick Answers: **119**
Detailed Answer: **133**

❍ **A.** Duration is measured by timing from the beginning of one contraction to the beginning of the next contraction.

❍ **B.** Duration is measured by timing from the end of one contraction to the beginning of the next contraction.

❍ **C.** Duration is measured by timing from the beginning of one contraction to the end of the same contraction.

❍ **D.** Duration is measured by timing from the peak of one contraction to the end of the same contraction.

Quick Check

106. The physician has ordered an intravenous infusion of Pitocin for the induction of labor. When caring for the obstetric client receiving intravenous Pitocin, the nurse should monitor for:

Quick Answers: **119**
Detailed Answer: **133**

- ❍ **A.** Maternal hypoglycemia
- ❍ **B.** Fetal bradycardia
- ❍ **C.** Maternal hyperreflexia
- ❍ **D.** Fetal movement

107. A client with diabetes visits the prenatal clinic at 28 weeks gestation. Which statement is true regarding insulin needs during pregnancy?

Quick Answers: **119**
Detailed Answer: **133**

- ❍ **A.** Insulin requirements moderate as the pregnancy progresses.
- ❍ **B.** A decreased need for insulin occurs during the second trimester.
- ❍ **C.** Elevations in human chorionic gonadotrophin decrease the need for insulin.
- ❍ **D.** Fetal development depends on adequate insulin regulation.

108. A client in the prenatal clinic is assessed to have a blood pressure of 180/96. The nurse should give priority to:

Quick Answers: **119**
Detailed Answer: **134**

- ❍ **A.** Providing a calm environment
- ❍ **B.** Obtaining a diet history
- ❍ **C.** Administering an analgesic
- ❍ **D.** Assessing fetal heart tones

109. A primigravida, age 42, is 6 weeks pregnant. Based on the client's age, her infant is at risk for:

Quick Answers: **119**
Detailed Answer: **134**

- ❍ **A.** Down syndrome
- ❍ **B.** Respiratory distress syndrome
- ❍ **C.** Turner's syndrome
- ❍ **D.** Pathological jaundice

110. A client with a missed abortion at 29 weeks gestation is admitted to the hospital. The client will most likely be treated with:

Quick Answers: **119**
Detailed Answer: **134**

- ❍ **A.** Magnesium sulfate
- ❍ **B.** Calcium gluconate
- ❍ **C.** Dinoprostone (Prostin E.)
- ❍ **D.** Bromocrystine (Pardel)

Quick Check

111. A client with preeclampsia has been receiving an infusion containing magnesium sulfate. Blood pressure is 160/80, deep tendon reflexes are 1 plus, and urinary output for the past hour is 100mL. The nurse should:

Quick Answers: **119**
Detailed Answer: **134**

❍ **A.** Continue the infusion of magnesium sulfate while monitoring the client's blood pressure

❍ **B.** Stop the infusion of magnesium sulfate and contact the physician

❍ **C.** Slow the infusion rate and turn the client on her left side

❍ **D.** Administer calcium gluconate and continue to monitor the blood pressure

112. Which statement describes the inheritance pattern of autosomal recessive disorders?

Quick Answers: **119**
Detailed Answer: **134**

❍ **A.** An affected newborn has unaffected parents.

❍ **B.** An affected newborn has one affected parent.

❍ **C.** Affected parents have a one in four chance of passing on the defective gene.

❍ **D.** Affected parents have unaffected children who are carriers.

113. A pregnant client, age 32, asks the nurse why her doctor has recommended a serum alpha fetoprotein. The nurse should explain that the doctor has recommended the test:

Quick Answers: **119**
Detailed Answer: **134**

❍ **A.** Because it is a state law

❍ **B.** To detect cardiovascular defects

❍ **C.** Because of her age

❍ **D.** To detect neurological defects

114. A client with hypothyroidism asks the nurse if she will still need to take thyroid medication during the pregnancy. The nurse's response is based on the knowledge that:

Quick Answers: **119**
Detailed Answer: **134**

❍ **A.** There is no need to take thyroid medication because the fetus's thyroid produces thyroid-stimulating hormones.

❍ **B.** Regulation of thyroid medication is more difficult because the thyroid gland increases in size during pregnancy.

❍ **C.** It is more difficult to maintain thyroid regulation during pregnancy due to a slowing of metabolism.

❍ **D.** Fetal growth is arrested if thyroid medication is continued during pregnancy.

Quick Check

115. The nurse is responsible for performing a neonatal assessment on a full-term infant. At 1 minute, the nurse could expect to find:

Quick Answers: **119**
Detailed Answer: **134**

- ❍ **A.** An apical pulse of 100
- ❍ **B.** Absence of tonus
- ❍ **C.** Cyanosis of the feet and hands
- ❍ **D.** Jaundice of the skin and sclera

116. A client with sickle cell anemia is admitted to the labor and delivery unit during the first phase of labor. The nurse should anticipate the client's need for:

Quick Answers: **119**
Detailed Answer: **135**

- ❍ **A.** Supplemental oxygen
- ❍ **B.** Fluid restriction
- ❍ **C.** Blood transfusion
- ❍ **D.** Delivery by Caesarean section

117. A client with diabetes has an order for ultrasonography. Preparation for an ultrasound includes:

Quick Answers: **119**
Detailed Answer: **135**

- ❍ **A.** Increasing fluid intake
- ❍ **B.** Limiting ambulation
- ❍ **C.** Administering an enema
- ❍ **D.** Withholding food for 8 hours

118. An infant who weighs 8 pounds at birth would be expected to weigh how many pounds at 1 year?

Quick Answers: **119**
Detailed Answer: **135**

- ❍ **A.** 14 pounds
- ❍ **B.** 16 pounds
- ❍ **C.** 18 pounds
- ❍ **D.** 24 pounds

119. A pregnant client with a history of alcohol addiction is scheduled for a nonstress test. The nonstress test:

Quick Answers: **119**
Detailed Answer: **135**

- ❍ **A.** Determines the lung maturity of the fetus
- ❍ **B.** Measures the activity of the fetus
- ❍ **C.** Shows the effect of contractions on the fetal heart rate
- ❍ **D.** Measures the neurological well-being of the fetus

Quick Check

120. A full-term male has hypospadias. Which statement describes hypospadias?

Quick Answers: **119**
Detailed Answer: **135**

- ❍ **A.** The urethral opening is absent.
- ❍ **B.** The urethra opens on the dorsal side of the penis.
- ❍ **C.** The penis is shorter than usual.
- ❍ **D.** The urethra opens on the ventral side of the penis.

121. A gravida III para II is admitted to the labor unit. Vaginal exam reveals that the client's cervix is 8cm dilated withcomplete effacement. The priority nursing diagnosis at this time is:

Quick Answers: **119**
Detailed Answer: **135**

- ❍ **A.** Alteration in coping related to pain
- ❍ **B.** Potential for injury related to precipitate delivery
- ❍ **C.** Alteration in elimination related to anesthesia
- ❍ **D.** Potential for fluid volume deficit related to NPO status

122. The client with varicella will most likely have an order for which category of medication?

Quick Answers: **119**
Detailed Answer: **135**

- ❍ **A.** Antibiotics
- ❍ **B.** Antipyretics
- ❍ **C.** Antivirals
- ❍ **D.** Anticoagulants

123. A client is admitted with complaints of chest pain. Which of the following drug orders should the nurse question?

Quick Answers: **119**
Detailed Answer: **135**

- ❍ **A.** Nitroglycerin
- ❍ **B.** Ampicillin
- ❍ **C.** Propranolol
- ❍ **D.** Verapamil

124. Which of the following instructions should be included in the teaching for the client with rheumatoid arthritis?

Quick Answers: **119**
Detailed Answer: **135**

- ❍ **A.** Avoid exercise because it fatigues the joints.
- ❍ **B.** Take prescribed anti-inflammatory medications with meals.
- ❍ **C.** Alternate hot and cold packs to affected joints.
- ❍ **D.** Avoid weight-bearing activity.

Quick Check

135. The nurse is providing postpartum teaching for a mother planning to breastfeed her infant. Which of the client's statements indicates the need for additional teaching?

Quick Answers: **119**
Detailed Answer: **137**

- ❍ **A.** "I'm wearing a support bra."
- ❍ **B.** "I'm expressing milk from my breast."
- ❍ **C.** "I'm drinking four glasses of fluid during a 24-hour period."
- ❍ **D.** "While I'm in the shower, I'll allow the water to run over my breasts."

136. Damage to the VII cranial nerve results in:

Quick Answers: **119**
Detailed Answer: **137**

- ❍ **A.** Facial pain
- ❍ **B.** Absence of ability to smell
- ❍ **C.** Absence of eye movement
- ❍ **D.** Tinnitus

137. A client is receiving Pyridium (phenazopyridine hydrochloride) for a urinary tract infection. The client should be taught that the medication can:

Quick Answers: **119**
Detailed Answer: **137**

- ❍ **A.** Cause diarrhea
- ❍ **B.** Change the color of her urine
- ❍ **C.** Cause mental confusion
- ❍ **D.** Cause changes in taste

138. Which of the following test should be performed before beginning a prescription of Accutane?

Quick Answers: **119**
Detailed Answer: **137**

- ❍ **A.** Check the calcium level
- ❍ **B.** Perform a pregnancy test
- ❍ **C.** Monitor apical pulse
- ❍ **D.** Obtain a creatinine level

139. A client with AIDS is taking Zovirax (acyclovir). Which nursing intervention is most critical during the administration of acyclovir?

Quick Answers: **119**
Detailed Answer: **137**

- ❍ **A.** Limiting the client's activity
- ❍ **B.** Encouraging a high-carbohydrate diet
- ❍ **C.** Utilizing an incentive spirometer to improve respiratory function
- ❍ **D.** Encouraging fluids

Quick Check

140. A client is admitted for an MRI (magnetic resonance imaging). The nurse should question the client regarding:

Quick Answers: **119**
Detailed Answer: **137**

- ❍ **A.** Hearing loss
- ❍ **B.** A titanium hip replacement
- ❍ **C.** Allergies to antibiotics
- ❍ **D.** Inability to move his feet

141. The nurse is caring for the client receiving Amphotericin B. Which of the following indicates that the client has experienced toxicity to this drug?

Quick Answers: **119**
Detailed Answer: **137**

- ❍ **A.** Changes in vision
- ❍ **B.** Nausea
- ❍ **C.** Urinary frequency
- ❍ **D.** Changes in skin color

142. The nurse should visit which of the following clients first?

Quick Answers: **119**
Detailed Answer: **137**

- ❍ **A.** The client with diabetes who has a blood glucose of 95mg/dL
- ❍ **B.** The client with hypertension being maintained on Lisinopril
- ❍ **C.** The client with chest pain and a history of angina
- ❍ **D.** The client with Raynaud's disease

143. A client with cystic fibrosis is taking pancreatic enzymes. The nurse should administer this medication:

Quick Answers: **119**
Detailed Answer: **137**

- ❍ **A.** Once per day in the morning
- ❍ **B.** Three times per day with meals
- ❍ **C.** Once per day at bedtime
- ❍ **D.** Four times per day

144. Cataracts result in opacity of the crystalline lens. Which of the following best explains the functions of the lens?

Quick Answers: **119**
Detailed Answer: **138**

- ❍ **A.** The lens controls stimulation of the retina.
- ❍ **B.** The lens orchestrates eye movement.
- ❍ **C.** The lens focuses light rays on the retina.
- ❍ **D.** The lens magnifies small objects.

Quick Check

145. A client who has glaucoma is to have miotic eyedrops instilled in both eyes. The nurse knows that the purpose of the medication is to:

Quick Answers: **119**
Detailed Answer: **138**

❍ **A.** Anesthetize the cornea

❍ **B.** Dilate the pupils

❍ **C.** Constrict the pupils

❍ **D.** Paralyze the muscles of accommodation

146. A client with a severe corneal ulcer has an order for Gentamycin gtt. q 4 hours and Neomycin 1 gtt q 4 hours. Which of the following schedules should be used when administering the drops?

Quick Answers: **119**
Detailed Answer: **138**

❍ **A.** Allow 5 minutes between the two medications.

❍ **B.** The medications may be used together.

❍ **C.** The medications should be separated by a cycloplegic drug.

❍ **D.** The medications should not be used in the same client.

147. The client with colorblindness will most likely have problems distinguishing which of the following colors?

Quick Answers: **119**
Detailed Answer: **138**

❍ **A.** Orange

❍ **B.** Violet

❍ **C.** Red

❍ **D.** White

148. The client with a pacemaker should be taught to:

Quick Answers: **119**
Detailed Answer: **138**

❍ **A.** Report ankle edema

❍ **B.** Check his blood pressure daily

❍ **C.** Refrain from using a microwave oven

❍ **D.** Monitor his pulse rate

149. The client with enuresis is being taught regarding bladder retraining. The nurse should advise the client to refrain from drinking after:

Quick Answers: **119**
Detailed Answer: **138**

❍ **A.** 1900

❍ **B.** 1200

❍ **C.** 1000

❍ **D.** 0700

Quick Check

150. Which of the following diet instructions should be given to the client with recurring urinary tract infections?

Quick Answers: **119**
Detailed Answer: **138**

- ❍ **A.** Increase intake of meats
- ❍ **B.** Avoid citrus fruits
- ❍ **C.** Perform pericare with hydrogen peroxide
- ❍ **D.** Drink a glass of cranberry juice every day

151. The physician has prescribed NPH insulin for a client with diabetes mellitus. Which statement indicates that the client knows when the peak action of the insulin occurs?

Quick Answers: **119**
Detailed Answer: **138**

- ❍ **A.** "I will make sure I eat breakfast within 2 hours of taking my insulin."
- ❍ **B.** "I will need to carry candy or some form of sugar with me all the time."
- ❍ **C.** "I will eat a snack around three o'clock each afternoon."
- ❍ **D.** "I can save my dessert from supper for a bedtime snack."

152. A client with rheumatoid arthritis is receiving Methotrexate. After reviewing the client's chart, the physician orders Wellcovorin (leucovorin calcium). The rationale for administering leucovorin calcium to a client receiving Methotrexate is to:

Quick Answers: **119**
Detailed Answer: **138**

- ❍ **A.** Treat iron-deficiency anemia caused by chemotherapeutic agents
- ❍ **B.** Create a synergistic effect that shortens treatment time
- ❍ **C.** Increase the number of circulating neutrophils
- ❍ **D.** Reverse drug toxicity and prevent tissue damage

153. A client tells the nurse that she is allergic to eggs, dogs, rabbits, and chicken feathers. Which order should the nurse question?

Quick Answers: **119**
Detailed Answer: **138**

- ❍ **A.** TB skin test
- ❍ **B.** Rubella vaccine
- ❍ **C.** ELISA test
- ❍ **D.** Chest x-ray

Quick Check

154. The physician has prescribed rantidine (Zantac) for a client with erosive gastritis. The nurse should administer the medication:

Quick Answers: **119**
Detailed Answer: **139**

- ❍ **A.** 30 minutes before meals
- ❍ **B.** With each meal
- ❍ **C.** In a single dose at bedtime
- ❍ **D.** 60 minutes after meals

155. A client is admitted to the hospital following a gunshot wound to the abdomen. A temporary colostomy is performed, and the physician writes an order to irrigate the proximal end of the colostomy. The nurse is aware that the proximal end of a double-barrel colostomy is the end that:

Quick Answers: **119**
Detailed Answer: **139**

- ❍ **A.** Is the opening on the client's left side
- ❍ **B.** Is the opening on the distal end on the client's left side
- ❍ **C.** Is the opening on the client's right side
- ❍ **D.** Is the opening on the distal right side

156. When the nurse checks the fundus of a client on the first postpartum day, she notes that the fundus is firm, at the level of the umbilicus, and is displaced to the right. The next action the nurse should take is to:

Quick Answers: **119**
Detailed Answer: **139**

- ❍ **A.** Check the client for bladder distention
- ❍ **B.** Assess the blood pressure for hypotension
- ❍ **C.** Determine whether an oxytoxic drug was given
- ❍ **D.** Check for the expulsion of small clots

157. The physician has ordered a CAT (computerized axial tomography) scan for a client with a possible cerebral aneurysm. Which information is most important to the nurse who is preparing the client for the CAT scan? The client:

Quick Answers: **119**
Detailed Answer: **139**

- ❍ **A.** Is having her menstrual period
- ❍ **B.** Has a history of claustrophobia
- ❍ **C.** Is allergic to oysters
- ❍ **D.** Has sensory deafness

158. A 6-month-old client is placed on strict bed rest following a hernia repair. Which toy is best suited to the client?

Quick Answers: **119**
Detailed Answer: **139**

- ❍ **A.** Colorful crib mobile
- ❍ **B.** Hand-held electronic games
- ❍ **C.** Cars in a plastic container
- ❍ **D.** 30-piece jigsaw puzzle

Quick Check

159. The nurse is preparing to discharge a client with a long history of polio. The nurse should tell the client that:

Quick Answers: **119**
Detailed Answer: **139**

- ❍ **A.** Taking a hot bath will decrease stiffness and spasticity.
- ❍ **B.** A schedule of strenuous exercise will improve muscle strength.
- ❍ **C.** Rest periods should be scheduled throughout the day.
- ❍ **D.** Visual disturbances may be corrected with prescription glasses.

160. A client on the postpartum unit has a proctoepisiotomy. The nurse should anticipate administering which medication?

Quick Answers: **119**
Detailed Answer: **139**

- ❍ **A.** Dulcolax suppository
- ❍ **B.** Docusate sodium (Colace)
- ❍ **C.** Methyergonovine maleate (Methergine)
- ❍ **D.** Methylphenidate (Ritalin)

161. A client with pancreatic cancer has an infusion of TPN (Total Parenteral Nutrition). The doctor has ordered a sliding scale insulin. The most likely explanation for this order is:

Quick Answers: **119**
Detailed Answer: **139**

- ❍ **A.** Total Parenteral Nutrition leads to negative nitrogen balance and elevated glucose levels.
- ❍ **B.** Total Parenteral Nutrition cannot be managed with oral hypoglycemics.
- ❍ **C.** Total Parenteral Nutrition is a high-glucose solution that often elevates the blood glucose levels.
- ❍ **D.** Total Parenteral Nutrition leads to further pancreatic disease.

162. An adolescent primigravida who is 10 weeks pregnant attends the antepartal clinic for her first check-up. To develop a teaching plan, the nurse should initially assess:

Quick Answers: **119**
Detailed Answer: **139**

- ❍ **A.** The client's knowledge of the signs of preterm labor
- ❍ **B.** The client's feelings about the pregnancy
- ❍ **C.** Whether the client was using a method of birth control
- ❍ **D.** The client's thought about future children

Quick Check

173. The nurse is caring for a client admitted with multiple trauma. Fractures include the pelvis, femur, and ulna. Which finding should be reported to the physician immediately?

Quick Answers: **119**
Detailed Answer: **141**

- ❍ **A.** Hematuria
- ❍ **B.** Muscle spasms
- ❍ **C.** Dizziness
- ❍ **D.** Nausea

174. A client is brought to the emergency room by the police. He is combative and yells, "I have to get out of here; they are trying to kill me." Which assessment is most likely correct in relation to this statement?

Quick Answers: **119**
Detailed Answer: **141**

- ❍ **A.** The client is experiencing an auditory hallucination.
- ❍ **B.** The client is having a delusion of grandeur.
- ❍ **C.** The client is experiencing paranoid delusions.
- ❍ **D.** The client is intoxicated.

175. The nurse is performing tracheostomy care. If the client coughs out the inner cannula, the nurse should:

Quick Answers: **119**
Detailed Answer: **141**

- ❍ **A.** Call the doctor
- ❍ **B.** Replace the inner cannula with a new one
- ❍ **C.** Hold open the stoma with forceps
- ❍ **D.** Begin rescue breathing

176. An infant's Apgar score is 9 at 5 minutes. The nurse is aware that the most likely cause for the deduction of one point is:

Quick Answers: **119**
Detailed Answer: **141**

- ❍ **A.** The baby is cold.
- ❍ **B.** The baby is experiencing bradycardia.
- ❍ **C.** The baby's hands and feet are blue.
- ❍ **D.** The baby is lethargic.

177. The primary reason for rapid continuous rewarming of the area affected by frostbite is to:

Quick Answers: **119**
Detailed Answer: **141**

- ❍ **A.** Lessen the amount of cellular damage
- ❍ **B.** Prevent the formation of blisters
- ❍ **C.** Promote movement
- ❍ **D.** Prevent pain and discomfort

Quick Check

178. A client recently started on hemodialysis wants to know how the dialysis will take the place of his kidneys. The nurse's response is based on the knowledge that hemodialysis works by:

Quick Answers: **119**
Detailed Answer: **141**

❍ **A.** Passing water through the dialyzing membrane

❍ **B.** Eliminating plasma proteins from the blood

❍ **C.** Lowering the pH by removing nonvolatile acids

❍ **D.** Filtering waste through a dialyzing membrane

179. During a home visit, a client with AIDS tells the nurse that he has been exposed to measles. Which action by the nurse is most appropriate?

Quick Answers: **119**
Detailed Answer: **141**

❍ **A.** Administering an antibiotic

❍ **B.** Contacting the physician for an order for immune globulin

❍ **C.** Administering an antiviral

❍ **D.** Telling the client that he should remain in isolation for 2 weeks

180. A client hospitalized with MRSA (methicillin-resistant staph aureus) is placed on contact precautions. Which statement is true regarding precautions for infections spread by contact?

Quick Answers: **119**
Detailed Answer: **141**

❍ **A.** The client should be placed in a room with negative pressure.

❍ **B.** Infection requires close contact; therefore, the door may remain open.

❍ **C.** Transmission is highly likely, so the client should wear a mask at all times.

❍ **D.** Infection requires skin-to-skin contact and is prevented by handwashing, gloves, and a gown.

181. A client with an above-the-knee amputation is being taught methods to prevent hip-flexion deformities. Which instruction should be given to the client?

Quick Answers: **119**
Detailed Answer: **142**

❍ **A.** "Lie supine with the head elevated on two pillows."

❍ **B.** "Lie prone every 4 hours during the day for 30 minutes."

❍ **C.** "Lie on your side with your head elevated."

❍ **D.** "Lie flat during the day."

Quick Check

191. The nurse is educating the lady's club in self-breast exam. The nurse is aware that most malignant breast masses occur in the Tail of Spence. On the diagram, place an X on the Tail of Spence.

Quick Answers: **120**
Detailed Answer: **143**

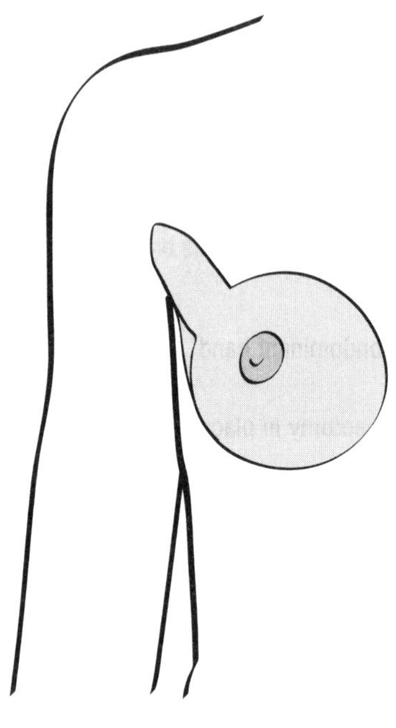

192. The toddler is admitted with a cardiac anomaly. The nurse is aware that the infant with a ventricular septal defect will:

Quick Answers: **120**
Detailed Answer: **143**

❍ **A.** Tire easily
❍ **B.** Grow normally
❍ **C.** Need more calories
❍ **D.** Be more susceptible to viral infections

193. A pregnant client with a history of alcohol addiction is scheduled for a nonstress test. The nonstress test:

Quick Answers: **120**
Detailed Answer: **143**

❍ **A.** Determines the lung maturity of the fetus
❍ **B.** Measures the activity of the fetus
❍ **C.** Shows the effect of contractions on fetal heart rate
❍ **D.** Measures the neurological well-being of the fetus

Quick Check

Quick Answers: **120**
Detailed Answer: **143**

194. The nurse is evaluating the client who is dilated 8cm. The following graph is noted on the monitor. Which action should be taken first by the nurse?

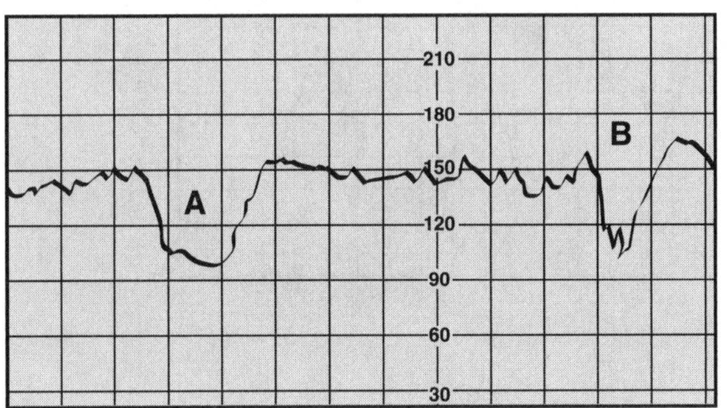

Fetal Heart Rate

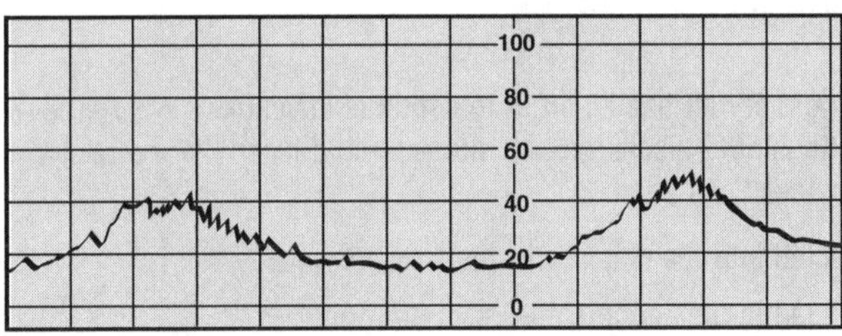

Uterine Contractions

❍ **A.** Instructing the client to push
❍ **B.** Performing a vaginal exam
❍ **C.** Turning off the Pitocin infusion
❍ **D.** Placing the client in a semi-Fowler's position

Quick Check

195. The nurse notes the following on the ECG monitor. The nurse would evaluate the cardiac arrhythmia as:

Quick Answers: **120**
Detailed Answer: **143**

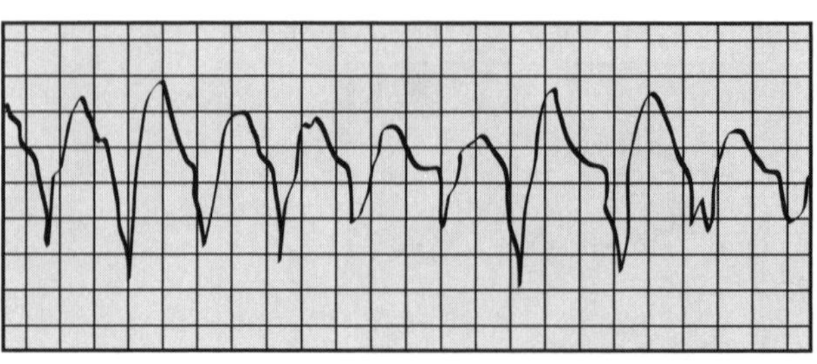

❍ **A.** Atrial flutter
❍ **B.** A sinus rhythm
❍ **C.** Ventricular tachycardia
❍ **D.** Atrial fibrillation

196. A client with clotting disorder has an order to continue Lovenox (enoxaparin) injections after discharge. The nurse should teach the client that Lovenox injections should:

Quick Answers: **120**
Detailed Answer: **144**

❍ **A.** Be injected into the deltoid muscle
❍ **B.** Be injected in the abdomen
❍ **C.** Aspirate after the injection
❍ **D.** Clear the air from the syringe before injections

197. The nurse has a pre-op order to administer Valium (diazepam) 10mg and Phenergan (promethazine) 25mg. The correct method of administering these medications is to:

Quick Answers: **120**
Detailed Answer: **144**

❍ **A.** Administer the medications together in one syringe
❍ **B.** Administer the medications separately
❍ **C.** Administer the Valium, wait 5 minutes, and administer the Phenergan
❍ **D.** Question the order because they cannot be given to the same client

Quick Check

198. A client with frequent urinary tract infections asks the nurse how she can prevent the reoccurrence. The nurse should teach the client to:

Quick Answers: **120**
Detailed Answer: **144**

- ❍ **A.** Douche after intercourse
- ❍ **B.** Void every 3 hours
- ❍ **C.** Obtain a urinalysis monthly
- ❍ **D.** Wipe from back to front after voiding

199. Which task should be assigned to the nursing assistant?

Quick Answers: **120**
Detailed Answer: **144**

- ❍ **A.** Placing the client in seclusion
- ❍ **B.** Emptying the Foley catheter of the preeclamptic client
- ❍ **C.** Feeding the client with dementia
- ❍ **D.** Ambulating the client with a fractured hip

200. The client has recently returned from having a thyroidectomy. The nurse should keep which of the following at the bedside?

Quick Answers: **120**
Detailed Answer: **144**

- ❍ **A.** A tracheotomy set
- ❍ **B.** A padded tongue blade
- ❍ **C.** An endotracheal tube
- ❍ **D.** An airway

Quick Check Answer Key

1. B
2. B
3. B
4. C
5. D
6. A
7. B
8. C
9. C
10. B
11. D
12. A
13. C
14. B
15. A
16. D
17. B
18. C
19. A
20. C
21. C
22. D
23. B
24. D
25. D
26. B
27. D
28. D
29. A
30. B
31. A
32. A
33. D
34. D
35. B
36. B
37. B
38. B
39. D
40. B
41. A
42. C
43. C
44. B
45. C
46. A
47. B
48. C
49. D
50. C
51. B
52. D
53. B
54. D
55. B
56. B
57. D
58. D
59. C
60. D
61. C
62. B
63. C
64. C
65. D
66. C
67. B
68. B
69. C
70. B
71. B
72. A
73. D
74. A
75. A
76. B
77. A
78. B
79. C
80. B
81. B
82. B
83. B
84. A
85. A
86. A
87. C

88. B
89. A
90. B
91. B
92. B
93. D
94. A
95. A
96. A
97. A
98. C
99. B
100. A
101. C
102. B
103. D
104. C
105. C
106. B
107. D
108. A
109. A
110. C
111. A
112. C
113. D
114. B
115. C
116. A
117. A
118. D
119. B
120. B
121. A
122. C
123. B
124. D
125. B
126. B
127. B
128. A
129. D
130. A
131. B
132. B
133. B
134. B
135. C
136. A
137. B
138. B
139. D
140. A
141. D
142. C
143. B
144. C
145. C
146. A
147. B
148. D
149. A
150. D
151. C
152. D
153. B
154. B
155. C
156. A
157. C
158. C
159. C
160. B
161. C
162. B
163. A
164. A
165. B
166. B
167. A
168. C
169. A
170. C
171. C
172. C
173. A
174. C
175. B
176. C
177. A
178. D
179. B
180. D
181. B
182. A
183. C

184. A

185. A

186. B

187. B

188. A

189. D

190. A

191. See diagram in "Answers and Rationales"

192. A

193. B

194. C

195. C

196. B

197. B

198. B

199. C

200. A

Answers and Rationales

1. **Answer B is correct.** Any lesion should be reported to the doctor. This can indicate a herpes lesion. Clients with open lesions related to herpes are delivered by Cesarean section because there is a possibility of transmission of the infection to the fetus with direct contact to lesions. It is not enough to document the finding, so answer A is incorrect. The physician must make the decision to perform a C-section, making answer C incorrect. It is not enough to continue primary care, so answer D is incorrect.

2. **Answer B is correct.** The client with HPV is at higher risk for cervical and vaginal cancer related to this STI. She is not at higher risk for the other cancers mentioned in answers A, C, and D, so those are incorrect.

3. **Answer B is correct.** A lesion that is painful is most likely a herpetic lesion. A chancre lesion associated with syphilis is not painful, so answer A is incorrect. In answer C, candidiasis is a yeast infection and does not present with a lesion, but it is exhibited by a white, cheesy discharge. Condylomata lesions are painless warts, so answer D is incorrect.

4. **Answer C is correct.** FTA is the only answer choice for treponema pallidum. Answers A and B are incorrect because VDRL and RPR are screening tests for syphilis but are not conclusive of the disease; they only indicate exposure to the disease. The Thayer-Martin culture is a test for gonorrhea, so answer D is incorrect.

5. **Answer D is correct.** The criteria for HELLP is hemolysis, elevated liver enzymes, and low platelet count. In answer A, an elevated blood glucose level is not associated with HELLP. Platelets are decreased in HELLP syndrome, not elevated, as stated in answer B. The creatinine levels are elevated in renal disease and are not associated with HELLP syndrome, as stated in answer C.

6. **Answer A is correct.** The answer can only be A because the other methods elicit different reflexes. Answer B elicits the triceps reflex, answer C elicits the patella reflex, and answer D elicits the radial nerve.

7. **Answer B is correct.** Brethine is used cautiously because it raises the blood glucose levels. Answers A, C, and D are all medications that are commonly used in the diabetic client, so there is no need to question the order for these medications.

8. **Answer C is correct.** When the L/S ratio reaches 2:1, the lungs are considered to be mature. The infant will most likely be small for gestational age and will not be at risk for birth trauma, so answer B is incorrect. The L/S ratio does not indicate congenital anomalies, as stated in answer A, and the infant is not at risk for intrauterine growth retardation, as stated in answer D.

9. **Answer C is correct.** Jitteriness is a sign of seizure in the neonate. Answers A, B, and D are incorrect because crying, wakefulness, and yawning are expected in the newborn.

10. **Answer B is correct.** The client is expected to become sleepy, have hot flashes, and experience lethargy. A decreasing urinary output, absence of the knee jerk reflex, and decreased respirations are signs of toxicity and are not expected side effects of magnesium sulfate. Therefore, answers A, C, and D are incorrect.

11. **Answer D is correct.** If the client experiences hypotension after an injection of epidural anesthetic, the nurse should turn him to the left side if possible, apply oxygen by mask, and speed the IV infusion. Epinephrine, not Benedryl, in answer B, should be kept for emergency administration. A is incorrect because placing the client in Trendelenburg position (head down) will allow the anesthesia to move up above the respiratory center, thereby decreasing the diaphragm's ability to move up and down, ventilating the client. Answer C is incorrect because the oxygen should be applied by mask, not cannula.

12. **Answer A is correct.** Cancer of the pancreas frequently leads to severe nausea and vomiting. Answers B, C, and D are incorrect because although they are a concern to the client, they are not the priority nursing diagnosis.

13. **Answer C is correct.** Measuring the girth daily with a paper tape measure and marking the area that is measured is the most objective method of estimating ascites. Inspection, in answer A, and checking for fluid waves, in answer D, are more subjective and not correct. Palpation of the liver will not tell the amount of ascites, so answer B is incorrect.

14. **Answer B is correct.** The vital signs indicate hypovolemic shock, so checking for fluid volume deficit is the appropriate action. Answers A, C, and D do not indicate cerebral tissue perfusion, airway clearance, or sensory perception alterations, and are incorrect.

15. **Answer A is correct.** The client with hemophilia is likely to experience bleeding episodes if he participates in contact sports. Drinking several carbonated drinks per day, as in answer B, has no bearing on the hemophiliac's condition. Having two sisters with sickle cell, as in answer C, is not information that would cause concern. Taking acetaminophen for pain, as in answer D, is an accepted practice and does not cause concern.

16. **Answer D is correct.** The client with neutropenia should not have visitors with any type of infection, so the best action by the nurse is to give the visitor a mask and a gown. Asking the visitor to wash his hands is good but will not help prevent the infection from spreading by droplets; therefore, answer A is incorrect. Answer B is incorrect because documenting the visitor's condition is not enough action for the nurse to take. Answer C is incorrect because asking the visitor to leave and not return until the client's white blood cell count is 1,000 is an insuffient intervention. The normal WBC is 5,000–10,000, so a WBC of 1,000 is not high enough to prevent the client from contracting infections.

17. **Answer B is correct.** For some clients with trauma to the neck, the answer would be A; however, in this situation, it is incorrect because lowering the head of the bed could further interfere with the airway. Increasing the infusion and placing the client in supine position is better. If atropine is administered to the client, it should be given IV, not IM, and there is no need for this action at present, as stated in answer C. Answer D is not necessary at this time.

18. **Answer C is correct.** When a chest tube is removed, the hole should be immediately covered with a Vaseline gauze to prevent air from rushing into the chest and causing the lung to collapse. The doctor, not the nurse, will order a chest x-ray; therefore, answer A is incorrect. Taking the BP in answer B is good but is not the priority action.

Answer D is incorrect because the Valsalva maneuver is done during removal of the tube, not afterward.

19. **Answer A is correct.** The normal international normalizing ratio (INR) is 2–3. A 9 might indicate spontaneous bleeding. Answer B is an incorrect action at this time. Answer C is incorrect because just instructing the client regarding his medication is not enough. Answer D is incorrect because increasing the frequency of neurological assessment will not prevent bleeding caused by the prolonged INR.

20. **Answer C is correct.** The food with the most calcium is the yogurt. The others are good choices, but not as good as the yogurt, which has approximately 400mg of calcium. Therefore, answers A, B, and D are incorrect.

21. **Answer C is correct.** The client receiving magnesium sulfate should have a Foley catheter in place, and the hourly intake and output should be checked because a sign of toxicity to magnesium sulfate is oliguria. There is no need to refrain from checking the blood pressure in the left arm, as stated in answer A. A padded tongue blade should be kept in the room at the bedside, just in case of a seizure, but this is not related to the magnesium sulfate infusion, so this makes answer B incorrect. Answer D is incorrect because just darkening the room will not prevent toxicity, although it might help with the headache associated with preeclampsia.

22. **Answer D is correct.** If the client's mother refuses to sign for the child's treatment, the doctor should be notified. Because the client is a minor, the court might order treatment. Answer A is incorrect because simply documenting the statement is not enough. Answer B is incorrect because it is not the nurse's responsibility to try to persuade the mother to allow the blood transfusion. Answer C is incorrect because the consequences of the denial of a blood transfusion are not known.

23. **Answer B is correct.** The nurse should be most concerned with laryngeal edema because of the area of burn. The next priority should be answer A, hypovolemia. Hypernatremia and hyperkalemia, as stated in answers C and D, are incorrect because the client will most likely experience hyponatremia and hypokalemia.

24. **Answer D is correct.** The client with anorexia shows the most improvement by weight gain. Selecting a balanced diet, as in answer A, is of little use if the client does not eat the diet. The hematocrit in answer B is incorrect because although it might improve by several means, such as blood transfusion, it does not indicate improvement in the anorexic condition. The tissue turgor indicates fluid stasis, not improvement of anorexia; therefore, answer C is incorrect.

25. **Answer D is correct.** Paresthesia, in answer D, is not normal and might indicate compartment syndrome. At this time, pain beneath the cast is normal, so answer A is incorrect. The client's toes should be warm to the touch and pulses should be present. Because answers B and C are normal findings, these answers are incorrect.

26. **Answer B is correct.** It is normal for the client to have a warm sensation when dye is injected. Answer A is incorrect because the client should not have a cold extremity. This indicates peripheral vascular disease. Answer C is incorrect because extreme chest pain can be related to a myocardial infarction. The pain is not normal. Answer D is incorrect because itching is a sign of an allergic reaction. Also, the itching will most likely be on the chest and skin folds.

27. **Answer D is correct.** It is not necessary to wear gloves to take the vital signs of the client under normal circumstances. If the client has active infection with methicillin-resistant staphylococcus aureus, gloves should be worn. The other answer choices indicate knowledge of infection control by the actions, so answers A, B, and C are incorrect.

28. **Answer D is correct.** During ECT, the client will have a grand mal seizure. This indicates completion of the electroconvulsive therapy. Answer A is incorrect because clients are frequently given medication that will cause drowsiness or sleep. Answer B is incorrect because vomiting is not a sign that the ECT has been effective. Answer C is incorrect because tachycardia might be present, but it is not a sign that the ECT has been effective.

29. **Answer A is correct.** Infection with pinworms begins when the eggs are ingested or inhaled. The eggs hatch in the upper intestine and mature in 2–8 weeks. The females then mate and migrate out the anus, where they lay up to 17,000 eggs. This causes intense itching. The mother should be told to use a flashlight to examine the rectal area about 2–3 hours after the child is asleep. Placing clear tape on a tongue blade will allow the eggs to adhere to the tape. The specimen should then be brought in to be evaluated. There is no need to scrape the skin, as stated in answer B. Collecting a stool specimen in the afternoon will probably not reveal the eggs because the worms often are not detected during the day; therefore, answer C is incorrect. Answer D is incorrect because eggs are not located in the hair.

30. **Answer B is correct.** Erterobiasis, or pinworms, is treated with Vermox (mebendazole) or Antiminth (pyrantel pamoate). The entire family should be treated to ensure that no eggs remain. The family should then be tested again in 2 weeks to ensure that no eggs remain. Answer A is incorrect because children less than 10 can be treated with Vermox. Answer C is incorrect because a single treatment is usually sufficient. Answer D is incorrect because there is no need for IV antibiotics for the client with pinworms.

31. **Answer A is correct.** The pregnant nurse should not be assigned to any client with radioactivity present. The client receiving linear accelerator therapy in answer A travels to the radium department for therapy; thus, the radiation stays in the department. The client himself is not radioactive. The client in answer B poses a risk to the pregnant client because the implant stays with the patient. The client in answer C is radioactive in very small doses. For approximately 72 hours, the client should dispose of urine and feces in special containers and use plastic spoons and forks. The client in answer D is also radioactive in small amounts, especially upon return from the procedure. Thus, answers B, C, and D are all incorrect.

32. **Answer A is correct.** The client with Cushing's syndrome has adrenocortical hypersecretion. This increase in the level of cortisone causes the client to be immune suppressed, and he should not have a roommate because of the possibility of infection. In answer B, the client with diabetes poses no risk to other clients. The client in answer C has an increase in growth hormone and poses no risk to himself or others. The client in answer D has hyperthyroidism or myxedema and so poses no risk to others or himself.

33. **Answer D is correct.** Malpractice is failing to perform or performing an act that causes harm to the client, making answer D correct. In answer A, negligence is failing to

perform care for the client. In answer B, a tort is a wrongful act committed to the client or his belongings. Answer C is incorrect because assault is willfully hitting or restraining the client.

34. **Answer D is correct.** The licensed practical nurse should not be assigned to begin a blood transfusion. The licensed practical nurse can insert a Foley catheter, as stated in answer A; discontinue a nasogastric tube, as stated in answer B; and collect sputum specimen, as stated in answer C. Thus, answers A, B, and C are all incorrect.

35. **Answer B is correct.** The vital signs are abnormal and should be reported to the doctor immediately. To continue to monitor the vital signs, as in answer A, could result in deterioration of the client's condition. Asking the client how he feels in answer C will provide only subjective data. The nurse in answer D is not the best nurse to assign because this client is unstable.

36. **Answer B is correct.** The nurse in answer B has the most experience in knowing possible complications involving preeclampsia. The nurse in answer A is a new nurse to the unit and so should not be assigned to this client; the nurses in answers C and D have no experience with the postpartum client, so neither should be assigned to this client.

37. **Answer B is correct.** An inaccurate narcotic count on the unit should be reported to the state Board of Nursing because narcotics are controlled substances. Answers A, C, and D are incorrect because they are of little concern to the state board. Although they are important functions, these actions would be resolved within the hospital.

38. **Answer B is correct.** After discussing with the nurse and documenting the incident, filing a formal reprimand is the first action for the charge nurse to take. If the nurse continues following an incorrect procedure that causes, or could cause, harm to the client, termination might be needed. The Joint Commission on Accreditation of Hospitals will probably be interested in the actions in answers A and C, but this is not the immediate action to take. The failure of the nursing assistant to care for the client with hepatitis might result in termination, but this is not of interest to the Joint Commission; therefore, answer D is incorrect.

39. **Answer D is correct.** The client with multiple sclerosis should receive priority because of the IV cortisone treatment. This client is at highest risk for complications. The clients in answers A and B are more stable and are not the priority. The client with MRSA (methicillin-resistant staphylococcus aureus) is being treated with antibiotics, but there is no data to indicate that the nurse should see this client first, so answer C is incorrect.

40. **Answer B is correct.** The two clients who can share a room are the pregnant client and the client with a broken arm and facial lacerations because these clients are stable. The other clients in answers A needs to be placed in separate rooms because the schizophrenic will further upset the client with an ulcerative colitis. Answer C is incorrect because this child is terminal and he should not be placed in the room with the client with a frontal head injury. Answer D is incorrect because the chest pain may be related to a myocardial infarction.

41. **Answer A is correct.** Before instilling eyedrops, the nurse should cleanse the area with water. A 6-year-old child is not developmentally ready to instill his own eyedrops, so answer B is incorrect. Although the mother of the child may instill the eyedrops, the

area must be cleansed before administration, so answer C is incorrect. The eye might appear to be clear, but the nurse should instill the eyedrops, as ordered, so answer D is incorrect.

42. **Answer C is correct.** The comment of most concern is answer C because hot dogs are commonly the cause of choking in children. There is no reason for concern in the comments in answers A, B, or D; therefore, these are incorrect.

43. **Answer C is correct.** There is no reason to tell the parents to leave because this might cause the child to become more agitated, making answer A incorrect. Removing his toys may also cause him to fret and make the examination more difficult, so answer B is incorrect. Answer D is incorrect because telling him that the behavior is inappropriate will not help because the child is too young to understand.

44. **Answer B is correct.** Hearing aids should be stored in a cool place in order to preserve the life of the battery. Answer A is incorrect because the mold should be cleaned daily. Answer C is incorrect because the hearing aid should not be cleaned with a toothpick. Answer D is incorrect because changing the batteries weekly is not necessary.

45. **Answer C is correct.** A risk for aspiration is the best answer because aspiration of blood can lead to airway obstruction. Answer A does not apply to a child who has undergone a tonsillectomy because there is no alteration in body image. Answer B is incorrect because impaired verbal communication might be true but is not the highest priority. Pain is an issue, but not the highest priority, so answer D is incorrect.

46. **Answer A is correct.** If the child has bacterial pneumonia, a high fever is usually present. Bacterial pneumonia usually presents with a productive cough, not a nonproductive cough, so answer B is incorrect. Rhinitis is often seen with viral pneumonia, not bacterial pneumonia, so answer C is incorrect. Vomiting and diarrhea are usually not seen with pneumonia, so answer D is incorrect.

47. **Answer B is correct.** For a child with LTB and the possibility of complete obstruction of the airway, emergency intubation equipment should always be kept at the bedside. Intravenous supplies and fluid will not treat an obstruction, so answers A and C are incorrect. Answer D is incorrect because although supplemental oxygen is needed, the child will need to be intubated for it to help.

48. **Answer C is correct.** Exophthalmos (protrusion of eyeballs) often occurs with hyperthyroidism. The client with hyperthyroidism will often exhibit tachycardia, increased appetite, and weight loss, not bradycardia, decreased appetite, or weight gain, so answers A, B, and D are incorrect.

49. **Answer D is correct.** The child with celiac disease should be on a gluten-free diet. Answer D is the only choice of foods that do not contain gluten, so answers A, B, and C are incorrect.

50. **Answer C is correct.** The child with an oxygen saturation level of 78% is hypoxic. He will require oxygen therapy. Checking the arterial blood gases in answer A is good but is not the highest priority and will not correct the problem. If the nurse does nothing, as in answer B, the client's condition will most likely continue to decline. Answer D is incorrect because assessing the pulse will probably reveal tachycardia, but this is not the highest priority.

51. **Answer B is correct.** Normal amniotic fluid is straw colored and odorless. An amniotomy is an artificial rupture of membranes. Fetal heart tones of 160 indicate tachycardia, so answer A is incorrect. Greenish fluid is indicative of meconium, so answer C is incorrect. If the nurse notes the umbilical cord, the client is experiencing a prolapsed cord. This would need to be reported immediately; therefore, answer D is incorrect.

52. **Answer D is correct.** Dilation of 3cm is the end of the latent phase of labor, so a request for an epidural would be expected. Answer A is a vague answer, and answer B would indicate the end of the first stage of labor, or complete dilation. Answer C indicates the transition phase and, thus, is incorrect.

53. **Answer B is correct.** The normal fetal heart rate is 120–160bpm; 100–110bpm is bradycardia. The first action would be to turn the client to the left side and apply oxygen. Answer A is not indicated at this time. Answer C is not the best action for clients experiencing bradycardia. There is no data to indicate the need to move the client to the delivery room at this time, so answer D is incorrect.

54. **Answer D is correct.** The expected effect of Pitocin is cervical dilation. Pitocin causes more intense contractions, which can increase the pain, so answer A is incorrect. Cervical effacement is caused by pressure on the presenting part, so answer B is incorrect. Answer C is incorrect because the word *infrequent* indicates irregular contractions.

55. **Answer B is correct.** A breach presentation calls for applying a fetal heart monitor. Answer A is incorrect because there is no need to prepare for a Caesarean section at this time. Answer C is incorrect because placing the client in Trendelenburg position is also not an indicated action. Answer D is incorrect because there is no need for an ultrasound based on the finding.

56. **Answer B is correct. Answer B is correct.** There are only a few reasons to apply an internal monitor: if the fetus is in distress or if the fetal heart tones cannot be assessed using the external monitor. Answer A is incorrect because cervical dilation is not a reason to apply an internal monitor. Answer C is incorrect because the fact that the fetus is at 0 station is not a reason to apply an internal monitor. Answer D is also incorrect because noting contractions every 3 minutes is not a reason to apply an internal monitor. It is not necessary for a scalp electrode placement, as long as the membranes are still intact.

57. **Answer D is correct.** Clients admitted in labor are told not to eat during labor, to avoid nausea and vomiting. Ice chips may be allowed, but this amount of fluid is not sufficient to prevent dehydration. Answer A is incorrect because impaired gas exchange related to hyperventilation is not a risk to the client. Answer B is incorrect because alteration in oxygen perfusion related to maternal position is not a problem encountered by the client at the end of the early phase of labor. Answer C is incorrect because not all clients have fetal monitoring.

58. **Answer D is correct.** This information indicates a late deceleration. This type of deceleration is caused by uteroplacental lack of oxygen. Answer A is incorrect because decelerations are not caused by fetal sleep, answer B results in a variable deceleration, and answer C is indicative of an early deceleration.

appropriate size for gestation, so answer C is incorrect. Growth retardation is associated with smoking, but this does not affect the infant length, making answer D incorrect.

75. **Answer A is correct.** To provide protection against antibody production, RhoGam should be given within 72 hours. Answers B, C and D are incorrect because they would be given too late to provide antibody protection. RhoGam can also be given during pregnancy.

76. **Answer B is correct.** When the membranes rupture, there is often a transient drop in the fetal heart tones. The heart tones should return to baseline quickly. Any alteration in fetal heart tones, such as bradycardia or tachycardia, should be reported. After the fetal heart tones are assessed, the nurse should evaluate the cervical dilation, as stated in answer A; vital signs, as stated in answer C; and level of discomfort, as stated in answer D.

77. **Answer A is correct.** The active phase of labor begins when the client is dilated 4–7cm. Answer B refers to the latent or early phase of labor, from 1cm to 3cm dilation. Answer C refers to the transition phase of labor, from 8cm to 10cm dilation. Answer D refers to the early phase of labor, from 1cm to 3cm dilation.

78. **Answer B is correct.** The infant of a mother with narcotic addiction will undergo withdrawal. Snugly wrapping the infant in a blanket will help prevent the muscle irritability that these babies often experience. Teaching the mother to provide tactile stimulation or provide for early infant stimulation, in answers A and C, is incorrect because he is irritable and needs quiet and little stimulation at this time. Placing the infant in an infant seat is incorrect because this will also cause movement that can increase muscle irritability; thus, answer D is incorrect.

79. **Answer C is correct.** Following epidural anesthesia, the client should be checked for hypotension and signs of shock every 5 minutes for 15 minutes. The client can be checked for cervical dilation later, after she is stable, so answer A is incorrect. The client should not be positioned supine because the anesthesia can move above the respiratory center and the client can stop breathing, making answer B incorrect. Fetal heart tones should be assessed after the blood pressure is checked, so answer D is incorrect.

80. **Answer B is correct.** The best way to prevent post-operative wound infection is handwashing. Use of prescribed antibiotics will treat infection, not prevent infections, so answer A is incorrect. Wearing a mask and asking the client to cover her mouth are good practices but will not prevent wound infections; thus, answers C and D are incorrect.

81. **Answer B is correct.** The client with a hip fracture will most likely have disalignment. Answer A is incorrect because all fractures experience pain. Coolness of the extremity and the absence of pulses are indicative of compartment syndrome or peripheral vascular disease, not a fractured hip, so answers C and D are incorrect.

82. **Answer B is correct.** After menopause, women lack hormones necessary to absorb and utilize calcium. Doing weight-bearing exercises and taking calcium supplements can help prevent osteoporosis, but these are not the most likely causes, so answers A and C are incorrect. Body types that frequently experience osteoporosis are thin Caucasian females, but they are not *most* likely to cause osteoporosis, so answer D is incorrect.

83. **Answer B is correct.** The infant's hips should be off the bed approximately 15° in Bryant's traction. Answers A and C are incorrect because they do not indicate that the traction is working correctly. Answer D is incorrect because Bryant's traction is skin traction, not skeletal traction.

84. **Answer A is correct.** Balanced skeletal traction uses pins and screws. A Steinman pin goes through large bones and is used to stabilize large bones such as the femur. Answer B is incorrect because only the affected leg is in traction. Kirschner wires are used to stabilize small bones, such as fingers and toes, so answer C is incorrect. Answer D is incorrect because this type of traction is not used for fractured hips.

85. **Answer A is correct.** Bleeding is a common complication of orthopedic surgery. The blood-collection device should be checked frequently to ensure that the client is not hemorrhaging. Answer B is incorrect because the client's pain should be assessed, but this is not life-threatening. Answer C is incorrect because the nutritional status should be assessed later. An immobilizer is not used, so answer D is incorrect.

86. **Answer A is correct.** The client's family member should be taught to flush the tube after each feeding and clamp the tube. The placement should be checked before feedings, so answer B is incorrect. Indigestion can occur with the PEG tube just as it can occur with any client, so there is no need to call the doctor, as suggested in answer C. Medications can be ordered for this, but it is not a reason for alarm. A percutaneous endoscopy gastrotomy tube is used for clients who have experienced difficulty swallowing. The tube is inserted directly into the stomach and does not require swallowing, so answer D is incorrect.

87. **Answer C is correct.** The client with a total knee replacement should be assessed for anemia. A hemaglobin of 6g/dL is extremely low and might require a blood transfusion (the normal is 14–18g/dL). Bleeding on the dressing of 2cm is not extreme, so answer A is incorrect. Circle the bleeding, write the date and time on the dressing, and chart the finding. If the drainage continues to enlarge, notify the doctor. A low-grade temperature is not unusual after surgery, so answer B is incorrect. Recheck the temperature in 1 hour. If the temperature rises above 101°F, report this finding to the doctor. Tylenol will probably be ordered. Voiding after surgery is not uncommon and is not a sign of immediate danger, so answer D is incorrect. Ensure that the client is well hydrated and monitored.

88. **Answer B is correct.** Plumbism is lead poisoning. If the parents have stained glass as a hobby, there is a danger that the lead used to adhere stained glass can drop in the work area where the child can consume the lead beads. Other factors associated with the consumption of lead are eating from pottery made in Central America or Mexico that is unfired. In answer A, there is no data to suggest that the child is drinking from pottery bought in Central America. Answer C is incorrect because the child in this situation lives in a house built in 1990. Lead was taken out of paint in 1976. Answer D is unrelated to plumbism.

89. **Answer A is correct.** An abduction pillow will help to prevent adduction of the hip joint. The client should be taught to avoid crossing the legs. Answer B is incorrect because the client should not flex the hip more than 90°; the straight chair would potentiate the flexion of the hip more than 90°. Answer C is incorrect because the client should use a walker, not crutches, to ambulate. Answer D is incorrect because a hard mattress is best, not a soft one.

90. **Answer B is correct.** A PTT of 300 is extremely prolonged and can indicate bleeding. Answers A, C, and D are incorrect because there is no need to report a PT of 20, a Protime of 30 seconds, or an INR of 3 because these are within normal findings.

91. **Answer B is correct.** Narcan is the antidote for narcotic overdose. If hypoxia occurs, the client should have oxygen administered by mask, not cannula, so answer A is incorrect. There is no data to support administering blood products or cardioresuscitation, so answers C and D are incorrect.

92. **Answer B is correct.** The 6-year-old should have a roommate as close to the same age as possible. The client in answer A is 16 and a female. The client in answer C is closest to the client's age, but the 10-year-old with sarcoma has cancer and will be treated with chemotherapy that makes him immune suppressed. The 6-year-old with osteomylitis is infected, so answer D is incorrect.

93. **Answer D is correct.** Plaquenil can cause color blindness, and therefore requires that the client's vision be evaluated every six months. Answer A is incorrect because there is no need to take the medication with milk. Answers B and C are incorrect because these actions are unnecessary. Answer C is incorrect because there is no need to remain upright for 30 minutes after taking the medication.

94. **Answer D is correct.** A plaster-of-Paris cast takes 24 hours to dry, and the client should not bear weight for 24 hours. The cast should be handled with the palms, not the fingertips, so answer A is incorrect. Answer B is incorrect because bivalving a cast is done for compartment syndrome and is not routine. The client should be told not to dry the cast with a hair dryer because this causes hot spots and could burn the client, so answer C is incorrect.

95. **Answer A is correct.** There is no reason that the client's friends should not be allowed to autograph the cast; it will not harm the cast in any way. This makes answers B, C, and D incorrect.

96. **Answer A is correct.** The nurse is performing the pin care correctly when she uses sterile gloves and Q-tips. The nurse can assist her co-worker by opening any packages of sterile dressings that are needed. Answers B, C, and D are incorrect. The nurse should use sterile gloves, not clean gloves, for pin care, a licensed practical nurse can perform pin care, and there is no need to clean the weights.

97. **Answer A is correct.** A body cast or spica cast extends from the upper abdomen to the knees or below. Bowel sounds should be checked to ensure that the client is not experiencing a paralytic illeus. Checking the blood pressure is a treatment for any client but is not specific to a spica cast, so answer B is incorrect. Answers C and D are incorrect because they are not concerns associated with a body cast or spica cast.

98. **Answer C is correct.** Halo traction will be ordered for the client with a cervical fracture. Russell's traction is used for bones of the lower extremities, as is Buck's traction, so answers A and B are incorrect. Cruchfield tongs are used while in the hospital and the client is immobile, so answer D is incorrect.

99. **Answer B is correct.** The controller for the continuous passive-motion device should be placed distal to the site to prevent the client from being able to turn off the machine. If the client is allowed to have the control close by, he might be tempted to turn off the machine and stop the passive motion. This treatment is often painful, so

the nurse should offer pain medication before the treatment. Answer A is incorrect because the client cannot ambulate during the therapy. Answer C is incorrect because pain is expected and is not a reason to turn off the machine. Answer D is incorrect because the continuous passive-motion machine does not alleviate the need for physical therapy.

100. **Answer A is correct.** The client's palms should rest lightly on the handles. The elbows should be flexed no more than 30° but should not be extended, so answer B is incorrect. The client should walk to the middle of the walker, not to the front of the walker, so answer C is incorrect. The client should be taught not to carry the walker, so answer D is incorrect.

101. **Answer C is correct.** The client with a prolapsed cord should be treated by elevating the hips and covering the cord with a moist, sterile saline gauze. The nurse should use her fingers to push up on the presenting part until a Caesarean section can be performed. Do not attempt to replace the cord, as stated in answer A. Answer B is incorrect because turning the client to the left side will not help take pressure off the cord. Answer D is incorrect because the cord should be covered with a moist, sterile gauze, not dry gauze.

102. **Answer B is correct.** Chest tubes work to reinflate the lung and drain serous fluid. The tube does not equalize expansion of the lungs, so answer A is incorrect. Pain is associated with collapse of the lung, and insertion of chest tubes is painful, so answer C is incorrect. Answer D is true but is not the primary rationale for performing chest tube insertion.

103. **Answer D is correct.** Success with breastfeeding depends on many factors, but the most dependable reason for success is desire and willingness to continue the breastfeeding until the infant and mother have time to adapt. The educational level, infant's birth weight, and size of the mother's breast have nothing to do with success, so answers A, B, and C are incorrect.

104. **Answer C is correct.** Green-tinged amniotic fluid is indicative of meconium staining. This finding indicates fetal distress. The presence of scant bloody discharge is normal, as are frequent urination and moderate uterine contractions, so answers A, B, and D are incorrect.

105. **Answer C is correct.** Duration is measured from the beginning of one contraction to the end of the same contraction. Answer A is related to frequency. Answer B is incorrect because we do not measure from the end of the contraction to the beginning of the contraction. Duration also is not measured from the peak of the contraction to the end, as stated in answer D.

106. **Answer B is correct.** The client receiving Pitocin should be monitored for decelerations. There is no association with Pitocin use and hypoglycemia, maternal hyperreflexia, or fetal movement, so answers A, C, and D are incorrect.

107. **Answer D is correct.** During pregnancy, insulin needs increase during the second and third trimesters; they do not decrease, as suggested in answer B. Insulin requirements do not moderate as the pregnancy progresses, so answer A is incorrect. Elevated human chorionic gonadotrophin elevate insulin needs; they do not decrease insulin needs. Thus, answer C is incorrect. Fetal development does depend on adequate nutrition and insulin regulation.

108. Answer A is correct. A calm environment is needed to prevent seizure activity. Any stimulation can precipitate seizures. Assessing the fetal heart tones is important but is not the highest priority in this situation, so answer D is incorrect. Obtaining a diet history should be done later, so answer B is incorrect. Administering an analgesic is not indicated because there is no data in the stem to indicate pain, so answer C is incorrect.

109. Answer A is correct. The client who is age 42 is at risk for fetal anomalies such as Down syndrome and other chromosomal aberrations. She is not at higher risk for respiratory distress syndrome or pathological jaundice, as stated in answers B and D. Turner's syndrome, in answer C, is a genetic disorder that is not associated with age factors in pregnancy.

110. Answer C is correct. The client with a missed abortion will have induction of labor. Prostin E. is a form of prostaglandin used to soften the cervix. Magnesium sulfate is used for preterm labor and preeclampsia, not to induce labor, so answer A is incorrect. Calcium gluconate is the antidote for magnesium sulfate and is not used for this client, so answer B is incorrect. Pardel is dopamine receptor stimulant used to treat Parkinson's disease; it was used at one time to dry up breast milk but is no longer used in obstetrics, so answer D is incorrect.

111. Answer A is correct. The client's blood pressure is within normal limits. The urinary output is also within normal limits. The only alteration from normal is the decreased deep tendon reflexes. The nurse should continue to monitor the blood pressure and check the magnesium level. The therapeutic level is 4.8–9.6mg/dL. There is no need to stop the infusion at this time or slow the rate, as stated in answers B and C. Calcium gluconate is the antidote for magnesium sulfate, but there is no data to indicate toxicity, so answer D is incorrect.

112. Answer C is correct. Autosomal recessive disorders can be passed from the parents to the infant if each parent passes the defective gene. If both parents pass the trait, the child will get two abnormal genes, and the disease results. The parents can also pass the trait to the infant. Answer A is incorrect because, to have an affected newborn, the parents must be carriers. Answer B is incorrect because both parents must be carriers. Answer D is incorrect because the parents can have affected children.

113. Answer D is correct. Alpha fetoprotein is a screening test done to detect neural tube defects such as spina bifida. The test is not mandatory, as stated in answer A; it does not indicate cardiovascular defects, as suggested in answer B; and her age has no bearing on the need for the test, as suggested in answer C.

114. Answer B is correct. During pregnancy, the thyroid gland triples in size. This makes it more difficult to regulate thyroid medication. Answer A is incorrect because there might be a need for thyroid medication during pregnancy. Answer C is incorrect because the thyroid function does not slow. Answer D is incorrect because fetal growth is not arrested if thyroid medication is continued.

115. Answer C is correct. Cyanosis of the feet and hands is acrocyanosis. This is a normal finding 1 minute after birth. Answers A and B are incorrect because an apical pulse should be 120–160 and the baby should have muscle tone. Jaundice immediately after birth is pathological jaundice and is abnormal, so answer D is incorrect.

116. **Answer A is correct.** Clients with sickle cell crises are treated with heat, hydration, oxygen, and pain relief. Fluids are increased, not decreased, so answer B is incorrect. Answer C is incorrect because blood transfusions are usually not required. Answer D is incorrect because these clients can be delivered vaginally.

117. **Answer A is correct.** Before ultrasonography, the client should be taught to drink plenty of fluids and not void. The client may ambulate, so answer B is incorrect. An enema is not needed, and there is no need to withhold food for 8 hours, so answers C and D are incorrect.

118. **Answer D is correct.** By 1 year of age, the infant is expected to triple his birth weight. Answers A, B, and C are incorrect because these weights are too low.

119. **Answer B is correct.** A nonstress test is done to evaluate periodic movements of the fetus. It is not done to evaluate lung maturity. Answer A is incorrect because a nonstress test does not measure lung maturity. An oxytocin challenge test shows the effect of contractions on fetal heart rate; this makes answer C incorrect. A nonstress test does not measure the neurological well-being of the fetus, so answer D is incorrect.

120. **Answer B is correct.** Hypospadia is a condition in which the urethra opens on the dorsal side of the penis. Answer A is incorrect because there is an opening. Answer C is incorrect because the penis is the correct size. Answer D is incorrect because the opening is on the dorsal side, not the ventral side.

121. **Answer A is correct.** Transition is the time during labor when the client loses concentration due to intense contractions. Potential for injury related to precipitate delivery has nothing to do with the dilation of the cervix, so answer B is incorrect. There is no data to indicate that the client has had anesthesia or fluid volume deficit, so answers C and D are incorrect.

122. **Answer C is correct.** Varicella is chicken pox. This herpes virus is treated with antiviral medications. The client is not treated with antibiotics or anticoagulants, so answers A and D are incorrect. The client might have a fever before the rash appears, but when the rash appears, the temperature is usually gone; thus, answer B is incorrect.

123. **Answer B is correct.** Clients with chest pain can be treated with nitroglycerin, a beta blocker such as propanolol, or Varapamil, so answers A, C, and D are incorrect. There is no indication for an antibiotic such as ampicillin.

124. **Answer B is correct.** Clients with rheumatoid arthritis should exercise, but not to the point of pain and not when inflammation is present, so answer A is incorrect. Anti-inflammatory drugs should be taken with meals because they cause stomach upset. Alternating heat and cold is not necessary, so answer C is incorrect. Warm, moist soaks are useful to decrease pain. Weight-bearing activities such as walking are useful, so answer D is incorrect.

125. **Answer D is correct.** Morphine is contraindicated in clients with gallbladder disease and pancreatitis because morphine causes spasms of the Sphenter of Oddi. Meperidine, Mylanta, and Cimetadine can be taken by the client with pancreatitis, so answers A, B, and C are incorrect.

144. **Answer C is correct.** The lens allows light to pass through the pupil and focus light on the retina. The lens does not stimulate the retina (answer A), assist with eye movement (answer B), or magnify small objects (answer D).

145. **Answer C is correct.** Miotic eyedrops constrict the pupil and allow aqueous humor to drain out of the Canal of Schlemm. Answer A is incorrect because miotics do not anesthetize the cornea. Answer B is incorrect because miotics do not dilate the pupil; they constrict the pupil. Answer D is incorrect because miotics do not paralyze the muscles of the eye.

146. **Answer A is correct.** When using eyedrops, allow 5 minutes between medications. Answer B is incorrect because the two medications should not be used simultaneously. Answer C is incorrect because there is no need for the client to also use a cycloplegic. Answer D is incorrect because these drugs can be used by the same client.

147. **Answer B is correct.** Clients with colorblindness will most likely have problems distinguishing violets, blues, and greens. The other colors are less commonly affected, so answers A, C, and D are incorrect.

148. **Answer D is correct.** The client with a pacemaker should be taught to count and record his pulse rate. Answer A is incorrect because ankle edema is a sign of right-sided congestive heart failure, not pacemaker malfunction. Although this is not normal, it is often present in clients with heart disease. If the edema is present in the hands and face, it should be reported. Answer B is incorrect because checking the blood pressure daily is not necessary for these clients. The client with a pacemaker can use a microwave oven, but he should stand about 5 feet from the oven while it is operating; thus, answer C is incorrect.

149. **Answer A is correct.** Clients who are being retrained for bladder control should be taught to withhold fluids after about 7 p.m., or 1900. The other hours are too early in the day, so answers B, C, and D are incorrect.

150. **Answer D is correct.** Cranberry juice is more alkaline and, when metabolized by the body, is excreted with acidic urine. Bacteria does not grow freely in acidic urine. Answer A, increasing intake of meats, is not associated with urinary tract infections. Answer B is incorrect because the client does not have to avoid citrus fruits. Pericare should be done, but not with hydrogen peroxide, so answer C is incorrect.

151. **Answer C is correct.** NPH insulin peaks in 8–12 hours, so a snack should be offered at that time. NPH insulin onsets in 90–120 minutes, so answer A is incorrect. Answer B is untrue because NPH insulin is time released and does not usually cause sudden hypoglycemia. Answer D is incorrect, but the client should eat a bedtime snack.

152. **Answer D is correct.** Methotrexate is a folic acid antagonist. Leucovorin is the drug given for toxicity to this drug. Answers A, B, and C are incorrect because the drug is not used to treat iron-deficiency anemia, create a synergistic effects, or increase the number of circulating neutrophils.

153. **Answer B is correct.** The client who is allergic to dogs, eggs, rabbits, and chicken feathers is most likely allergic to the rubella vaccine. The client who is allergic to neomycin is also at risk. Answers A, C, and D are incorrect because there is no danger to the client if he has an order for a TB skin test, ELISA test, or chest x-ray.

154. Answer B is correct. Zantac (rantidine) is a histamine blocker. This drug should be given with meals, for optimal effect. It should not be given before meals, so answer A is incorrect. Tagamet (cimetidine) is a histamine blocker that can be given in one dose at bedtime, so answer C is incorrect. These drugs should not be given after meals, so answer D is incorrect.

155. Answer C is correct. The proximal end of the double-barrel colostomy is the end toward the small intestines. This end is on the client's right side. The distal end, in answers A, B, and D, is on the client's left side.

156. Answer A is correct. If the nurse checks the fundus and finds it to be displaced to the right or left, this is an indication of a full bladder. Answer B is incorrect because this finding is not associated with hypotension or clots. Oxytoxic drugs (Pitocin) are used to contract the uterus, but the fact that the client did or did not receive Pitocin does not help with the plan of action; therefore, answer C is incorrect. Answer D is incorrect because expulsion of small clots is normal; it has nothing to do with displacement to the right.

157. Answer C is correct. Answer C is correct because a history of allergies to oysters may indicate a potential allergy to the dye used in the contrast medium. Answer A is incorrect because the client can have a CAT scan if she is having her menses. Answer B is incorrect because a history of claustrophobia is not related to having a CAT scan. Answer D is incorrect because a client with sensory hearing loss can have a CAT scan.

158. Answer C is correct. Answer A is incorrect because a 6-month-old is too old for the colorful mobile. Answers B and D are incorrect because he is too young to play with the electronic game or the 30-piece jigsaw puzzle. The best toy for this age is the cars in a plastic container.

159. Answer C is correct. The client with polio has muscle weakness. Periods of rest throughout the day will conserve the client's energy. Answer A is incorrect because taking a *hot* bath can cause burns; however, a warm bath would be helpful. Answer B is incorrect because strenuous exercises are not advisable. Answer D is incorrect because visual disturbances are directly associated with polio; however, there is no guarantee that these visual disturbances can be corrected by glasses.

160. Answer B is correct. The client with a protoepisiotomy will need stool softeners such as docusate sodium. Answer A is incorrect because suppositories are given only with an order from the doctor. Answer C is incorrect because Methergine (methylergonovine) is a drug used to contract the uterus. Answer D is incorrect because Ritalin (methylphenidate) is a drug given for hyperactivity.

161. Answer C is correct. Total Parenteral Nutrition is a high-glucose solution. This therapy often causes the glucose levels to be elevated. Because this is a common complication, insulin might be ordered. Answer A is incorrect because TPN is used to treat negative nitrogen balance; it will not lead to negative nitrogen balance. Answer B is incorrect because Total Parenteral Nutrition can be managed with oral hypoglycemic drugs, but it is difficult. Answer D is incorrect because Total Parenteral Nutrition will not lead to further pancreatic disease.

162. Answer B is correct. The client who is 10 weeks pregnant should be assessed to determine how she feels about the pregnancy. Answer A is incorrect because it is too early to discuss preterm labor. Answer C is incorrect because it is too late to discuss whether she was using a method of birth control. Answer D is incorrect because now is not the time to discuss future children; this can be done after the client delivers.

163. **Answer A is correct.** Demerol and Phenergan are given for their synergistic effect. *Synergistic* means that one drug increases the effectiveness of the other. Demerol is a narcotic analgesic, and Phenergan is an antianxiety, antiemetic medication. Answer B is incorrect because they are not given for the agonist effect; an agonist is a medication that works with chemicals or substances in the blood, such as hormones. Answer C is incorrect because they are not given together to cause extrapyramidal effects. Answer D is incorrect because antagonists work against one another.

164. **Answer A is correct.** A thyroid scan with contrast uses a dye, so the client should be assessed for allergies to iodine. The client will not have a bolus of fluid, will not be asleep, and will not have a urinary catheter inserted, so answers B, C, and D are incorrect.

165. **Answer B is correct.** RhoGam is used to prevent formation of Rh antibodies. It does not provide immunity to Rh isoenzymes, eliminate circulating Rh antibodies, or convert the Rh factor from negative to positive, so answers A, C, and D are incorrect.

166. **Answer B is correct.** A client with a fractured foot often has a short leg cast applied to stabilize the fracture. Answer A is incorrect because a spica cast is used to stabilize a fractured pelvis or vertebral fracture. Answer C is incorrect because Kirschner wires are used to stabilize small bones such as toes. Answer D is incorrect because the client will most likely have a cast application.

167. **Answer A is correct.** A Trendelenburg test is done to determine muscle weakness. The Trendelenburg sign is positive if the client cannot stand on one leg without having pelvic weakness. The test is not done to determine fluid volume, as stated in answer B, or to determine the client's ability to concentrate, as stated in answer C. Answer D is incorrect because the Trendelenburg test does not check for dexterity.

168. **Answer C is correct.** Immunosuppressants are used to prevent antibody formation. Answer A is incorrect because antivirals are not used in this client. Answer B is not correct because antibiotics do not prevent organ rejection. Answer D is incorrect because analgesics do not prevent rejection.

169. **Answer A is correct.** Before cataract removal, the client will have Mydriatic drops instilled to dilate the pupil. This will facilitate removal of the lens. Answer B is incorrect because miotics constrict the pupil and are not used in cataract clients. Answer C is incorrect because a laser is not used to smooth and reshape the lens. The diseased lens is removed. Answer D is incorrect because a silicone oil is not injected in this client.

170. **Answer C is correct.** Answers A and B are not recommended because placing mirrors and pictures in several locations tends to cause agitation. Answer C is correct because placing simple signs that indicate the location of rooms where the client sleeps, eats, and bathes will help the client be more independent. Answer D is incorrect because alternating healthcare workers also confuses the client and leads to further confusion.

171. **Answer C is correct.** A Jackson-Pratt drain is a serum-collection device commonly used in abdominal surgery. Answers A, B, and D are incorrect because a Jackson-Pratt

drain will not prevent the need for dressing changes, reduce edema of the incision, or keep the common bile duct open. A t-tube is used to keep the common bile duct open.

172. Answer C is correct. Head lag is associated with the pre-term newborn and is an expected finding in the newborn less than 36 weeks gestation. Answer A is incorrect because the presence of Mongolian spots are not associated with the pre-term newborn. Answers B and D are findings associated with the full-term newborn, therefore they are incorrect.

173. Answer A is correct. Hematuria in a client with a pelvic fracture can indicate trauma to the bladder or impending bleeding disorders. Answers B, C, and D are incorrect because it is not unusual for the client to complain of muscles spasms, dizziness, or nausea following multiple traumas.

174. Answer C is correct. The statement "They are trying to kill me" indicates paranoid delusions. There is no data to indicate that the client is hearing voices, as stated in answer A. Delusions of grandeur are fixed beliefs that the client is superior or perhaps a famous person, so answer B is incorrect. There is no data to indicate that the client is intoxicated, so answer D is incorrect.

175. Answer B is correct. Because there is an inner and an outer cannula, the nurse should simply replace the old one with a new, sterile one. Answer A is incorrect because there is no need to call the doctor. Answer C is incorrect because there is no need to hold open the stoma because there is an out cannula. Answer D is incorrect because there is no data to support the lack of respirations in the client.

176. Answer C is correct. Infants with a 9 Apgar at 5 minutes most likely have acryocyanosis, a normal physiologic adaptation to birth. Answer A is incorrect because it is most likely not related to the infant being cold. Answer B is incorrect because there is no evidence that the baby has bradycardia. Answer D is incorrect because there is no evidence that the baby is lethargic.

177. Answer A is correct. The primary reason for rapid, continuous rewarming of an area affected by frostbite is to lessen cellular damage. Answers B, C, and D are not primary reasons for rapid continuous rewarming, therefore they are incorrect.

178. Answer D is correct. Hemodialysis works by using a dialyzing membrane to filter waste that has accumulated in the blood. Answer A is incorrect because it does not pass *water* through a dialyzing membrane. Answer B is not correct because hemodialysis does not eliminate plasma protein from the blood. Answer C is incorrect because it does not lower the pH.

179. Answer B is correct. The client who is immune-suppressed and exposed to measles should be treated with medications to boost his immunity to the virus. An antibiotic or antiviral will not protect the client, so answers A and C are incorrect. Answer D is incorrect because it is too late to place the client in isolation.

180. Answer D is correct. The client with MRSA should be placed in isolation. Gloves, a gown, and a mask should be used when caring for the client. The door should remain closed, but a negative-pressure room is not necessary, so answers A and B are incorrect. MRSA is spread by contact with blood or body fluid, or by touch to the skin of the client. MRSA is cultured from the nasal passages of the client, so the client should be instructed to cover the nose and mouth when he sneezes or coughs. Answer C is incorrect because it is not necessary for the client to wear the mask at all times. The nurse should wear the mask.

181. Answer B is correct. To prevent hip-flexion deformities, the client should be instructed to lie prone every 4 hours for 30 minutes during the day. This will force the leg to extend to 0 and prevent the contracture. Answer A, C, and D are incorrect because lying on his back or side, or flat will not help.

182. Answer A is correct. During a Whipple procedure, the head of the pancreas, a portion of the stomach, the jejunum, and a portion of the stomach are removed and reanastomosed. Answer B is incorrect because the proximal third of the small intestine is not removed. The entire stomach is not removed, as in answer C, and the esophagus also is not removed, as in answer D.

183. Answer C is correct. Pepper is not processed and contains bacteria. Answer A is incorrect because fruits can be eaten; they should be cooked or washed and peeled. Answers B and D are allowed.

184. Answer A is correct. Coumadin (sodium warfarin) is an anticoagulant. One of the tests for bleeding time is a Protime. This test should be done monthly. Answer B is incorrect because eating more fruits and vegetables is not necessary, and dark-green vegetables contain vitamin K that increases clotting. Answer C is incorrect because drinking more liquids is not necessary. Answer D is not correct because avoiding crowds is also not necessary.

185. Answer A is correct. The client having removal of a central venous catheter should be told to hold his breath and bear down. This is known as the Valsalva maneuver. This prevents air from entering the line. Answers B, C, and D are incorrect because they will not facilitate removal.

186. Answer B is correct. Clients with a history of streptococcal infections might have antibodies that render the streptokinase ineffective. Answer A is incorrect because there is no reason to assess the client for allergies to pineapples or bananas. There is no correlation to the use of phenytoin and streptokinase, so answer C is incorrect. A history of alcohol abuse is also not a factor in the order for streptokinase, so answer D is incorrect.

187. Answer B is correct. The client who is immune-suppressed and has bone marrow suppression should be taught not to floss his teeth. Answer A is incorrect because using oils and cream-based soaps is allowed. Answer C is incorrect because the client can eat salt. An electric razor is the best way to shave, so answer D is incorrect.

188. Answer A is correct. The best method and safest way to change the ties of a tracheotomy is to apply the new ones before removing the old ones. Answer B is not enough action. Having a helper is good, but the helper might not prevent the client from coughing out the tracheotomy. Answer C is not the best way to prevent the client from coughing out the tracheotomy. Answer D is incorrect because asking the doctor to suture the tracheotomy in place is not appropriate.

189. Answer D is correct. The output of 300mL is indicative of hemorrhage and should be reported immediately. Answer A is incorrect because turning the client to the left side will not help. Milking the tube is done only with an order and will not help in this situation, so answer B is incorrect. Slowing the intravenous infusion is inappropriate. The infusion should be increased, so answer C is incorrect.

190. Answer A is correct. The infant with tetrology of falot has five heart defects. He will be treated with digoxin to slow and strengthen the heart. Epinephrine, aminophyline, and atropine will speed the heart rate and are not used in this client, so answers B, C, and D are incorrect.

191. See diagram. The Tail of Spence is located in the upper outer quadrant of the breast.

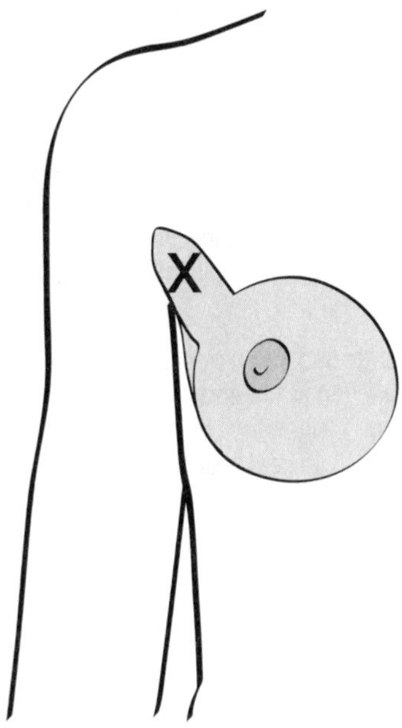

192. Answer A is correct. The toddler with a ventricular septal defect will tire easily. Answer B is incorrect because he will be small for his age. He will not need more calories, so answer C is incorrect. He will be susceptible to bacterial infection, but he will be no more susceptible to viral infections than other children, so answer D is incorrect.

193. Answer B is correct. A nonstress test determines periodic movement of the fetus. It does not determine lung maturity, show contractions, or measure neurological well-being, so answers A, C, and D are incorrect.

194. Answer C is correct. The monitor indicates variable decelerations caused by cord compression. If Pitocin is infusing, the nurse should turn off the Pitocin. Instructing the client to push is incorrect because pushing might increase the decelerations and because the client is 8cm dilated. Performing a vaginal exam should be done after turning off the Pitocin. Therefore, answers A, B, and D are incorrect.

195. Answer C is correct. The graft indicates ventricular tachycardia. The others are not noted on the ECG strip, so answers A, B, and D are incorrect.

196. **Answer B is correct.** Answer A is incorrect because Lovenox injections should be given in the abdomen. Answers C and D are incorrect because the client should not aspirate after the injection or clear the air from the syringe before injection.

197. **Answer B is correct.** Answer A is incorrect because Valium (diazepam) is not administered with other medications. Both medications can be given to the same client, so answer D is incorrect. Answer C is not necessary, therefore is incorrect.

198. **Answer B is correct.** Voiding every 3 hours prevents stagnant urine from collecting in the bladder, where bacteria can grow. Answer A is incorrect because douching is not recommended. Answer C is incorrect because obtaining a urinalysis monthly is not necessary. Answer D is incorrect because the client should practice wiping from front to back after voiding and bowel movements.

199. **Answer C is correct.** Of these clients, the one who should be assigned to the care of the nursing assistant is the client with dementia. An RN or the physician can place the client in seclusion, so answer A is incorrect. Answer B is incorrect because the nurse should empty the Foley catheter of the preeclamptic client because the client is unstable. Answer D is incorrect because a nurse or physical therapist should ambulate the client with a fractured hip.

200. **Answer A is correct.** The client who has recently had a thyroidectomy is at risk for tracheal edema. If the client experiences tracheal edema, the endotracheal tube or airway will not correct the problem, so answers C and D will not work. A padded tongue blade is used for seizures and is not used for the client with tracheal edema, so answer D is incorrect.

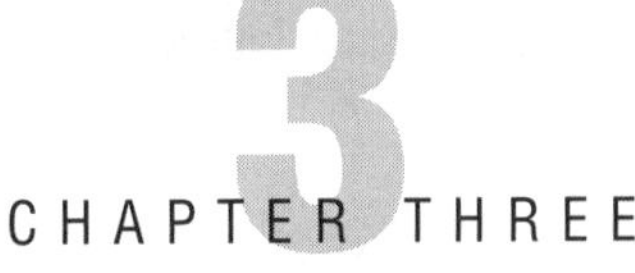

CHAPTER THREE

Practice Exam 3 and Rationales

Quick Check

1. A client hospitalized with severe depression and suicidal ideation refuses to talk with the nurse. The nurse recognizes that the suicidal client has difficulty:

Quick Answers: **187**
Detailed Answer: **190**

   - ❍ **A.** Expressing feelings of low self-worth
   - ❍ **B.** Discussing remorse and guilt for actions
   - ❍ **C.** Displaying dependence on others
   - ❍ **D.** Expressing anger toward others

2. A client receiving HydroDIURIL (hydrochlorothiazide) is instructed to increase her dietary intake of potassium. The best snack for the client requiring increased potassium is:

Quick Answers: **187**
Detailed Answer: **190**

   - ❍ **A.** Pear
   - ❍ **B.** Apple
   - ❍ **C.** Orange
   - ❍ **D.** Banana

3. The nurse is caring for a client following removal of the thyroid. Immediately post-op, the nurse should:

Quick Answers: **187**
Detailed Answer: **190**

   - ❍ **A.** Maintain the client in a semi-Fowler's position with the head and neck supported by pillows
   - ❍ **B.** Encourage the client to turn her head side to side, to promote drainage of oral secretions
   - ❍ **C.** Maintain the client in a supine position with sandbags placed on either side of the head and neck
   - ❍ **D.** Encourage the client to cough and breathe deeply every 2 hours, with the neck in a flexed position

Quick Check

4. A client hospitalized with chronic dyspepsia is diagnosed with gastric cancer. Which of the following is associated with an increased incidence of gastric cancer?

Quick Answers: **187**
Detailed Answer: **190**

❍ **A.** Dairy products
❍ **B.** Carbonated beverages
❍ **C.** Refined sugars
❍ **D.** Luncheon meats

5. A client is sent to the psychiatric unit for forensic evaluation after he is accused of arson. His tentative diagnosis is antisocial personality disorder. In reviewing the client's record, the nurse could expect to find:

Quick Answers: **187**
Detailed Answer: **190**

❍ **A.** A history of consistent employment
❍ **B.** A below-average intelligence
❍ **C.** A history of cruelty to animals
❍ **D.** An expression of remorse for his actions

6. The licensed vocational nurse may not assume the primary care for a client:

Quick Answers: **187**
Detailed Answer: **190**

❍ **A.** In the fourth stage of labor
❍ **B.** Two days post-appendectomy
❍ **C.** With a venous access device
❍ **D.** With bipolar disorder

7. The physician has ordered dressings with mafenide acetate (Sulfamylon) cream for a client with full-thickness burns of the hands and arms. Before dressing changes, the nurse should give priority to:

Quick Answers: **187**
Detailed Answer: **190**

❍ **A.** Administering pain medication
❍ **B.** Checking the adequacy of urinary output
❍ **C.** Requesting a daily complete blood count
❍ **D.** Obtaining a blood glucose by finger stick

8. The nurse is teaching a group of parents about gross motor development of the toddler. Which behavior is an example of the normal gross motor skill of a toddler?

Quick Answers: **187**
Detailed Answer: **190**

❍ **A.** She can pull a toy behind her.
❍ **B.** She can copy a horizontal line.
❍ **C.** She can build a tower of eight blocks.
❍ **D.** She can broad-jump.

Quick Check

9. A client hospitalized with a fractured mandible is to be discharged. Which piece of equipment should be kept on the client with a fractured mandible?

Quick Answers: 187
Detailed Answer: 190

- ❍ **A.** Wire cutters
- ❍ **B.** Oral airway
- ❍ **C.** Pliers
- ❍ **D.** Tracheostomy set

10. The nurse is to administer digoxin (Lanoxin) elixir to a 6-month-old with a congenital heart defect. The nurse auscultates an apical pulse rate of 100. The nurse should:

Quick Answers: 187
Detailed Answer: 190

- ❍ **A.** Record the heart rate and call the physician
- ❍ **B.** Record the heart rate and administer the medication
- ❍ **C.** Administer the medication and recheck the heart rate in 15 minutes
- ❍ **D.** Hold the medication and recheck the heart rate in 30 minutes

11. A mother of a 3-year-old hospitalized with lead poisoning asks the nurse to explain the treatment for her daughter. The nurse's explanation is based on the knowledge that lead poisoning is treated with:

Quick Answers: 187
Detailed Answer: 191

- ❍ **A.** Gastric lavage
- ❍ **B.** Chelating agents
- ❍ **C.** Antiemetics
- ❍ **D.** Activated charcoal

12. An 18-month-old is scheduled for a cleft palate repair. The usual type of restraints for the child with a cleft palate repair are:

Quick Answers: 187
Detailed Answer: 191

- ❍ **A.** Elbow restraints
- ❍ **B.** Full arm restraints
- ❍ **C.** Wrist restraints
- ❍ **D.** Mummy restraints

13. A client with glaucoma has been prescribed Timoptic (timolol) eyedrops. Timoptic should be used with caution in the client with a history of:

Quick Answers: 187
Detailed Answer: 191

- ❍ **A.** Diabetes
- ❍ **B.** Gastric ulcers
- ❍ **C.** Emphysema
- ❍ **D.** Pancreatitis

Quick Check

14. An elderly client who experiences nighttime confusion wanders from his room into the room of another client. The nurse can best help decrease the client's confusion by:

Quick Answers: **187**
Detailed Answer: **191**

❍ **A.** Assigning a nursing assistant to sit with him until he falls asleep

❍ **B.** Allowing the client to room with another elderly client

❍ **C.** Administering a bedtime sedative

❍ **D.** Leaving a nightlight on during the evening and night shifts

15. Which of the following is a common complaint of the client with end-stage renal failure?

Quick Answers: **187**
Detailed Answer: **191**

❍ **A.** Weight loss

❍ **B.** Itching

❍ **C.** Ringing in the ears

❍ **D.** Bruising

16. Which of the following medication orders needs further clarification?

Quick Answers: **187**
Detailed Answer: **191**

❍ **A.** Darvocet (propoxyphene) 65mg PO every 4–6 hrs. PRN

❍ **B.** Mysoline (primidone) 250mg PO TID

❍ **C.** Coumadin (warfarin sodium) 10mg PO

❍ **D.** Premarin (conjugated estrogen) .625mg PO daily

17. The best diet for the client with Meniere's syndrome is one that is:

Quick Answers: **187**
Detailed Answer: **191**

❍ **A.** High in fiber

❍ **B.** Low in sodium

❍ **C.** High in iodine

❍ **D.** Low in fiber

18. Which of the following findings is associated with right-sided heart failure?

Quick Answers: **187**
Detailed Answer: **191**

❍ **A.** Shortness of breath

❍ **B.** Nocturnal polyuria

❍ **C.** Daytime oliguria

❍ **D.** Crackles in the lungs

Quick Check

19. An 8-year-old admitted with an upper-respiratory infection has an order for O_2 saturation via pulse oximeter. To ensure an accurate reading, the nurse should:

- ❍ **A.** Place the probe on the child's abdomen
- ❍ **B.** Recalibrate the oximeter at the beginning of each shift
- ❍ **C.** Apply the probe and wait 15 minutes before obtaining a reading
- ❍ **D.** Place the probe on the child's finger

Quick Answers: **187**
Detailed Answer: **191**

20. An infant with Tetralogy of Fallot is discharged with a prescription for lanoxin elixir. The nurse should instruct the mother to:

- ❍ **A.** Administer the medication using a nipple
- ❍ **B.** Administer the medication using the calibrated dropper in the bottle
- ❍ **C.** Administer the medication using a plastic baby spoon
- ❍ **D.** Administer the medication in a baby bottle with 1oz. of water

Quick Answers: **187**
Detailed Answer: **191**

21. The client scheduled for electroconvulsive therapy tells the nurse, "I'm so afraid. What will happen to me during the treatment?" Which of the following statements is most therapeutic for the nurse to make?

- ❍ **A.** "You will be given medicine to relax you during the treatment."
- ❍ **B.** "The treatment will produce a controlled grand mal seizure."
- ❍ **C.** "The treatment might produce nausea and headache."
- ❍ **D.** "You can expect to be sleepy and confused for a time after the treatment."

Quick Answers: **187**
Detailed Answer: **191**

22. Which of the following skin lesions is associated with Lyme's disease?

- ❍ **A.** Bull's eye rash
- ❍ **B.** Papular crusts
- ❍ **C.** Bullae
- ❍ **D.** Plaques

Quick Answers: **187**
Detailed Answer: **191**

Quick Check

23. Which of the following snacks would be suitable for the child with gluten-induced enteropathy?

Quick Answers: **187**
Detailed Answer: **192**

- ❍ **A.** Soft oatmeal cookie
- ❍ **B.** Buttered popcorn
- ❍ **C.** Peanut butter and jelly sandwich
- ❍ **D.** Cheese pizza

24. A client with schizophrenia is receiving chlorpromazine (Thorazine) 400mg twice a day. An adverse side effect of the medication is:

Quick Answers: **187**
Detailed Answer: **192**

- ❍ **A.** Photosensitivity
- ❍ **B.** Elevated temperature
- ❍ **C.** Weight gain
- ❍ **D.** Elevated blood pressure

25. Which information should be given to the client taking phenytoin (Dilantin)?

Quick Answers: **187**
Detailed Answer: **192**

- ❍ **A.** Taking the medication with meals will increase its effectiveness.
- ❍ **B.** The medication can cause sleep disturbances.
- ❍ **C.** More frequent dental appointments will be needed for special gum care.
- ❍ **D.** The medication decreases the effects of oral contraceptives.

26. A client has returned to his room following an esophagoscopy. Before offering fluids, the nurse should give priority to assessing the client's:

Quick Answers: **187**
Detailed Answer: **192**

- ❍ **A.** Level of consciousness
- ❍ **B.** Gag reflex
- ❍ **C.** Urinary output
- ❍ **D.** Movement of extremities

27. Which instruction should be included in the discharge teaching for the client with cataract surgery?

Quick Answers: **187**
Detailed Answer: **192**

- ❍ **A.** Over-the-counter eyedrops can be used to treat redness and irritation.
- ❍ **B.** The eye shield should be worn at night.
- ❍ **C.** It will be necessary to wear special cataract glasses.
- ❍ **D.** A prescription for medication to control post-operative pain will be needed.

Quick Check

28. An 8-year-old is admitted with drooling, muffled phonation, and a temperature of 102°F. The nurse should immediately notify the doctor because the child's symptoms are suggestive of:

Quick Answers: **187**
Detailed Answer: **192**

❍ **A.** Strep throat
❍ **B.** Epiglottitis
❍ **C.** Laryngotracheobronchitis
❍ **D.** Bronchiolitis

29. Phototherapy is ordered for a newborn with physiologic jaundice. The nurse caring for the infant should:

Quick Answers: **187**
Detailed Answer: **192**

❍ **A.** Offer the baby sterile water between feedings of formula
❍ **B.** Apply an emollient to the baby's skin to prevent drying
❍ **C.** Wear a gown, gloves, and a mask while caring for the infant
❍ **D.** Place the baby on enteric isolation

30. A teen hospitalized with anorexia nervosa is now permitted to leave her room and eat in the dining room. Which of the following nursing interventions should be included in the client's plan of care?

Quick Answers: **187**
Detailed Answer: **192**

❍ **A.** Weighing the client after she eats
❍ **B.** Having a staff member remain with her for 1 hour after she eats
❍ **C.** Placing high-protein foods in the center of the client's plate
❍ **D.** Providing the client with child-size utensils

31. According to Erickson's stage of growth and development, the developmental task associated with middle childhood is:

Quick Answers: **187**
Detailed Answer: **192**

❍ **A.** Trust
❍ **B.** Initiative
❍ **C.** Independence
❍ **D.** Industry

32. The nurse should observe for side effects associated with the use of bronchodilators. A common side effect of bronchodilators is:

Quick Answers: **187**
Detailed Answer: **192**

❍ **A.** Tinnitus
❍ **B.** Nausea
❍ **C.** Ataxia
❍ **D.** Hypotension

Quick Check

33. The 5-minute Apgar of a baby delivered by C-section is recorded as 9. The most likely reason for this score is:

Quick Answers: 187
Detailed Answer: 193

❍ **A.** The mottled appearance of the trunk

❍ **B.** The presence of conjunctival hemorrhages

❍ **C.** Cyanosis of the hands and feet

❍ **D.** Respiratory rate of 20–28 per minute

34. A 5-month-old infant is admitted to the ER with a temperature of 103.6°F and irritability. The mother states that the child has been listless for the past several hours and that he had a seizure on the way to the hospital. A lumbar puncture confirms a diagnosis of bacterial meningitis. The nurse should assess the infant for:

Quick Answers: 187
Detailed Answer: 193

❍ **A.** Periorbital edema

❍ **B.** Tenseness of the anterior fontanel

❍ **C.** Positive Babinski reflex

❍ **D.** Negative scarf sign

35. A client with a bowel resection and anastamosis returns to his room with an NG tube attached to intermittent suction. Which of the following observations indicates that the nasogastric suction is working properly?

Quick Answers: 187
Detailed Answer: 193

❍ **A.** The client's abdomen is soft.

❍ **B.** The client is able to swallow.

❍ **C.** The client has active bowel sounds.

❍ **D.** The client's abdominal dressing is dry and intact.

36. The nurse is teaching the client with insulin-dependent diabetes the signs of hypoglycemia. Which of the following signs is associated with hypoglycemia?

Quick Answers: 187
Detailed Answer: 193

❍ **A.** Tremulousness

❍ **B.** Slow pulse

❍ **C.** Nausea

❍ **D.** Flushed skin

37. Which of the following symptoms is associated with exacerbation of multiple sclerosis?

Quick Answers: 187
Detailed Answer: 193

❍ **A.** Anorexia

❍ **B.** Seizures

❍ **C.** Diplopia

❍ **D.** Insomnia

Quick Check

38. Which of the following conditions is most likely related to the development of renal calculi?

Quick Answers: 187
Detailed Answer: 193

- A. Gout
- B. Pancreatitis
- C. Fractured femur
- D. Disc disease

39. A client with AIDS is admitted for treatment of wasting syndrome. Which of the following dietary modifications can be used to compensate for the limited absorptive capability of the intestinal tract?

Quick Answers: 187
Detailed Answer: 193

- A. Thoroughly cooking all foods
- B. Offering yogurt and buttermilk between meals
- C. Forcing fluids
- D. Providing small, frequent meals

40. The treatment protocol for a client with acute lymphocytic leukemia includes prednisone, methotrexate, and cimetadine. The purpose of the cimetadine is to:

Quick Answers: 187
Detailed Answer: 193

- A. Decrease the secretion of pancreatic enzymes
- B. Enhance the effectiveness of methotrexate
- C. Promote peristalsis
- D. Prevent a common side effect of prednisone

41. Which of the following meal choices is suitable for a 6-month-old infant?

Quick Answers: 187
Detailed Answer: 193

- A. Egg white, formula, and orange juice
- B. Apple juice, carrots, whole milk
- C. Rice cereal, apple juice, formula
- D. Melba toast, egg yolk, whole milk

42. The LPN is preparing to administer an injection of vitamin K to the newborn. The nurse should administer the injection in the:

Quick Answers: 187
Detailed Answer: 193

- A. Rectus femoris muscle
- B. Vastus lateralis muscle
- C. Deltoid muscle
- D. Dorsogluteal muscle

Quick Check

43. The physician has prescribed Cytoxan (cyclophosphamide) for a client with nephotic syndrome. The nurse should:

Quick Answers: **187**
Detailed Answer: **193**

- ❍ **A.** Encourage the client to drink extra fluids
- ❍ **B.** Request a low-protein diet for the client
- ❍ **C.** Bathe the client using only mild soap and water
- ❍ **D.** Provide additional warmth for swollen, inflamed joints

44. The nurse is caring for a client with detoxification from alcohol. Which medication is used in the treatment of alcohol withdrawal?

Quick Answers: **187**
Detailed Answer: **194**

- ❍ **A.** Antabuse (disulfiram)
- ❍ **B.** Romazicon (flumazenil)
- ❍ **C.** Dolophine (methodone)
- ❍ **D.** Ativan (lorazepam)

45. A client with insulin-dependent diabetes takes 20 units of NPH insulin at 7 a.m. The nurse should observe the client for signs of hypoglycemia at:

Quick Answers: **187**
Detailed Answer: **194**

- ❍ **A.** 8 a.m.
- ❍ **B.** 10 a.m.
- ❍ **C.** 3 p.m.
- ❍ **D.** 5 a.m.

46. The licensed practical nurse is assisting the charge nurse in planning care for a client with a detached retina. Which of the following nursing diagnoses should receive priority?

Quick Answers: **187**
Detailed Answer: **194**

- ❍ **A.** Alteration in comfort
- ❍ **B.** Alteration in mobility
- ❍ **C.** Alteration in skin integrity
- ❍ **D.** Alteration in O_2 perfusion

47. The primary purpose for using a CPM machine for the client with a total knee repair is to help:

Quick Answers: **187**
Detailed Answer: **194**

- ❍ **A.** Prevent contractures
- ❍ **B.** Promote flexion of the artificial joint
- ❍ **C.** Decrease the pain associated with early ambulation
- ❍ **D.** Alleviate lactic acid production in the leg muscles

Quick Check

48. Which of the following statements reflects Kohlberg's theory of the moral development of the preschool-age child?

Quick Answers: **187**
Detailed Answer: **194**

❍ **A.** Obeying adults is seen as correct behavior.

❍ **B.** Showing respect for parents is seen as important.

❍ **C.** Pleasing others is viewed as good behavior.

❍ **D.** Behavior is determined by consequences.

49. A toddler with otitis media has just completed antibiotic therapy. A recheck appointment should be made to:

Quick Answers: **187**
Detailed Answer: **194**

❍ **A.** Determine whether the ear infection has affected her hearing

❍ **B.** Make sure that she has taken all the antibiotic

❍ **C.** Document that the infection has completely cleared

❍ **D.** Obtain a new prescription in case the infection recurs

50. A factory worker is brought to the nurse's office after a metal fragment enters his right eye. The nurse should:

Quick Answers: **187**
Detailed Answer: **194**

❍ **A.** Cover the right eye with a sterile 4×4

❍ **B.** Attempt to remove the metal with a cotton-tipped applicator

❍ **C.** Flush the eye for 10 minutes with running water

❍ **D.** Cover both eyes and transport the client to the ER

51. The nurse is caring for a client with systemic lupus erythematosis (SLE). The major complication associated with systemic lupus erythematosis is:

Quick Answers: **187**
Detailed Answer: **194**

❍ **A.** Nephritis

❍ **B.** Cardiomegaly

❍ **C.** Desquamation

❍ **D.** Meningitis

52. Which diet is associated with an increased risk of colorectal cancer?

Quick Answers: **187**
Detailed Answer: **194**

❍ **A.** Low protein, complex carbohydrates

❍ **B.** High protein, simple carbohydrates

❍ **C.** High fat, refined carbohydrates

❍ **D.** Low carbohydrates, complex proteins

Quick Check

53. The nurse is caring for an infant following a cleft lip repair. While comforting the infant, the nurse should avoid:

 ❍ A. Holding the infant
 ❍ B. Offering a pacifier
 ❍ C. Providing a mobile
 ❍ D. Offering sterile water

Quick Answers: **187**
Detailed Answer: **194**

54. The physician has ordered Amoxil (amoxicillin) 500mg capsules for a client with esophageal varices. The nurse can best care for the client's needs by:

 ❍ A. Giving the medication as ordered
 ❍ B. Providing extra water with the medication
 ❍ C. Giving the medication with an antacid
 ❍ D. Requesting an alternate form of the medication

Quick Answers: **187**
Detailed Answer: **195**

55. The nurse is providing dietary instructions for a client with iron-deficiency anemia. Which food is a poor source of iron?

 ❍ A. Tomatoes
 ❍ B. Legumes
 ❍ C. Dried fruits
 ❍ D. Nuts

Quick Answers: **187**
Detailed Answer: **195**

56. The nurse is teaching a client with Parkinson's disease ways to prevent curvatures of the spine associated with the disease. To prevent spinal flexion, the nurse should tell the client to:

 ❍ A. Periodically lie prone without a neck pillow
 ❍ B. Sleep only in dorsal recumbent position
 ❍ C. Rest in supine position with his head elevated
 ❍ D. Sleep on either side but keep his back straight

Quick Answers: **187**
Detailed Answer: **195**

57. The nurse is planning dietary changes for a client following an episode of pancreatitis. Which diet is suitable for the client?

 ❍ A. Low calorie, low carbohydrate
 ❍ B. High calorie, low fat
 ❍ C. High protein, high fat
 ❍ D. Low protein, high carbohydrate

Quick Answers: **187**
Detailed Answer: **195**

Quick Check

58. A client with hypothyroidism frequently complains of feeling cold. The nurse should tell the client that she will be more comfortable if she:

Quick Answers: 187
Detailed Answer: 195

❍ **A.** Uses an electric blanket at night

❍ **B.** Dresses in extra layers of clothing

❍ **C.** Applies a heating pad to her feet

❍ **D.** Takes a hot bath morning and evening

59. A client has been hospitalized with a diagnosis of laryngeal cancer. Which factor is most significant in the development of laryngeal cancer?

Quick Answers: 187
Detailed Answer: 195

❍ **A.** A family history of laryngeal cancer

❍ **B.** Chronic inhalation of noxious fumes

❍ **C.** Frequent straining of the vocal cords

❍ **D.** A history of alcohol and tobacco use

60. The nurse is completing an assessment history of a client with pernicious anemia. Which complaint differentiates pernicious anemia from other types of anemia?

Quick Answers: 187
Detailed Answer: 195

❍ **A.** Difficulty in breathing after exertion

❍ **B.** Numbness and tingling in the extremities

❍ **C.** A faster-than-usual heart rate

❍ **D.** Feelings of lightheadedness

61. The chart of a client with schizophrenia states that the client has echolalia. The nurse can expect the client to:

Quick Answers: 187
Detailed Answer: 195

❍ **A.** Speak using words that rhyme

❍ **B.** Repeat words or phrases used by others

❍ **C.** Include irrelevant details in conversation

❍ **D.** Make up new words with new meanings

62. Which early morning activity helps to reduce the symptoms associated with rheumatoid arthritis?

Quick Answers: 187
Detailed Answer: 195

❍ **A.** Brushing the teeth

❍ **B.** Drinking a glass of juice

❍ **C.** Drinking a cup of coffee

❍ **D.** Brushing the hair

Quick Check

63. A newborn weighed 7 pounds at birth. At 6 months of age, the infant could be expected to weigh:

Quick Answers: **187**
Detailed Answer: **195**

- ❍ **A.** 14 pounds
- ❍ **B.** 18 pounds
- ❍ **C.** 25 pounds
- ❍ **D.** 30 pounds

64. A client with nontropical sprue has an exacerbation of symptoms. Which meal selection is responsible for the recurrence of the client's symptoms?

Quick Answers: **187**
Detailed Answer: **196**

- ❍ **A.** Tossed salad with oil and vinegar dressing
- ❍ **B.** Baked potato with sour cream and chives
- ❍ **C.** Cream of tomato soup and crackers
- ❍ **D.** Mixed fruit and yogurt

65. A client with congestive heart failure has been receiving Digoxin (lanoxin). Which finding indicates that the medication is having a desired effect?

Quick Answers: **187**
Detailed Answer: **196**

- ❍ **A.** Increased urinary output
- ❍ **B.** Stabilized weight
- ❍ **C.** Improved appetite
- ❍ **D.** Increased pedal edema

66. Which play activity is best suited to the gross motor skills of the toddler?

Quick Answers: **187**
Detailed Answer: **196**

- ❍ **A.** Coloring book and crayons
- ❍ **B.** Ball
- ❍ **C.** Building cubes
- ❍ **D.** Swing set

67. The physician has ordered Basalgel (aluminum carbonate gel) for a client with recurrent indigestion. The nurse should teach the client common side effects of the medication, which include:

Quick Answers: **187**
Detailed Answer: **196**

- ❍ **A.** Constipation
- ❍ **B.** Urinary retention
- ❍ **C.** Diarrhea
- ❍ **D.** Confusion

Quick Check

68. A client is admitted with suspected abdominal aortic aneurysm (AAA). A common complaint of the client with an abdominal aortic aneurysm is:

Quick Answers: **187**
Detailed Answer: **196**

❍ **A.** Loss of sensation in the lower extremities
❍ **B.** Back pain that lessens when standing
❍ **C.** Decreased urinary output
❍ **D.** Pulsations in the periumbilical area

69. A client is admitted with acute adrenal crisis. During the intake assessment, the nurse can expect to find that the client has:

Quick Answers: **187**
Detailed Answer: **196**

❍ **A.** Low blood pressure
❍ **B.** Slow, regular pulse
❍ **C.** Warm, flushed skin
❍ **D.** Increased urination

70. An elderly client is hospitalized for a transurethral prostatectomy. Which finding should be reported to the doctor immediately?

Quick Answers: **187**
Detailed Answer: **196**

❍ **A.** Hourly urinary output of 40–50cc
❍ **B.** Bright red urine with many clots
❍ **C.** Dark red urine with few clots
❍ **D.** Requests for pain med q 4 hrs.

71. A 9-year-old is admitted with suspected rheumatic fever. Which finding is suggestive of polymigratory arthritis?

Quick Answers: **187**
Detailed Answer: **196**

❍ **A.** Irregular movements of the extremities and facial grimacing
❍ **B.** Painless swelling over the extensor surfaces of the joints
❍ **C.** Faint areas of red demarcation over the back and abdomen
❍ **D.** Swelling, inflammation, and effusion of the joints

72. A child with croup is placed in a cool, high-humidity tent connected to room air. The primary purpose of the tent is to:

Quick Answers: **187**
Detailed Answer: **196**

❍ **A.** Prevent insensible water loss
❍ **B.** Provide a moist environment with oxygen at 30%
❍ **C.** Prevent dehydration and reduce fever
❍ **D.** Liquefy secretions and relieve laryngeal spasm

Quick Check

73. A client is admitted with a diagnosis of hypothyroidism. An initial assessment of the client would reveal:

Quick Answers: **187**
Detailed Answer: **196**

❍ **A.** Slow pulse rate, weight loss, diarrhea, and cardiac failure

❍ **B.** Weight gain, lethargy, slowed speech, and decreased respiratory rate

❍ **C.** Rapid pulse, constipation, and bulging eyes

❍ **D.** Decreased body temperature, weight loss, and increased respirations

74. Which statement describes the contagious stage of varicella?

Quick Answers: **187**
Detailed Answer: **197**

❍ **A.** The contagious stage is 1 day before the onset of the rash until the appearance of vesicles.

❍ **B.** The contagious stage lasts during the vesicular and crusting stages of the lesions.

❍ **C.** The contagious stage is from the onset of the rash until the rash disappears.

❍ **D.** The contagious stage is 1 day before the onset of the rash until all the lesions are crusted.

75. A client admitted to the psychiatric unit claims to be the Son of God and insists that he will not be kept away from his followers. The most likely explanation for the client's delusion is:

Quick Answers: **187**
Detailed Answer: **197**

❍ **A.** A religious experience

❍ **B.** A stressful event

❍ **C.** Low self-esteem

❍ **D.** Overwhelming anxiety

76. The nurse is caring for an 8-year-old following a routine tonsillectomy. Which finding should be reported immediately?

Quick Answers: **187**
Detailed Answer: **197**

❍ **A.** Reluctance to swallow

❍ **B.** Drooling of blood-tinged saliva

❍ **C.** An axillary temperature of 99°F

❍ **D.** Respiratory stridor

Quick Check

77. The nurse is admitting a client with a suspected duodenal ulcer. The client will most likely report that his abdominal discomfort lessens when he:

Quick Answers: 187
Detailed Answer: 197

- ❍ **A.** Skips a meal
- ❍ **B.** Rests in recumbent position
- ❍ **C.** Eats a meal
- ❍ **D.** Sits upright after eating

78. Which of the following meal selections is appropriate for the client with celiac disease?

Quick Answers: 187
Detailed Answer: 197

- ❍ **A.** Toast, jam, and apple juice
- ❍ **B.** Peanut butter cookies and milk
- ❍ **C.** Rice Krispies bar and milk
- ❍ **D.** Cheese pizza and Kool-Aid

79. A client with hyperthyroidism is taking lithium carbonate to inhibit thyroid hormone release. Which complaint by the client should alert the nurse to a problem with the client's medication?

Quick Answers: 187
Detailed Answer: 197

- ❍ **A.** The client complains of blurred vision.
- ❍ **B.** The client complains of increased thirst and increased urination.
- ❍ **C.** The client complains of increased weight gain over the past year.
- ❍ **D.** The client complains of changes in taste.

80. A 2-month-old infant has just received her first Tetramune injection. The nurse should tell the mother that the immunization:

Quick Answers: 187
Detailed Answer: 197

- ❍ **A.** Will need to be repeated when the child is 4 years of age
- ❍ **B.** Is given to determine whether the child is susceptible to pertussis
- ❍ **C.** Is one of a series of injections that protects against dpt and Hib
- ❍ **D.** Is a one-time injection that protects against MMR and varicella

Quick Check

81. The nurse is caring for a client hospitalized with bipolar disorder, manic phase. Which of the following snacks would be best for the client with mania?

- ❍ **A.** Potato chips
- ❍ **B.** Diet cola
- ❍ **C.** Apple
- ❍ **D.** Milkshake

Quick Answers: **187**
Detailed Answer: **197**

82. A 2-year-old is hospitalized with suspected intussusception. Which finding is associated with intussusception?

- ❍ **A.** "Currant jelly" stools
- ❍ **B.** Projectile vomiting
- ❍ **C.** "Ribbonlike" stools
- ❍ **D.** Palpable mass over the flank

Quick Answers: **187**
Detailed Answer: **197**

83. A client is being treated for cancer with linear acceleration radiation. The physician has marked the radiation site with a blue marking pen. The nurse should:

- ❍ **A.** Remove the unsightly markings with acetone or alcohol
- ❍ **B.** Cover the radiation site with loose gauze dressing
- ❍ **C.** Sprinkle baby powder over the radiated area
- ❍ **D.** Refrain from using soap or lotion on the marked area

Quick Answers: **187**
Detailed Answer: **197**

84. The nurse is caring for a client with acromegaly. Following a transphenoidal hypophysectomy, the nurse should:

- ❍ **A.** Monitor the client's blood sugar
- ❍ **B.** Suction the mouth and pharynx every hour
- ❍ **C.** Place the client in low Trendelenburg position
- ❍ **D.** Encourage the client to cough

Quick Answers: **187**
Detailed Answer: **197**

85. A client newly diagnosed with diabetes is started on Precose (acarbose). The nurse should tell the client that the medication should be taken:

- ❍ **A.** 1 hour before meals
- ❍ **B.** 30 minutes after meals
- ❍ **C.** With the first bite of a meal
- ❍ **D.** Daily at bedtime

Quick Answers: **187**
Detailed Answer: **198**

Quick Check

86. A client with a deep decubitus ulcer is receiving therapy in the hyperbaric oxygen chamber. Before therapy, the nurse should:

Quick Answers: **187**
Detailed Answer: **198**

- ❍ **A.** Apply a lanolin-based lotion to the skin
- ❍ **B.** Wash the skin with water and pat dry
- ❍ **C.** Cover the area with a petroleum gauze
- ❍ **D.** Apply an occlusive dressing to the site

87. A client with a laryngectomy returns from surgery with a nasogastric tube in place. The primary reason for placement of the nasogastric tube is to:

Quick Answers: **187**
Detailed Answer: **198**

- ❍ **A.** Prevent swelling and dysphagia
- ❍ **B.** Decompress the stomach via suction
- ❍ **C.** Prevent contamination of the suture line
- ❍ **D.** Promote healing of the oral mucosa

88. The chart indicates that a client has expressive aphasia following a stroke. The nurse understands that the client will have difficulty with:

Quick Answers: **188**
Detailed Answer: **198**

- ❍ **A.** Speaking and writing
- ❍ **B.** Comprehending spoken words
- ❍ **C.** Carrying out purposeful motor activity
- ❍ **D.** Recognizing and using an object correctly

89. A camp nurse is applying sunscreen to a group of children enrolled in swim classes. Chemical sunscreens are most effective when applied:

Quick Answers: **188**
Detailed Answer: **198**

- ❍ **A.** Just before sun exposure
- ❍ **B.** 5 minutes before sun exposure
- ❍ **C.** 15 minutes before sun exposure
- ❍ **D.** 30 minutes before sun exposure

90. A post-operative client has an order for Demerol (meperidine) 75mg and Phenergan (promethazine) 25mg IM every 3–4 hours as needed for pain. The combination of the two medications produces a/an:

Quick Answers: **188**
Detailed Answer: **198**

- ❍ **A.** Agonist effect
- ❍ **B.** Synergistic effect
- ❍ **C.** Antagonist effect
- ❍ **D.** Excitatory effect

Quick Check

91. Before administering a client's morning dose of Lanoxin (digoxin), the nurse checks the apical pulse rate and finds a rate of 54. The appropriate nursing intervention is to:

Quick Answers: **188**
Detailed Answer: **198**

❍ **A.** Record the pulse rate and administer the medication

❍ **B.** Administer the medication and monitor the heart rate

❍ **C.** Withhold the medication and notify the doctor

❍ **D.** Withhold the medication until the heart rate increases

92. What information should the nurse give a new mother regarding the introduction of solid foods for her infant?

Quick Answers: **188**
Detailed Answer: **198**

❍ **A.** Solid foods should not be given until the extrusion reflex disappears, at 8–10 months of age.

❍ **B.** Solid foods should be introduced one at a time, with 4- to 7-day intervals.

❍ **C.** Solid foods can be mixed in a bottle or infant feeder to make feeding easier.

❍ **D.** Solid foods should begin with fruits and vegetables.

93. A client with schizophrenia is started on Zyprexa (olanzapine). Three weeks later, the client develops severe muscle rigidity and elevated temperature. The nurse should give priority to:

Quick Answers: **188**
Detailed Answer: **198**

❍ **A.** Withholding all morning medications

❍ **B.** Ordering a CBC and CPK

❍ **C.** Administering prescribed anti-Parkinsonian medication

❍ **D.** Transferring the client to a medical unit

94. A client with human immunodeficiency syndrome has gastrointestinal symptoms, including diarrhea. The nurse should teach the client to avoid:

Quick Answers: **188**
Detailed Answer: **198**

❍ **A.** Calcium-rich foods

❍ **B.** Canned or frozen vegetables

❍ **C.** Processed meat

❍ **D.** Raw fruits and vegetables

95. A 4-year-old is admitted with acute leukemia. It will be most important to monitor the child for:

Quick Answers: **188**
Detailed Answer: **199**

❍ **A.** Abdominal pain and anorexia

❍ **B.** Fatigue and bruising

❍ **C.** Bleeding and pallor

❍ **D.** Petechiae and mucosal ulcers

Quick Check

96. A 5-month-old is diagnosed with atopic dermatitis. Nursing interventions will focus on:

- ❍ **A.** Preventing infection
- ❍ **B.** Administering antipyretics
- ❍ **C.** Keeping the skin free of moisture
- ❍ **D.** Limiting oral fluid intake

Quick Answers: **188**
Detailed Answer: **199**

97. The nurse is caring for a client with a history of diverticulitis. The client complains of abdominal pain, fever, and diarrhea. Which food was responsible for the client's symptoms?

- ❍ **A.** Mashed potatoes
- ❍ **B.** Steamed carrots
- ❍ **C.** Baked fish
- ❍ **D.** Whole-grain cereal

Quick Answers: **188**
Detailed Answer: **199**

98. The physician has scheduled a Whipple procedure for a client with pancreatic cancer. The nurse recognizes that the client's cancer is located in:

- ❍ **A.** The tail of the pancreas
- ❍ **B.** The head of the pancreas
- ❍ **C.** The body of the pancreas
- ❍ **D.** The entire pancreas

Quick Answers: **188**
Detailed Answer: **199**

99. A child with cystic fibrosis is being treated with inhalation therapy with Pulmozyme (dornase alfa). A side effect of the medication is:

- ❍ **A.** Weight gain
- ❍ **B.** Hair loss
- ❍ **C.** Sore throat
- ❍ **D.** Brittle nails

Quick Answers: **188**
Detailed Answer: **199**

100. The doctor has ordered Percocet (oxycodone) for a client following abdominal surgery. The primary objective of nursing care for the client receiving an opiate analgesic is to:

- ❍ **A.** Prevent addiction
- ❍ **B.** Alleviate pain
- ❍ **C.** Facilitate mobility
- ❍ **D.** Prevent nausea

Quick Answers: **188**
Detailed Answer: **199**

Quick Check

101. Which finding is the best indication that a client with ineffective airway clearance needs suctioning?

❍ **A.** Oxygen saturation
❍ **B.** Respiratory rate
❍ **C.** Breath sounds
❍ **D.** Arterial blood gases

Quick Answers: **188**
Detailed Answer: **199**

102. A client with tuberculosis has a prescription for Myambutol (ethambutol HCl). The nurse should tell the client to notify the doctor immediately if he notices:

❍ **A.** Gastric distress
❍ **B.** Changes in hearing
❍ **C.** Red discoloration of bodily fluids
❍ **D.** Changes in color vision

Quick Answers: **188**
Detailed Answer: **199**

103. The primary cause of anemia in a client with chronic renal failure is:

❍ **A.** Poor iron absorption
❍ **B.** Destruction of red blood cells
❍ **C.** Lack of intrinsic factor
❍ **D.** Insufficient erythropoietin

Quick Answers: **188**
Detailed Answer: **199**

104. Which of the following nursing interventions has the highest priority for the client scheduled for an intravenous pyelogram?

❍ **A.** Providing the client with a favorite meal for dinner
❍ **B.** Asking if the client has allergies to shellfish
❍ **C.** Encouraging fluids the evening before the test
❍ **D.** Telling the client what to expect during the test

Quick Answers: **188**
Detailed Answer: **199**

105. The doctor has prescribed aspirin 325mg daily for a client with transient ischemic attacks. The nurse knows that aspirin was prescribed to:

❍ **A.** Prevent headaches
❍ **B.** Boost coagulation
❍ **C.** Prevent cerebral anoxia
❍ **D.** Keep platelets from clumping together

Quick Answers: **188**
Detailed Answer: **199**

Quick Check

106. A client with tuberculosis who has been receiving combined therapy with INH and Rifampin asks the nurse how long he will have to take medication. The nurse should tell the client that:

Quick Answers: **188**
Detailed Answer: **199**

❍ **A.** Medication is rarely needed after 2 weeks.

❍ **B.** He will need to take medication the rest of his life.

❍ **C.** The course of combined therapy is usually 6 months.

❍ **D.** He will be re-evaluated in 1 month to see if further medication is needed.

107. Which development milestone puts the 4-month-old infant at greatest risk for injury?

Quick Answers: **188**
Detailed Answer: **199**

❍ **A.** Switching objects from one hand to another

❍ **B.** Crawling

❍ **C.** Standing

❍ **D.** Rolling over

108. A client taking Dilantin (phenytoin) for tonic-clonic seizures is preparing for discharge. Which information should be included in the client's discharge care plan?

Quick Answers: **188**
Detailed Answer: **200**

❍ **A.** The medication can cause dental staining.

❍ **B.** The client will need to avoid a high-carbohydrate diet.

❍ **C.** The client will need a regularly scheduled CBC.

❍ **D.** The medication can cause problems with drowsiness.

109. Assessment of a newborn male reveals that the infant has hypospadias. The nurse knows that:

Quick Answers: **188**
Detailed Answer: **200**

❍ **A.** The infant should not be circumcised.

❍ **B.** Surgical correction will be done by 6 months of age.

❍ **C.** Surgical correction is delayed until 6 years of age.

❍ **D.** The infant should be circumcised to facilitate voiding.

110. The nurse is providing dietary teaching for a client with elevated cholesterol levels. Which cooking oil is not suggested for the client on a low-cholesterol diet?

Quick Answers: **188**
Detailed Answer: **200**

❍ **A.** Safflower oil

❍ **B.** Sunflower oil

❍ **C.** Coconut oil

❍ **D.** Canola oil

Quick Check

111. The nurse is caring for a client with stage III Alzheimer's disease. A characteristic of this stage is:

- ❍ **A.** Memory loss
- ❍ **B.** Failing to recognize familiar objects
- ❍ **C.** Wandering at night
- ❍ **D.** Failing to communicate

Quick Answers: **188**
Detailed Answer: **200**

112. The doctor has prescribed Cortone (cortisone) for a client with systemic lupus erythematosis. Which instruction should be given to the client?

- ❍ **A.** Take the medication 30 minutes before eating.
- ❍ **B.** Report changes in appetite and weight.
- ❍ **C.** Wear sunglasses to prevent cataracts.
- ❍ **D.** Schedule a time to take the influenza vaccine.

Quick Answers: **188**
Detailed Answer: **200**

113. The nurse is caring for a client with an above-the-knee amputation (AKA). To prevent contractures, the nurse should:

- ❍ **A.** Place the client in a prone position 15–30 minutes twice a day
- ❍ **B.** Keep the foot of the bed elevated on shock blocks
- ❍ **C.** Place trochanter rolls on either side of the affected leg
- ❍ **D.** Keep the client's leg elevated on two pillows

Quick Answers: **188**
Detailed Answer: **200**

114. The mother of a 6-month-old asks when her child will have all his baby teeth. The nurse knows that most children have all their primary teeth by age:

- ❍ **A.** 12 months
- ❍ **B.** 18 months
- ❍ **C.** 24 months
- ❍ **D.** 30 months

Quick Answers: **188**
Detailed Answer: **200**

115. While caring for a client with cervical cancer, the nurse notes that the radioactive implant is lying in the bed. The nurse should:

- ❍ **A.** Place the implant in a biohazard bag and return it to the lab
- ❍ **B.** Give the client a pair of gloves and ask her to reinsert the implant
- ❍ **C.** Use tongs to pick up the implant and return it to a lead-lined container
- ❍ **D.** Discard the implant in the commode and double-flush

Quick Answers: **188**
Detailed Answer: **200**

Quick Check

116. The nurse is preparing to discharge a client following a laparoscopic cholecystectomy. The nurse should:

Quick Answers: 188
Detailed Answer: 200

- ❍ **A.** Tell the client to avoid a tub bath for 5 to 7 days
- ❍ **B.** Tell the client to expect clay-colored stools
- ❍ **C.** Tell the client that she can expect lower abdominal pain for the next week
- ❍ **D.** Tell the client that she can resume a regular diet immediately

117. A high school student returns to school following a 3-week absence due to mononucleosis. The school nurse knows it will be important for the client:

Quick Answers: 188
Detailed Answer: 200

- ❍ **A.** To drink additional fluids throughout the day
- ❍ **B.** To avoid contact sports for 1–2 months
- ❍ **C.** To have a snack twice a day to prevent hypoglycemia
- ❍ **D.** To continue antibiotic therapy for 6 months

118. A 6-year-old with cystic fibrosis has an order for pancreatic replacement. The nurse knows that the medication will be given:

Quick Answers: 188
Detailed Answer: 201

- ❍ **A.** At bedtime
- ❍ **B.** With meals and snacks
- ❍ **C.** Twice daily
- ❍ **D.** Daily in the morning

119. The doctor has prescribed a diet high in vitamin B12 for a client with pernicious anemia. Which foods are highest in B12?

Quick Answers: 188
Detailed Answer: 201

- ❍ **A.** Meat, eggs, dairy products
- ❍ **B.** Peanut butter, raisins, molasses
- ❍ **C.** Broccoli, cauliflower, cabbage
- ❍ **D.** Shrimp, legumes, bran cereals

120. A client with hypertension has begun an aerobic exercise program. The nurse should tell the client that the recommended exercise regimen should begin slowly and build up to:

Quick Answers: 188
Detailed Answer: 201

- ❍ **A.** 20–30 minutes three times a week
- ❍ **B.** 45 minutes two times a week
- ❍ **C.** 1 hour four times a week
- ❍ **D.** 1 hour two times a week

Quick Check

121. A client with breast cancer is returned to the room following a right total mastectomy. The nurse should:

- ❍ **A.** Elevate the client's right arm on pillows
- ❍ **B.** Place the client's right arm in a dependent sling
- ❍ **C.** Keep the client's right arm on the bed beside her
- ❍ **D.** Place the client's right arm across her body

Quick Answers: **188**
Detailed Answer: **201**

122. A neurological consult has been ordered for a pediatric client with suspected absence seizures. The client with absence seizures can be expected to have:

- ❍ **A.** Short, abrupt muscle contraction
- ❍ **B.** Quick, bilateral severe jerking movements
- ❍ **C.** Abrupt loss of muscle tone
- ❍ **D.** A brief lapse in consciousness

Quick Answers: **188**
Detailed Answer: **201**

123. A client with schizoaffective disorder is exhibiting Parkinsonian symptoms. Which medication is responsible for the development of Parkinsonian symptoms?

- ❍ **A.** Zyprexa (olanzapine)
- ❍ **B.** Cogentin (benzatropine mesylate)
- ❍ **C.** Benadryl (diphenhydramine)
- ❍ **D.** Depakote (divalproex sodium)

Quick Answers: **188**
Detailed Answer: **201**

124. Which activity is best suited to the 12-year-old with juvenile rheumatoid arthritis?

- ❍ **A.** Playing video games
- ❍ **B.** Swimming
- ❍ **C.** Working crossword puzzles
- ❍ **D.** Playing slow-pitch softball

Quick Answers: **188**
Detailed Answer: **201**

125. The glycosylated hemoglobin of a 40-year-old client with diabetes mellitus is 2.5%. The nurse understands that:

- ❍ **A.** The client can have a higher-calorie diet.
- ❍ **B.** The client has good control of her diabetes.
- ❍ **C.** The client requires adjustment in her insulin dose.
- ❍ **D.** The client has poor control of her diabetes.

Quick Answers: **188**
Detailed Answer: **201**

Quick Check

126. The physician has ordered Stadol (butorphanol) for a postoperative client. The nurse knows that the medication is having its intended effect if the client:

Quick Answers: **188**
Detailed Answer: **201**

- ❍ **A.** Is asleep 30 minutes after the injection
- ❍ **B.** Asks for extra servings on his meal tray
- ❍ **C.** Has an increased urinary output
- ❍ **D.** States that he is feeling less nauseated

127. The mother of a child with cystic fibrosis tells the nurse that her child makes "snoring" sounds when breathing. The nurse is aware that many children with cystic fibrosis have:

Quick Answers: **188**
Detailed Answer: **202**

- ❍ **A.** Choanal atresia
- ❍ **B.** Nasal polyps
- ❍ **C.** Septal deviations
- ❍ **D.** Enlarged adenoids

128. A client is hospitalized with hepatitis A. Which of the client's regular medications is contraindicated due to the current illness?

Quick Answers: **188**
Detailed Answer: **202**

- ❍ **A.** Prilosec (omeprazole)
- ❍ **B.** Synthroid (levothyroxine)
- ❍ **C.** Premarin (conjugated estrogens)
- ❍ **D.** Lipitor (atorvastatin)

129. The nurse has been teaching the role of diet in regulating blood pressure to a client with hypertension. Which meal selection indicates that the client understands his new diet?

Quick Answers: **188**
Detailed Answer: **202**

- ❍ **A.** Cornflakes, whole milk, banana, and coffee
- ❍ **B.** Scrambled eggs, bacon, toast, and coffee
- ❍ **C.** Oatmeal, apple juice, dry toast, and coffee
- ❍ **D.** Pancakes, ham, tomato juice, and coffee

130. An 18-month-old is being discharged following hypospadias repair. Which instruction should be included in the nurse's discharge teaching?

Quick Answers: **188**
Detailed Answer: **202**

- ❍ **A.** The child should not play on his rocking horse.
- ❍ **B.** Applying warm compresses to decrease pain.
- ❍ **C.** Diapering should be avoided for 1–2 weeks.
- ❍ **D.** The child will need a special diet to promote healing.

Quick Check

131. An obstetrical client calls the clinic with complaints of morning sickness. The nurse should tell the client to:

Quick Answers: **188**
Detailed Answer: **202**

❍ **A.** Keep crackers at the bedside for eating before she arises

❍ **B.** Drink a glass of whole milk before going to sleep at night

❍ **C.** Skip breakfast but eat a larger lunch and dinner

❍ **D.** Drink a glass of orange juice after adding a couple of teaspoons of sugar

132. The nurse has taken the blood pressure of a client hospitalized with methicillin-resistant staphylococcus aureus. Which action by the nurse indicates an understanding regarding the care of clients with MRSA?

Quick Answers: **188**
Detailed Answer: **202**

❍ **A.** The nurse leaves the stethoscope in the client's room for future use.

❍ **B.** The nurse cleans the stethoscope with alcohol and returns it to the exam room.

❍ **C.** The nurse uses the stethoscope to assess the blood pressure of other assigned clients.

❍ **D.** The nurse cleans the stethoscope with water, dries it, and returns it to the nurse's station.

133. The physician has discussed the need for medication with the parents of an infant with congenital hypothyroidism. The nurse can reinforce the physician's teaching by telling the parents that:

Quick Answers: **188**
Detailed Answer: **202**

❍ **A.** The medication will be needed only during times of rapid growth.

❍ **B.** The medication will be needed throughout the child's lifetime.

❍ **C.** The medication schedule can be arranged to allow for drug holidays.

❍ **D.** The medication is given one time daily every other day.

134. A client with diabetes mellitus has a prescription for Glucotrol XL (glipizide). The client should be instructed to take the medication:

Quick Answers: **188**
Detailed Answer: **202**

❍ **A.** At bedtime

❍ **B.** With breakfast

❍ **C.** Before lunch

❍ **D.** After dinner

Quick Check

135. The nurse is caring for a client admitted with suspected myasthenia gravis. Which finding is usually associated with a diagnosis of myasthenia gravis?

Quick Answers: 188
Detailed Answer: 202

❍ **A.** Visual disturbances, including diplopia
❍ **B.** Ascending paralysis and loss of motor function
❍ **C.** Cogwheel rigidity and loss of coordination
❍ **D.** Progressive weakness that is worse at the day's end

136. The nurse is teaching the parents of an infant with osteogenesis imperfecta. The nurse should tell the parents:

Quick Answers: 188
Detailed Answer: 202

❍ **A.** That the infant will need daily calcium supplements
❍ **B.** To lift the infant by the buttocks when diapering
❍ **C.** That the condition is a temporary one
❍ **D.** That only the bones are affected by the disease

137. Physician's orders for a client with acute pancreatitis include the following: strict NPO, NG tube to low intermittent suction. The nurse recognizes that these interventions will:

Quick Answers: 188
Detailed Answer: 203

❍ **A.** Reduce the secretion of pancreatic enzymes
❍ **B.** Decrease the client's need for insulin
❍ **C.** Prevent secretion of gastric acid
❍ **D.** Eliminate the need for analgesia

138. A client with diverticulitis is admitted with nausea, vomiting, and dehydration. Which finding suggests a complication of diverticulitis?

Quick Answers: 188
Detailed Answer: 203

❍ **A.** Pain in the left lower quadrant
❍ **B.** Boardlike abdomen
❍ **C.** Low-grade fever
❍ **D.** Abdominal distention

139. The diagnostic work-up of a client hospitalized with complaints of progressive weakness and fatigue confirms a diagnosis of myasthenia gravis. The medication used to treat myasthenia gravis is:

Quick Answers: 188
Detailed Answer: 203

❍ **A.** Prostigmin (neostigmine)
❍ **B.** Atropine (atropine sulfate)
❍ **C.** Didronel (etidronate)
❍ **D.** Tensilon (edrophonium)

Quick Check

140. A client with AIDS complains of a weight loss of 20 pounds in the past month. Which diet is suggested for the client with AIDS?

Quick Answers: **188**
Detailed Answer: **203**

- ❍ **A.** High calorie, high protein, high fat
- ❍ **B.** High calorie, high carbohydrate, low protein
- ❍ **C.** High calorie, low carbohydrate, high fat
- ❍ **D.** High calorie, high protein, low fat

141. The nurse is caring for a 4-year-old with cerebral palsy. Which nursing intervention will help ready the child for rehabilitative services?

Quick Answers: **188**
Detailed Answer: **203**

- ❍ **A.** Patching one of the eyes to strengthen the muscles
- ❍ **B.** Providing suckers and pinwheels to help strengthen tongue movement
- ❍ **C.** Providing musical tapes to provide auditory training
- ❍ **D.** Encouraging play with a video game to improve muscle coordination

142. At the 6-week check-up, the mother asks when she can expect the baby to sleep all night. The nurse should tell the mother that most infants begin to sleep all night by age:

Quick Answers: **188**
Detailed Answer: **203**

- ❍ **A.** 1 month
- ❍ **B.** 2 months
- ❍ **C.** 3–4 months
- ❍ **D.** 5–6 months

143. Which of the following pediatric clients is at greatest risk for latex allergy?

Quick Answers: **188**
Detailed Answer: **203**

- ❍ **A.** The child with a myelomeningocele
- ❍ **B.** The child with epispadias
- ❍ **C.** The child with coxa plana
- ❍ **D.** The child with rheumatic fever

144. The nurse is teaching the mother of a child with cystic fibrosis how to do chest percussion. The nurse should tell the mother to:

Quick Answers: **188**
Detailed Answer: **203**

- ❍ **A.** Use the heel of her hand during percussion
- ❍ **B.** Change the child's position every 20 minutes
- ❍ **C.** Do percussion after the child eats and at bedtime
- ❍ **D.** Use cupped hands during percussion

Quick Check

145. The nurse calculates the amount of an antibiotic for injection to be given to an infant. The amount of medication to be administered is 1.25mL. The nurse should:

Quick Answers: **188**
Detailed Answer: **203**

❍ **A.** Divide the amount into two injections and administer in each vastus lateralis muscle

❍ **B.** Give the medication in one injection in the dorsogluteal muscle

❍ **C.** Divide the amount in two injections and give one in the ventrogluteal muscle and one in the vastus lateralis muscle

❍ **D.** Give the medication in one injection in the ventrogluteal muscle

146. A client with schizophrenia is receiving depot injections of Haldol Deconate (haloperidol decanoate). The client should be told to return for his next injection in:

Quick Answers: **188**
Detailed Answer: **203**

❍ **A.** 1 week

❍ **B.** 2 weeks

❍ **C.** 4 weeks

❍ **D.** 6 weeks

147. A 3-year-old is immobilized in a hip spica cast. Which discharge instruction should be given to the parents?

Quick Answers: **188**
Detailed Answer: **204**

❍ **A.** Keep the bed flat, with a small pillow beneath the cast

❍ **B.** Provide crayons and a coloring book for play activity

❍ **C.** Increase her intake of high-calorie foods for healing

❍ **D.** Tuck a disposable diaper beneath the cast at the perineal opening

148. The nurse is caring for a client following the reimplantation of the thumb and index finger. Which finding should be reported to the physician immediately?

Quick Answers: **188**
Detailed Answer: **204**

❍ **A.** Temperature of 100°F

❍ **B.** Coolness and discoloration of the digits

❍ **C.** Complaints of pain

❍ **D.** Difficulty moving the digits

Quick Check

149. When assessing the urinary output of a client who has had extracorporeal lithotripsy, the nurse can expect to find:

Quick Answers: **188**
Detailed Answer: **204**

- ❍ **A.** Cherry-red urine that gradually becomes clearer
- ❍ **B.** Orange-tinged urine containing particles of calculi
- ❍ **C.** Dark red urine that becomes cloudy in appearance
- ❍ **D.** Dark, smoky-colored urine with high specific gravity

150. The physician has prescribed Cognex (tacrine) for a client with dementia. The nurse should monitor the client for adverse reactions, which include:

Quick Answers: **188**
Detailed Answer: **204**

- ❍ **A.** Hypoglycemia
- ❍ **B.** Jaundice
- ❍ **C.** Urinary retention
- ❍ **D.** Tinnitus

151. The physician has ordered a low-potassium diet for a child with acute glomerulonephritis. Which snack is suitable for the child with potassium restrictions?

Quick Answers: **188**
Detailed Answer: **204**

- ❍ **A.** Raisins
- ❍ **B.** Oranges
- ❍ **C.** Apricots
- ❍ **D.** Bananas

152. The physician has ordered a blood test for *H. pylori.* The nurse should prepare the client by:

Quick Answers: **188**
Detailed Answer: **204**

- ❍ **A.** Withholding intake after midnight
- ❍ **B.** Telling the client that no special preparation is needed
- ❍ **C.** Explaining that a small dose of radioactive isotope will be used
- ❍ **D.** Giving an oral suspension of glucose 1 hour before the test

153. The nurse is preparing to give an oral potassium supplement. The nurse should:

Quick Answers: **188**
Detailed Answer: **204**

- ❍ **A.** Give the medication without diluting it
- ❍ **B.** Give the medication with 4oz. of juice
- ❍ **C.** Give the medication with water only
- ❍ **D.** Give the medication on an empty stomach

Quick Check

154. The physician has ordered cultures for cytomegalovirus (CMV). Which statement is true regarding collection of cultures for cytomegalovirus?

Quick Answers: **188**
Detailed Answer: **204**

- ❍ **A.** Stool cultures are preferred for definitive diagnosis.
- ❍ **B.** Pregnant caregivers may obtain cultures.
- ❍ **C.** Collection of one specimen is sufficient.
- ❍ **D.** Accurate diagnosis depends on fresh specimens.

155. A pediatric client with burns to the hands and arms has dressing changes with Sulfamylon (mafenide acetate) cream. The nurse is aware that the medication:

Quick Answers: **188**
Detailed Answer: **204**

- ❍ **A.** Will cause dark staining of the surrounding skin
- ❍ **B.** Produces a cooling sensation when applied
- ❍ **C.** Can alter the function of the thyroid
- ❍ **D.** Produces a burning sensation when applied

156. The physician has ordered Dilantin (phenytoin) for a client with generalized seizures. When planning the client's care, the nurse should:

Quick Answers: **188**
Detailed Answer: **204**

- ❍ **A.** Maintain strict intake and output
- ❍ **B.** Check the pulse before giving the medication
- ❍ **C.** Administer the medication 30 minutes before meals
- ❍ **D.** Provide oral hygiene and gum care every shift

157. A client receiving chemotherapy for breast cancer has an order for Zofran (ondansetron) 8mg PO to be given 30 minutes before induction of the chemotherapy. The purpose of the medication is to:

Quick Answers: **188**
Detailed Answer: **204**

- ❍ **A.** Prevent anemia
- ❍ **B.** Promote relaxation
- ❍ **C.** Prevent nausea
- ❍ **D.** Increase neutrophil counts

158. The physician has ordered Cortisporin ear drops for a 2-year-old. To administer the ear drops, the nurse should:

Quick Answers: **188**
Detailed Answer: **205**

- ❍ **A.** Pull the ear down and back
- ❍ **B.** Pull the ear straight out
- ❍ **C.** Pull the ear up and back
- ❍ **D.** Leave the ear undisturbed

Quick Check

159. A client with schizophrenia has been taking Thorazine (chlorpromazine) 200mg four times a day. Which finding should be reported to the doctor immediately?

Quick Answers: **188**
Detailed Answer: **205**

- ❍ **A.** The client complains of thirst
- ❍ **B.** The client has gained 4 pounds in the past 2 months
- ❍ **C.** The client complains of a sore throat
- ❍ **D.** The client naps throughout the day

160. A client with iron-deficiency anemia is taking an oral iron supplement. The nurse should tell the client to take the medication with:

Quick Answers: **188**
Detailed Answer: **205**

- ❍ **A.** Orange juice
- ❍ **B.** Water only
- ❍ **C.** Milk
- ❍ **D.** Apple juice

161. A client is admitted with burns of the right arm, chest, and head. According to the Rule of Nines, the percent of burn injury is:

Quick Answers: **188**
Detailed Answer: **205**

- ❍ **A.** 18%
- ❍ **B.** 27%
- ❍ **C.** 36%
- ❍ **D.** 45%

162. A client who was admitted with chest pain and shortness of breath has a standing order for oxygen via mask. Standing orders for oxygen mean that the nurse can apply oxygen at:

Quick Answers: **188**
Detailed Answer: **205**

- ❍ **A.** 2L per minute
- ❍ **B.** 6L per minute
- ❍ **C.** 10L per minute
- ❍ **D.** 12L per minute

163. The nurse is caring for a client with an ileostomy. The nurse should pay careful attention to care around the stoma because:

Quick Answers: **188**
Detailed Answer: **205**

- ❍ **A.** Digestive enzymes cause skin breakdown.
- ❍ **B.** Stools are less watery and contain more solid matter.
- ❍ **C.** The stoma will heal more slowly than expected.
- ❍ **D.** It is difficult to fit the appliance to the stoma site.

Quick Check

164. The physician has ordered aspirin therapy for a client with severe rheumatoid arthritis. A sign of acute aspirin toxicity is:

Quick Answers: **188**
Detailed Answer: **205**

- ❍ **A.** Anorexia
- ❍ **B.** Diarrhea
- ❍ **C.** Tinnitus
- ❍ **D.** Pruritis

165. A client is admitted to the emergency room with symptoms of delirium tremens. After admitting the client to a private room, the priority nursing intervention is to:

Quick Answers: **188**
Detailed Answer: **205**

- ❍ **A.** Obtain a history of his alcohol use
- ❍ **B.** Provide seizure precautions
- ❍ **C.** Keep the room cool and dark
- ❍ **D.** Administer thiamine and zinc

166. The nurse is providing dietary teaching for a client with gout. Which dietary selection is suitable for the client with gout?

Quick Answers: **188**
Detailed Answer: **205**

- ❍ **A.** Broiled liver, macaroni and cheese, spinach
- ❍ **B.** Stuffed crab, steamed rice, peas
- ❍ **C.** Baked chicken, pasta salad, asparagus casserole
- ❍ **D.** Steak, baked potato, tossed salad

167. A newborn has been diagnosed with exstrophy of the bladder. The nurse should position the newborn:

Quick Answers: **188**
Detailed Answer: **205**

- ❍ **A.** Prone
- ❍ **B.** Supine
- ❍ **C.** On either side
- ❍ **D.** With the head elevated

168. The mother of a 3-month-old with esophageal reflux asks the nurse what she can do to lessen the baby's reflux. The nurse should tell the mother to:

Quick Answers: **188**
Detailed Answer: **205**

- ❍ **A.** Feed the baby only when he is hungry
- ❍ **B.** Burp the baby after the feeding is completed
- ❍ **C.** Place the baby supine with head elevated
- ❍ **D.** Burp the baby frequently throughout the feeding

Quick Check

169. A child is hospitalized with a fractured femur involving the epiphysis. Epiphyseal fractures are serious because:

Quick Answers: **188**
Detailed Answer: **206**

- ❍ **A.** Bone marrow is lost through the fracture site.
- ❍ **B.** Normal bone growth is affected.
- ❍ **C.** Blood supply to the bone is obliterated.
- ❍ **D.** Callus formation prevents bone healing.

170. Before administering a nasogastric feeding to a client hospitalized following a CVA, the nurse aspirates 40mL of residual. The nurse should:

Quick Answers: **188**
Detailed Answer: **206**

- ❍ **A.** Replace the aspirate and administer the feeding
- ❍ **B.** Discard the aspirate and withhold the feeding
- ❍ **C.** Discard the aspirate and begin the feeding
- ❍ **D.** Replace the aspirate and withhold the feeding

171. A client has an order for Dilantin (phenytoin) .2g orally twice a day. The medication is available in 100mg capsules. For the morning medication, the nurse should administer:

Quick Answers: **188**
Detailed Answer: **206**

- ❍ **A.** 1 capsule
- ❍ **B.** 2 capsules
- ❍ **C.** 3 capsules
- ❍ **D.** 4 capsules

172. The LPN is reviewing the lab results of an elderly client when she notes a specific gravity of 1.025. The nurse recognizes that:

Quick Answers: **188**
Detailed Answer: **206**

- ❍ **A.** The client has impaired renal function.
- ❍ **B.** The client has a normal specific gravity.
- ❍ **C.** The client has mild to moderate dehydration.
- ❍ **D.** The client has diluted urine from fluid overload.

173. A client with acute pancreatitis has requested pain medication. Which pain medication is indicated for the client with acute pancreatitis?

Quick Answers: **188**
Detailed Answer: **206**

- ❍ **A.** Demerol (meperidine)
- ❍ **B.** Toradol (ketorolac)
- ❍ **C.** Morphine (morphine sulfate)
- ❍ **D.** Codeine (codeine)

Quick Check

174. A client with a hiatal hernia has been taking magnesium hydroxide for relief of heartburn. Overuse of magnesium-based antacids can cause the client to have:

Quick Answers: **188**
Detailed Answer: **206**

❍ **A.** Constipation

❍ **B.** Weight gain

❍ **C.** Anorexia

❍ **D.** Diarrhea

175. When performing a newborn assessment, the nurse measures the circumference of the neonate's head and chest. Which assessment finding is expected in the normal newborn?

Quick Answers: **188**
Detailed Answer: **206**

❍ **A.** The head and chest circumference are the same.

❍ **B.** The head is 2cm larger than the chest.

❍ **C.** The head is 3cm smaller than the chest.

❍ **D.** The head is 4cm larger than the chest.

176. A client with a history of clots is receiving Lovenox (enoxaparin). Which drug is given to counteract the effects of enoxaparin?

Quick Answers: **188**
Detailed Answer: **206**

❍ **A.** Calcium gluconate

❍ **B.** Aquamephyton

❍ **C.** Methergine

❍ **D.** Protamine sulfate

177. The nurse is formulating a plan of care for a client with a cognitive disorder. Which activity is most appropriate for the client with confusion and short attention span?

Quick Answers: **188**
Detailed Answer: **206**

❍ **A.** Taking part in a reality-orientation group

❍ **B.** Participating in unit community goal setting

❍ **C.** Going on a field trip with a group of clients

❍ **D.** Meeting with an assertiveness training group

178. The mother of a child with hemophilia asks the nurse which over-the-counter medication is suitable for her child's joint discomfort. The nurse should tell the mother to purchase:

Quick Answers: **188**
Detailed Answer: **206**

❍ **A.** Advil (ibuprofen)

❍ **B.** Tylenol (acetaminophen)

❍ **C.** Aspirin (acetylsalicytic acid)

❍ **D.** Naproxen (naprosyn)

Quick Check

179. Which home remedy is suitable to relieve the itching associated with varicella?

Quick Answers: **188**
Detailed Answer: **206**

- ❍ **A.** Dusting the lesions with baby powder
- ❍ **B.** Applying gauze saturated in hydrogen peroxide
- ❍ **C.** Using cool compresses of normal saline
- ❍ **D.** Applying a paste of baking soda and water

180. The nurse is caring for a newborn with hypospadias. Which statement describes hypospadias?

Quick Answers: **188**
Detailed Answer: **207**

- ❍ **A.** The urinary meatus is located on the underside of the penis rather than the tip.
- ❍ **B.** The ureters allow a reflux of urine into the kidneys.
- ❍ **C.** The urinary meatus is located on the topside of the penis rather than the tip.
- ❍ **D.** The bladder lies outside the abdominal cavity.

181. The recommended time for daily administration of Tagamet (cimetidine) is:

Quick Answers: **188**
Detailed Answer: **207**

- ❍ **A.** Before breakfast
- ❍ **B.** Mid-afternoon
- ❍ **C.** After dinner
- ❍ **D.** At bedtime

182. Which statement best describes the difference between the pain of angina and the pain of myocardial infarction?

Quick Answers: **188**
Detailed Answer: **207**

- ❍ **A.** Pain associated with angina is relieved by rest.
- ❍ **B.** Pain associated with myocardial infarction is always more severe.
- ❍ **C.** Pain associated with angina is confined to the chest area.
- ❍ **D.** Pain associated with myocardial infarction is referred to the left arm.

183. The nurse is developing a bowel-retraining plan for a client with multiple sclerosis. Which measure is likely to be least helpful to the client:

Quick Answers: **188**
Detailed Answer: **207**

- ❍ **A.** Limiting fluid intake to 1000mL per day
- ❍ **B.** Providing a high-roughage diet
- ❍ **C.** Elevating the toilet seat for easy access
- ❍ **D.** Establishing a regular schedule for toileting

Quick Check

184. The nurse is providing dietary teaching for a client with Meniere's disease. Which statement indicates that the client understands the role of diet in triggering her symptoms?

Quick Answers: **189**
Detailed Answer: **207**

- ❍ **A.** "I can expect to see more problems with tinnitus if I eat a lot of dairy products."
- ❍ **B.** "I need to limit foods that taste salty or that contain a lot of sodium."
- ❍ **C.** "I can help control problems with vertigo if I avoid breads and cereals."
- ❍ **D.** "I need to eat fewer foods that are high in potassium, such as raisins and bananas."

185. The nurse is assessing a multigravida, 36 weeks gestation for symptoms of pregnancy-induced hypertension and preeclampsia. The nurse should give priority to assessing the client for:

Quick Answers: **189**
Detailed Answer: **207**

- ❍ **A.** Facial swelling
- ❍ **B.** Pulse deficits
- ❍ **C.** Ankle edema
- ❍ **D.** Diminished reflexes

186. An adolescent with borderline personality disorders is hospitalized with suicidal ideation and self-mutilation. Which goal is both therapeutic and realistic for this client?

Quick Answers: **189**
Detailed Answer: **207**

- ❍ **A.** The client will remain in her room when feeling overwhelmed by sadness.
- ❍ **B.** The client will request medication when feeling loss of emotional control.
- ❍ **C.** The client will leave group activities to pace when feeling anxious.
- ❍ **D.** The client will seek out a staff member to verbalize feelings of anger and sadness.

187. A client with angina has an order for nitroglycerin ointment. Before applying the medication, the nurse should:

Quick Answers: **189**
Detailed Answer: **207**

- ❍ **A.** Apply the ointment to the previous application
- ❍ **B.** Obtain both a radial and an apical pulse
- ❍ **C.** Remove the previously applied ointment
- ❍ **D.** Tell the client he will experience pain relief in 15 minutes

Quick Check

188. The nurse is caring for a client who is unconscious following a fall. Which comment by the nurse will help the client become reoriented when he regains consciousness?

Quick Answers: **189**
Detailed Answer: **207**

- ❍ **A.** "I am your nurse and I will be taking care of you today."
- ❍ **B.** "Can you tell me your name and where you are?"
- ❍ **C.** "I know you are confused right now, but everything will be alright."
- ❍ **D.** "You were in an accident that hurt your head. You are in the hospital."

189. Following a generalized seizure, the nurse can expect the client to:

Quick Answers: **189**
Detailed Answer: **207**

- ❍ **A.** Be unable to move the extremities
- ❍ **B.** Be drowsy and prone to sleep
- ❍ **C.** Remember events before the seizure
- ❍ **D.** Have a drop in blood pressure

190. A client with oxylate renal calculi should be taught to limit his intake of foods such as:

Quick Answers: **189**
Detailed Answer: **208**

- ❍ **A.** Strawberries
- ❍ **B.** Oranges
- ❍ **C.** Apples
- ❍ **D.** Pears

191. A 6-year-old is diagnosed with Legg-Calve Perthes disease of the right femur. An important part of the child's care includes instructing the parents:

Quick Answers: **189**
Detailed Answer: **208**

- ❍ **A.** To increase the amount of dietary protein
- ❍ **B.** About exercises to strengthen affected muscles
- ❍ **C.** About relaxation exercises to minimize pain in the joints
- ❍ **D.** To prevent weight bearing on the affected leg

192. The nurse is assessing an infant with Hirschsprung's disease. The nurse can expect the infant to:

Quick Answers: **189**
Detailed Answer: **208**

- ❍ **A.** Weigh less than expected for height and age
- ❍ **B.** Have infrequent bowel movements
- ❍ **C.** Exhibit clubbing of the fingers and toes
- ❍ **D.** Have hyperactive deep tendon reflexes

Quick Check

193. The physician has prescribed supplemental iron for a prenatal client. The nurse should tell the client to take the medication with:

Quick Answers: **189**
Detailed Answer: **208**

- ❍ **A.** Milk, to prevent stomach upset
- ❍ **B.** Tomato juice, to increase absorption
- ❍ **C.** Oatmeal, to prevent constipation
- ❍ **D.** Water, to increase serum iron levels

194. The nurse is teaching a client with a history of obesity and hypertension regarding dietary requirements during pregnancy. Which statement indicates that the client needs further teaching?

Quick Answers: **189**
Detailed Answer: **208**

- ❍ **A.** "I need to reduce my daily intake to 1,200 calories a day."
- ❍ **B.** "I need to drink at least a quart of milk a day."
- ❍ **C.** "I shouldn't add salt when I am cooking."
- ❍ **D.** "I need to eat more protein and fiber each day."

195. An elderly client is admitted to the psychiatric unit from the nursing home. Transfer information indicates that the client has become confused and disoriented, with behavioral problems. The client will also likely show a loss of ability in:

Quick Answers: **189**
Detailed Answer: **208**

- ❍ **A.** Speech
- ❍ **B.** Judgment
- ❍ **C.** Endurance
- ❍ **D.** Balance

196. The physician has ordered an external monitor for a laboring client. If the fetus is in the left occipital posterior (LOP) position, the nurse knows that the ultrasound transducer will be located:

Quick Answers: **189**
Detailed Answer: **208**

- ❍ **A.** Near the symphysis pubis
- ❍ **B.** Near the umbilicus
- ❍ **C.** Over the fetal back
- ❍ **D.** Over the fetal abdomen

197. A client develops tremors while withdrawing from alcohol. Which medication is routinely administered to lessen physiological effects of alcohol withdrawal?

Quick Answers: **189**
Detailed Answer: **208**

- ❍ **A.** Dolophine (methodone)
- ❍ **B.** Klonopin (clonazepam)
- ❍ **C.** Narcan (naloxone)
- ❍ **D.** Antabuse (disulfiram)

Quick Check

198. A client with Type II diabetes has an order for regular insulin 10 units SC each morning. The client's breakfast should be served within:

- ❍ **A.** 15 minutes
- ❍ **B.** 20 minutes
- ❍ **C.** 30 minutes
- ❍ **D.** 45 minutes

Quick Answers: **189**
Detailed Answer: **208**

199. A 10-year-old has an order for Demerol (meperidine) 35mg IM for pain. The medication is available as Demerol 50mg per mL. How much should the nurse administer?

- ❍ **A.** .5mL
- ❍ **B.** .6mL
- ❍ **C.** .7mL
- ❍ **D.** .8mL

Quick Answers: **189**
Detailed Answer: **208**

200. Which antibiotic is contraindicated for the treatment of infections in infants and young children?

- ❍ **A.** Tetracyn (tetracycline)
- ❍ **B.** Amoxil (amoxicillin)
- ❍ **C.** Cefotan (cefotetan)
- ❍ **D.** E-Mycin (erythromycin)

Quick Answers: **189**
Detailed Answer: **208**

Quick Check Answer Key

1. D
2. D
3. A
4. D
5. C
6. C
7. A
8. A
9. A
10. B
11. B
12. A
13. C
14. D
15. B
16. C
17. B
18. B
19. D
20. B
21. A
22. A
23. B
24. B
25. C
26. B
27. B
28. B
29. A
30. B
31. D
32. B
33. C
34. B
35. A
36. A
37. C
38. A
39. D
40. D
41. C
42. B
43. A
44. D
45. C
46. B
47. B
48. D
49. C
50. D
51. A
52. C
53. B
54. D
55. A
56. A
57. B
58. B
59. D
60. B
61. B
62. C
63. A
64. C
65. A
66. B
67. A
68. D
69. A
70. B
71. D
72. D
73. B
74. D
75. C
76. D
77. C
78. C
79. B
80. C
81. D
82. A
83. D
84. A
85. C
86. B
87. C

88. A
89. D
90. B
91. C
92. B
93. C
94. D
95. C
96. A
97. D
98. B
99. C
100. B
101. C
102. D
103. D
104. C
105. D
106. C
107. D
108. C
109. A
110. C
111. B
112. D
113. A
114. D
115. C
116. A
117. B
118. B
119. A
120. A
121. A
122. D
123. A
124. B
125. B
126. A
127. B
128. D
129. C
130. A
131. A
132. A
133. B
134. B
135. D
136. B
137. A
138. B
139. A
140. D
141. B
142. C
143. A
144. D
145. A
146. C
147. D
148. B
149. A
150. B
151. C
152. B
153. B
154. D
155. D
156. D
157. C
158. A
159. C
160. A
161. B
162. B
163. A
164. C
165. B
166. D
167. C
168. D
169. B
170. A
171. B
172. B
173. A
174. D
175. B
176. D
177. A
178. B
179. D
180. A
181. D
182. A
183. A

184. B

185. A

186. D

187. C

188. D

189. B

190. A

191. D

192. B

193. B

194. A

195. B

196. C

197. B

198. C

199. C

200. A

Answers and Rationales

1. **Answer D is correct.** The suicidal client has difficulty expressing anger toward others. The depressed suicidal client frequently expresses feelings of low self-worth, feelings of remorse and guilt, and a dependence on others; therefore, answers A, B, and C are incorrect.

2. **Answer D is correct.** Answers A, B, and C are incorrect because they contain lower amounts of potassium. (Note that the banana contains 450mg K+, the orange contains 235mg K+, the pear contains 208mg K+, and the apple contains 165mg K+.)

3. **Answer A is correct.** Following a thyroidectomy, the client should be placed in semi-Fowler's position to decrease swelling that would place pressure on the airway. Answers B, C, and D are incorrect because they would increase the chances of post-operative complications that include bleeding, swelling, and airway obstruction.

4. **Answer D is correct.** Luncheon meats contain preservatives such as nitrites that have been linked to gastric cancer. Answers A, B, and C have not been found to increase the risk of gastric cancer; therefore, they are incorrect.

5. **Answer C is correct.** A history of cruelty to people and animals, truancy, setting fires, and lack of guilt or remorse are associated with a diagnosis of conduct disorder in children, which becomes a diagnosis of antisocial personality disorder in adults. Answer A is incorrect because the client with antisocial personality disorder does not hold consistent employment. Answer B is incorrect because the IQ is usually higher than average. Answer D is incorrect because of a lack of guilt or remorse for wrong-doing.

6. **Answer C is correct.** The licensed vocational nurse may not assume primary care of the client with a central venous access device. The licensed vocational nurse may care for the client in labor, the client post-operative client, and the client with bipolar disorder; therefore, answers A, B, and D are incorrect.

7. **Answer A is correct.** Sulfamylon (mafenide acetate) produces a painful sensation when applied to the burn wound; therefore, the client should receive pain medication before dressing changes. Answers B, C, and D do not pertain to dressing changes for the client with burns, so they are incorrect.

8. **Answer A is correct.** According to the Denver Developmental Screening Test, the child can pull a toy behind her by age 2 years. Answers B, C, and D are not accomplished until ages 4–5 years; therefore, they are incorrect.

9. **Answer A is correct.** The client with a fractured mandible should keep a pair of wire cutters with him at all times to release the device in case of choking or aspiration. Answer B is incorrect because the wires would prevent insertion of an oral airway. Answer C is incorrect because it would be of no use in releasing the wires. Answer D is incorrect because it would be used only as a last resort in case of airway obstruction.

10. **Answer B is correct.** The infant's apical heart rate is within the accepted range for administering the medication. Answers A, C, and D are incorrect because the apical heart rate is suitable for giving the medication.

11. **Answer B is correct.** Chelating agents are used to treat the client with poisonings from heavy metals such as lead and iron. Answers A and D are used to remove noncorrosive poisons; therefore, they are incorrect. Answer C prevents vomiting; therefore, it is an incorrect response.

12. **Answer A is correct.** The least restrictive restraint for the infant with cleft lip and cleft palate repair is elbow restraints. Answers B, C, and D are more restrictive and unnecessary; therefore, they are incorrect.

13. **Answer C is correct.** Beta blockers such as timolol (Timoptic) can cause bronchospasms in the client with chronic obstructive lung disease. Timoptic is not contraindicated for use in clients with diabetes, gastric ulcers, or pancreatitis; therefore, answers A, B, and C are incorrect.

14. **Answer D is correct.** Leaving a nightlight on during the evening and night shifts helps the client remain oriented to the environment and fosters independence. Answers A and B will not decrease the client's confusion. Answer C will increase the likelihood of confusion in an elderly client.

15. **Answer B is correct.** Pruritis or itching is caused by the presence of uric acid crystals on the skin, which is common in the client with end-stage renal failure. Answers A, C, and D are not associated with end-stage renal failure.

16. **Answer C is correct.** There is no specified time or frequency for the ordered medication. Answers A, B, and D contain specified time and frequency, therefore they do not require further clarification.

17. **Answer B is correct.** A low-sodium diet is best for the client with Meniere's syndrome. Answers A, C, and D do not relate to the care of the client with Meniere's syndrome; therefore, they are incorrect.

18. **Answer B is correct.** Increased voiding at night is a symptom of right-sided heart failure. Answers A and D are incorrect because they are symptoms of left-sided heart failure. Answer C does not relate to the client's diagnosis; therefore, it is incorrect.

19. **Answer D is correct.** The pulse oximeter should be placed on the child's finger or earlobe because blood flow to these areas is most accessible for measuring oxygen concentration. Answer A is incorrect because the probe cannot be secured to the abdomen. Answer B is incorrect because it should be recalibrated before application. Answer C is incorrect because a reading is obtained within seconds, not minutes.

20. **Answer B is correct.** The medication should be administered using the calibrated dropper that comes with the medication. Answers A and C are incorrect because part or all of the medication could be lost during administration. Answer D is incorrect because part or all of the medication will be lost if the child does not finish the bottle.

21. **Answer A is correct.** The client will receive medication that relaxes skeletal muscles and produces mild sedation. Answers B and D are incorrect because such statements increase the client's anxiety level. Nausea and headache are not associated with ECT; therefore, answer C is incorrect.

22. **Answer A is correct.** Lyme's disease produces a characteristic annular or circular rash sometimes described as a "bull's eye" rash. Answers B, C, and D are incorrect because they are not symptoms associated with Lyme's disease.

23. **Answer B is correct.** The client with gluten-induced enteropathy experiences symptoms after ingesting foods containing wheat, oats, barley, or rye. Corn or millet are substituted in the diet. Answers A, C, and D are incorrect because they contain foods that worsen the client's condition.

24. **Answer B is correct.** Neuroleptic malignant syndrome is an adverse reaction that is characterized by extreme elevations in temperature. Answers A and C are incorrect because they are expected side effects. Elevations in blood pressure are associated with reactions between foods containing tyramine and MAOI; therefore, answer D is incorrect.

25. **Answer C is correct.** Gingival hyperplasia is a side effect of phenytoin. The client will need more frequent dental visits. Answers A, B, and D do not apply to the medication; therefore, they are incorrect.

26. **Answer B is correct.** The client's gag reflex is depressed before having an EGD. The nurse should give priority to checking for the return of the gag reflex before offering the client oral fluids. Answer A is incorrect because conscious sedation is used. Answers C and D are not affected by the procedure; therefore, they are incorrect.

27. **Answer B is correct.** The eye shield should be worn at night or when napping, to prevent accidental trauma to the operative eye. Prescription eyedrops, not over-the-counter eyedrops, are ordered for the client; therefore, Answer A is incorrect. The client might or might not require glasses following cataract surgery; therefore, answer C is incorrect. Answer D is incorrect because cataract surgery is pain free.

28. **Answer B is correct.** The child's symptoms are consistent with those of epiglottitis, an infection of the upper airway that can result in total airway obstruction. Symptoms of strep throat, laryngotracheobronchitis, and bronchiolitis are different than those presented by the client; therefore, answers A, C, and D are incorrect.

29. **Answer A is correct.** Providing additional fluids will help the newborn eliminate excess bilirubin in the stool and urine. Answer B is incorrect because oils and lotions should not be used with phototherapy. Physiologic jaundice is not associated with infection; therefore, answers C and D are incorrect.

30. **Answer B is correct.** Having a staff member remain with the client for 1 hour after meals will help prevent self-induced vomiting. Answer A is incorrect because the client will weigh more after meals, which can undermine treatment. Answer C is incorrect because the client will need a balanced diet and excess protein might not be well tolerated at first. Answer D is incorrect because it treats the client as a child rather than as an adult.

31. **Answer D is correct.** According to Erikson's Psychosocial Developmental Theory, the developmental task of middle childhood is industry versus inferiority. Answer A is incorrect because it is the developmental task of infancy. Answer B is incorrect because it is the developmental task of the school-age child. Answer C is incorrect because it is not one of Erikson's developmental stages.

32. **Answer B is correct.** A side effect of bronchodilators is nausea. Answers A and C are not associated with bronchodilators; therefore, they are incorrect. Answer D is incorrect because hypotension is a sign of toxicity, not a side effect.

33. **Answer C is correct.** Although cyanosis of the hands and feet is common in the newborn, it accounts for an Apgar score of less than 10. Answer B suggests cooling, which is not scored by the Apgar. Answer B is incorrect because conjunctival hemorrhages are not associated with the Apgar. Answer D is incorrect because it is within normal range as measured by the Apgar.

34. **Answer B is correct.** Tenseness of the anterior fontanel indicates an increase in intracranial pressure. Answer A is incorrect because periorbital edema is not associated with meningitis. Answer C is incorrect because a positive Babinski reflex is normal in the infant. Answer D is incorrect because it relates to the preterm infant, not the infant with meningitis.

35. **Answer A is correct.** Nasogastric suction decompresses the stomach and leaves the abdomen soft and nondistended. Answer B is incorrect because it does not relate to the effectiveness of the NG suction. Answer C is incorrect because it relates to peristalsis, not the effectiveness of the NG suction. Answer D is incorrect because it relates to wound healing, not the effectiveness of the NG suction.

36. **Answer A is correct.** Tremulousness is an early sign of hypoglycemia. Answers B, C, and D are incorrect because they are symptoms of hyperglycemia.

37. **Answer C is correct.** The most common sign associated with exacerbation of multiple sclerosis is double vision. Answers A, B, and D are not associated with a diagnosis of multiple sclerosis; therefore, they are incorrect.

38. **Answer A is correct.** Gout and renal calculi are the result of increased amounts of uric acid. Answer B is incorrect because it does not contribute to renal calculi. Answers C and D can result from decreased calcium levels. Renal calculi are the result of excess calcium; therefore, answers C and D are incorrect.

39. **Answer D is correct.** Providing small, frequent meals will improve the client's appetite and help reduce nausea. Answer A is incorrect because it does not compensate for limited absorption. Foods and beverages containing live cultures are discouraged for the immune-compromised client; therefore, answer B is incorrect. Answer C is incorrect because forcing fluids will not compensate for limited absorption of the intestine.

40. **Answer D is correct.** A common side effect of prednisone is gastric ulcers. Cimetadine is given to help prevent the development of ulcers. Answers A, B, and C do not relate to the use of cimetadine; therefore, they are incorrect.

41. **Answer C is correct.** Rice cereal, apple juice, and formula are suitable foods for the 6-month-old infant. Whole milk, orange juice, and eggs are not suitable for the young infant; therefore, they are incorrect.

42. **Answer B is correct.** The nurse should administer the injection in the vastus lateralis muscle. Answers A and C are not as well developed in the newborn; therefore, they are incorrect. Answer D is incorrect because the dorsogluteal muscle is not used for IM injections until the child is 3 years of age.

43. **Answer A is correct.** The client taking Cytoxan should increase his fluid intake to prevent hemorrhagic cystitis. Answers B, C, and D do not relate to the question; therefore, they are incorrect.

44. **Answer D is correct.** Benzodiazepines are ordered for the client in alcohol withdrawal to prevent delirium tremens. Answer A is incorrect because it is a medication used in aversive therapy to maintain sobriety. Answer B is incorrect because it is used for the treatment of benzodiazepine overdose. Answer C is incorrect because it is the treatment for opiate withdrawal.

45. **Answer C is correct.** The client taking NPH insulin should have a snack midafternoon to prevent hypoglycemia. Answers A and B are incorrect because the times are too early for symptoms of hypoglycemia. Answer D is incorrect because the time is too late and the client would be in severe hypoglycemia.

46. **Answer B is correct.** The client with a detached retina will have limitations in mobility before and after surgery. Answer A is incorrect because a detached retina produces no pain or discomfort. Answers C and D do not apply to the client with a detached retina; therefore, they are incorrect.

47. **Answer B is correct.** The primary purpose for the continuous passive-motion machine is to promote flexion of the artificial joint. The device should be placed at the foot of the client's bed. Answers A, C, and D do not describe the purpose of the CPM machine; therefore, they are incorrect.

48. **Answer D is correct.** According to Kohlberg, in the preconventional stage of development, the behavior of the preschool child is determined by the consequences of the behavior. Answers A, B, and C describe other stages of moral development; therefore, they are incorrect.

49. **Answer C is correct.** The client should be assessed following completion of antibiotic therapy to determine whether the infection has cleared. Answer A would be done if there are repeated instances of otitis media; therefore, it is incorrect. Answer B is incorrect because it will not determine whether the child has taken the medication. Answer D is incorrect because the purpose of the recheck is to determine whether the infection is gone.

50. **Answer D is correct.** The nurse should cover both of the client's eyes and transport him immediately to the ER or the doctor's office. Answers A, B, and D are incorrect because they increase the risk of further damage to the eye.

51. **Answer A is correct.** The major complication of SLE is lupus nephritis, which results in end-stage renal disease. SLE affects the musculoskeletal, integumentary, renal, nervous, and cardiovascular systems, but the major complication is renal involvement; therefore, answers B and D are incorrect. Answer C is incorrect because the SLE produces a "butterfly" rash, not desquamation.

52. **Answer C is correct.** A diet that is high in fat and refined carbohydrates increases the risk of colorectal cancer. High fat content results in an increase in fecal bile acids, which facilitate carcinogenic changes. Refined carbohydrates increase the transit time of food through the gastrointestinal tract and increase the exposure time of the intestinal mucosa to cancer-causing substances. Answers A, B, and D do not relate to the question; therefore, they are incorrect.

53. **Answer B is correct.** The nurse should avoid giving the infant a pacifier or bottle because sucking is not permitted. Holding the infant cradled in the arms, providing a

mobile, and offering sterile water using a Breck feeder are permitted; therefore, answers A, C, and D are incorrect.

54. Answer D is correct. The client with esophageal varices can develop spontaneous bleeding from the mechanical irritation caused by taking capsules; therefore, the nurse should request the medication in a suspension. Answer A is incorrect because it does not best meet the client's needs. Answer B is incorrect because it is not the best means of preventing bleeding. Answer C is incorrect because the medications should not be given with milk or antacids.

55. Answer A is correct. Tomatoes are a poor source of iron, although they are an excellent source of vitamin C, which increases iron absorption. Answers B, C, and D are good sources of iron; therefore, they are incorrect.

56. Answer A is correct. Periodically lying in a prone position without a pillow will help prevent the flexion of the spine that occurs with Parkinson's disease. Answers B and C flex the spine; therefore, they are incorrect. Answer D is not realistic because of position changes during sleep; therefore, it is incorrect.

57. Answer B is correct. The client recovering from pancreatitis needs a diet that is high in calories and low in fat. Answers A, C, and D are incorrect because they can increase the client's discomfort.

58. Answer B is correct. Dressing in layers and using extra covering will help decrease the feeling of being cold that is experienced by the client with hypothyroidism. Decreased sensation and decreased alertness are common in the client with hypothyroidism; therefore, the use of electric blankets and heating pads can result in burns, making answers A and C incorrect. Answer D is incorrect because the client with hypothyroidism has dry skin, and a hot bath morning and evening would make her condition worse.

59. Answer D is correct. A history of frequent alcohol and tobacco use is the most significant factor in the development of cancer of the larynx. Answers A, B, and C are also factors in the development of laryngeal cancer, but they are not the most significant; therefore, they are incorrect.

60. Answer B is correct. Numbness and tingling in the extremities is common in the client with pernicious anemia, but not those with other types of anemia. Answers A, C, and D are incorrect because they are symptoms of all types of anemia.

61. Answer B is correct. The client with echolalia repeats words or phrases used by others. Answer A is incorrect because it refers to clang association. Answer C is incorrect because it refers to circumstantiality. Answer D is incorrect because it refers to neologisms.

62. Answer C is correct. Holding a cup of coffee or hot chocolate helps to relieve the pain and stiffness of the hands. Answers A, B, and D do not relieve the symptoms of rheumatoid arthritis; therefore, they are incorrect.

63. Answer A is correct. The infant's birth weight should double by 6 months of age. Answers B, C, and D are incorrect because they are greater than the expected weight gain by 6 months of age.

64. **Answer C is correct.** Symptoms associated with nontropical sprue and celiac disease are caused by the ingestion of gluten, which is found in wheat, oats, barley, and rye. Creamed soup and crackers contain gluten. Answers A, B, and D do not contain gluten; therefore, they are incorrect.

65. **Answer A is correct.** Lanoxin (digoxin) slows and strengthens the contraction of the heart. An increase in urinary output shows that the medication is having a desired effect by eliminating excess fluid from the body. Answer B is incorrect because the weight would decrease. Answer C might occur but is not directly related to the question; therefore, it is incorrect. Answer D is incorrect because pedal edema would decrease, not increase.

66. **Answer B is correct.** The toddler has gross motor skills suited to playing with a ball, which can be kicked forward or thrown overhand. Answers A and C are incorrect because they require fine motor skills. Answer D is incorrect because the toddler lacks gross motor skills for play on the swing set.

67. **Answer A is correct.** Antacids containing aluminum and calcium tend to cause constipation. Answer A refers to the side effects of anticholinergic medications used to treat ulcers; therefore, it is incorrect. Answer C refers to antacids containing magnesium; therefore, it is incorrect. Answer D refers to dopamine antagonists used to treat ulcers; therefore, it is incorrect.

68. **Answer D is correct.** The client with an abdominal aortic aneurysm frequently complains of pulsations or "feeling my heart beat" in the abdomen. Answers A and C are incorrect because they occur with rupture of the aneurysm. Answer B is incorrect because back pain is not affected by changes in position.

69. **Answer A is correct.** The client with acute adrenal crisis has symptoms of hypovolemia and shock; therefore, the blood pressure would be low. Answer B is incorrect because the pulse would be rapid and irregular. Answer C is incorrect because the skin would be cool and pale. Answer D is incorrect because the urinary output would be decreased.

70. **Answer B is correct.** Bright red bleeding with many clots indicates arterial bleeding that requires surgical intervention. Answer A is within normal limits; therefore, it is incorrect. Answer C indicates venous bleeding, which can be managed by nursing intervention; therefore, it is incorrect. Answer D does not indicate excessive need for pain management that requires the doctor's attention; therefore, it is incorrect.

71. **Answer D is correct.** The child with polymigratory arthritis will exhibit swollen, painful joints. Answer B is incorrect because it describes subcutaneous nodules. Answer C is incorrect because it describes erythema marginatum. Answer A is incorrect because it describes Syndeham's chorea.

72. **Answer D is correct.** The primary reason for placing a child with croup under a mist tent is to liquefy secretions and relieve laryngeal spasms. Answer A is incorrect because it does not prevent insensible water loss. Answer B is incorrect because the oxygen concentration is too high. Answer C is incorrect because the mist tent does not prevent dehydration or reduce fever.

73. **Answer B is correct.** Symptoms of hypothyroidism include weight gain, lethargy, slow speech, and decreased respirations. Answers A and D do not describe symptoms

associated with myxedema; therefore, they are incorrect. Answer C describes symptoms associated with Graves's disease; therefore, it is incorrect.

74. **Answer D is correct.** The contagious stage of varicella begins 24 hours before the onset of the rash and lasts until all the lesions are crusted. Answers A, B, and C are inaccurate regarding the time of contagion; therefore, they are incorrect.

75. **Answer C is correct.** Delusions of grandeur are associated with low self-esteem. Answer A is incorrect because conversion is expressed as sensory or motor deficits. Answers B and D can cause an increase in the client's delusions but do not explain their purpose; therefore, they are incorrect.

76. **Answer D is correct.** Respiratory stridor is a symptom of partial airway obstruction. Answers A, B, and C are expected with a tonsillectomy; therefore, they are incorrect.

77. **Answer C is correct.** Pain associated with duodenal ulcers is lessened if the client eats a meal or snack. Answer A is incorrect because it makes the pain worse. Answer B refers to dumping syndrome; therefore, it is incorrect. Answer D refers to gastroesophageal reflux; therefore, it is incorrect.

78. **Answer C is correct.** Foods containing rice or millet are permitted on the diet of the client with celiac disease. Answers A, B, and D are not permitted because they contain flour made from wheat, which exacerbates the symptoms of celiac disease; therefore, they are incorrect.

79. **Answer B is correct.** Increased thirst and increased urination are signs of lithium toxicity. Answers A and D do not relate to the medication; therefore, they are incorrect. Answer C is an expected side effect of the medication; therefore, it is incorrect.

80. **Answer C is correct.** The immunization protects the child against diphtheria, pertussis, tetanus, and *H. influenza b.* Answer A is incorrect because a second injection is given before 4 years of age. Answer B is not a true statement; therefore, it is incorrect. Answer D is incorrect because it is not a one-time injection, nor does it protect against measles, mumps, rubella, or varicella.

81. **Answer D is correct.** The milkshake will provide needed calories and nutrients for the client with mania. Answers A and B are incorrect because they are high in sodium, which causes the client to excrete the lithium. Answer C has some nutrient value, but not as much as the milkshake.

82. **Answer A is correct.** The child with intussusception has stools that contain blood and mucus, which are described as "currant jelly" stools. Answer B is a symptom of pyloric stenosis; therefore, it is incorrect. Answer C is a symptom of Hirschsprung's; therefore, it is incorrect. Answer D is a symptom of Wilms tumor; therefore, it is incorrect.

83. **Answer D is correct.** The nurse should not use water, soap, or lotion on the area marked for radiation therapy. Answer A is incorrect because it would remove the marking. Answers B and C are not necessary for the client receiving radiation; therefore, they are incorrect.

84. **Answer A is correct.** Growth hormone levels generally fall rapidly after a hypophysectomy, allowing insulin levels to rise. The result is hypoglycemia. Answer B is incorrect because it traumatizes the oral mucosa. Answer C is incorrect because the client's

head should be elevated to reduce pressure on the operative site. Answer D is incorrect because it increases pressure on the operative site that can lead to a leak of cerebral spinal fluid.

85. **Answer C is correct.** Precose (acarbose) is to be taken with the first bite of a meal. Answers A, B, and D are incorrect because they specify the wrong schedule for medication administration.

86. **Answer B is correct.** The client going for therapy in the hyperbaric oxygen chamber requires no special skin care; therefore, washing the skin with water and patting it dry are suitable. Lotions, petroleum products, perfumes, and occlusive dressings interfere with oxygenation of the skin; therefore, answers A, C, and D are incorrect.

87. **Answer C is correct.** The primary reason for the NG to is to allow for nourishment without contamination of the suture line. Answer A is not a true statement; therefore, it is incorrect. Answer B is incorrect because there is no mention of suction. Answer D is incorrect because the oral mucosa was not involved in the laryngectomy.

88. **Answer A is correct.** The client with expressive aphasia has trouble forming words that are understandable. Answer B is incorrect because it describes receptive aphasia. Answer C refers to apraxia; therefore, it is incorrect. Answer D is incorrect because it refers to agnosia.

89. **Answer D is correct.** Sunscreens of at least an SPF of 15 should be applied 20–30 minutes before going into the sun. Answers A, B, and C are incorrect because they do not allow sufficient time for sun protection.

90. **Answer B is correct.** The combination of the two medications produces an effect greater than that of either drug used alone. Agonist effects are similar to those produced by chemicals normally present in the body; therefore, answer A is incorrect. Antagonist effects are those in which the actions of the drugs oppose one another; therefore, answer C is incorrect. Answer D is incorrect because the drugs would have a combined depressing, not excitatory, effect.

91. **Answer C is correct.** The medication should be withheld and the doctor should be notified. Answers A, B, and D are incorrect because they do not provide for the client's safety.

92. **Answer B is correct.** Solid foods should be added to the diet one at a time, with 4- to 7-day intervals between new foods. The extrusion reflex fades at 3–4 months of age; therefore, answer A is incorrect. Answer C is incorrect because solids should not be added to the bottle and the use of infant feeders is discouraged. Answer D is incorrect because the first food added to the infant's diet is rice cereal.

93. **Answer C is correct.** The client's symptoms suggest an adverse reaction to the medication known as neuroleptic malignant syndrome. Answers A, B, and D are not appropriate.

94. **Answer D is correct.** The client with HIV should adhere to a low-bacteria diet by avoiding raw fruits and vegetables. Answers A, B, and C are incorrect because they are permitted in the client's diet.

95. **Answer C is correct.** The child with leukemia has low platelet counts, which contribute to spontaneous bleeding. Answers A, B, and D, common in the child with leukemia, are not life-threatening.

96. **Answer A is correct.** The nurse should prevent the infant with atopic dermatitis (eczema) from scratching, which can lead to skin infections. Answer B is incorrect because fever is not associated with atopic dermatitis. Answers C and D are incorrect choices because they increase dryness of the skin, which worsens the symptoms of atopic dermatitis.

97. **Answer D is correct.** Symptoms associated with diverticulitis are usually reported after eating popcorn, celery, raw vegetables, whole grains, and nuts. Answers A, B, and C are incorrect because they are allowed in the diet of the client with diverticulitis.

98. **Answer B is correct.** The Whipple procedure is performed for cancer located in the head of the pancreas. Answers A, C, and D are not correct because of the location of the cancer.

99. **Answer C is correct.** Side effects of Pulmozyme include sore throat, hoarseness, and laryngitis. Answers A, B, and D are not associated with the use of Pulmozyme; therefore, they are incorrect.

100. **Answer B is correct.** The nurse should be concerned with alleviating the client's pain. Answers A, C, and D are not primary objectives in the care of the client receiving an opiate analgesic; therefore, they are incorrect.

101. **Answer C is correct.** Changes in breath sounds are the best indication of the need for suctioning in the client with ineffective airway clearance. Answers A, B, and D are incorrect because they can be altered by other conditions.

102. **Answer D is correct.** An adverse reaction to Myambutol is change in visual acuity or color vision. Answer A is incorrect because it does not relate to the medication. Answer C is incorrect because it is an adverse reaction to Streptomycin. Answer C is incorrect because it is a side effect of Rifampin.

103. **Answer D is correct.** Insufficient erythropoietin production is the primary cause of anemia in the client with chronic renal failure. Answers A, B, and C do not relate to the anemia seen in the client with chronic renal failure; therefore, they are incorrect.

104. **Answer C is correct.** The contrast media used during an intravenous pyelogram contains iodine, which can result in an anaphylactic reaction. Answers A, B, and D do not relate specifically to the test; therefore, they are incorrect.

105. **Answer D is correct.** Aspirin prevents the platelets from clumping together to prevent clots. Answer A is incorrect because the low-dose aspirin will not prevent headaches. Answers B and C are untrue statements; therefore, they are incorrect.

106. **Answer C is correct.** The usual course of treatment using a combined therapy with INH and Rifampin is 6 months. Answers A and D are incorrect because the treatment time is too brief. Answer B is incorrect because the medication is not needed for life.

107. **Answer D is correct.** At 4 months of age, the infant can roll over, which makes it vulnerable to falls from dressing tables or beds without rails. Answer A is incorrect

because it does not prove a threat to safety. Answers B and C are incorrect choices because the 4-month-old is not capable of crawling or standing.

108. **Answer C is correct.** Adverse side effects of Dilantin include agranulocytosis and aplastic anemia; therefore, the client will need frequent CBCs. Answer A is incorrect because the medication does not cause dental staining. Answer B is incorrect because the medication does not interfere with the metabolism of carbohydrates. Answer D is incorrect because the medication does not cause drowsiness.

109. **Answer A is correct.** The infant with hypospadias should not be circumcised because the foreskin is used in reconstruction. Answer B and C are incorrect because reconstruction is done between 16 and 18 months of age, before toilet training. Answer D is incorrect because the infant with hypospadias should not be circumcised.

110. **Answer C is correct.** Coconut oil is high in saturated fat and is not appropriate for the client on a low-cholesterol diet. Answers A, B, and D are incorrect because they are suggested for the client with elevated cholesterol levels.

111. **Answer B is correct.** In stage III of Alzheimer's disease, the client develops agnosia, or failure to recognize familiar objects. Answer A is incorrect because it appears in stage I. Answer C is incorrect because it appears in stage II. Answer D is incorrect because it appears in stage IV.

112. **Answer D is correct.** The client taking steroid medication should receive an annual influenza vaccine. Answer A is incorrect because the medication should be taken with food. Answer B is incorrect because increased appetite and weight gain are expected side effects of the medication. Answer C is incorrect because wearing sunglasses will not prevent cataracts.

113. **Answer A is correct.** The client with an above-the-knee amputation should be placed prone 15–30 minutes twice a day to prevent contractures. Answers B and D are incorrect choices because elevating the extremity after the first 24 hours will promote the development of contractures. Use of a trochanter roll will prevent rotation of the extremity but will not prevent contractures; therefore, answer D is incorrect.

114. **Answer D is correct.** All 20 primary, or deciduous, teeth should be present by age 30 months. Answers A, B, and C are incorrect because the ages are wrong.

115. **Answer C is correct.** The radioactive implant should be picked up with tongs and returned to the lead-lined container. Answer A is incorrect because radioactive materials are placed in lead-lined containers, not plastic ones, and are returned to the radiation department, not the lab. Answer B is incorrect because the client should not touch the implant or try to reinsert it. Answer D is incorrect because the implant should not be placed in the commode for disposal.

116. **Answer A is correct.** Following a laparoscopic cholecystectomy, the client should avoid a tub bath for 5 to 7 days. Answer B is incorrect because the stools should not be clay colored. Answer C is incorrect because pain is usually located in the shoulders. Answer D is incorrect because the client should not resume a regular diet until clear liquids have been tolerated.

117. **Answer B is correct.** The client recovering from mononucleosis should avoid contact sports and other activities that could result in injury or rupture of the spleen. Answer A

is incorrect because the client does not need additional fluids. Hypoglycemia is not associated with mononucleosis; therefore, answer C is incorrect. Answer D is incorrect because antibiotics are not usually indicated in the treatment of mononucleosis.

118. **Answer B is correct.** Pancreatic enzyme replacement is given with each meal and each snack. Answers A, C, and D do not specify a relationship to meals; therefore, they are incorrect.

119. **Answer A is correct.** Meat, eggs, and dairy products are foods high in vitamin B12. Answer B is incorrect because peanut butter, raisins, and molasses are sources rich in iron. Answer C is incorrect because broccoli, cauliflower, and cabbage are all sources rich in vitamin K. Answer D is incorrect because shrimp, legumes, and bran cereals are high in magnesium.

120. **Answer A is correct.** The client's aerobic workout should be 20–30 minutes long three times a week. Answers B, C, and D exceed the recommended time for the client beginning an aerobic program; therefore, they are incorrect.

121. **Answer A is correct.** A total mastectomy involves removal of the entire breast and some or all of the axillary lymph nodes. Following surgery, the client's right arm should be elevated on pillows, to facilitate lymph drainage. Answers B, C, and D are incorrect because they would not help facilitate lymph drainage and would create increased edema in the affected extremity.

122. **Answer D is correct.** Absence seizures, formerly known as petit mal seizures, are characterized by a brief lapse in consciousness accompanied by rapid eye blinking, lip smacking, and minor myoclonus of the upper extremities. Answer A refers to myoclonic seizures; therefore, it is incorrect. Answer B refers to tonic clonic, formerly known as grand mal, seizures; therefore, it is incorrect. Answer C refers to atonic seizures; therefore, it is incorrect.

123. **Answer A is correct.** A side effect of antipsychotic medication, such as Zyprexa, is the development of Parkinsonian symptoms. Answers B and C are incorrect choices because they are used to reverse Parkinsonian symptoms in the client taking antipsychotic medication. Answer D is incorrect because the medication is an anticonvulsant used to stabilize mood. Parkinsonian symptoms are not associated with anticonvulsant medication.

124. **Answer B is correct.** Exercises that provide light passive resistance are best for the child with rheumatoid arthritis. Answers A and C require movement of the hands and fingers that might be too painful for the child with juvenile rheumatoid arthritis; therefore, they are incorrect. Answer D is incorrect because it requires the use of larger joints affected by the disease.

125. **Answer B is correct.** The client's diabetes is well under control. Answer A is incorrect because it will lead to elevated blood sugar levels and poorer control of the client's diabetes. Answer C is incorrect because the diet and insulin dose are appropriate for the client. Answer D is incorrect because the desired range for glycosylated hemoglobin in the adult client is 2.5%–5.9%.

126. **Answer A is correct.** Stadol reduces the perception of pain, which allows the postoperative client to rest. Answers B and C are not affected by the medication; therefore,

they are incorrect. Relief of pain generally results in less nausea, but it is not the intended effect of the medication; therefore, answer D is incorrect.

127. **Answer B is correct.** Children with cystic fibrosis are susceptible to chronic sinusitis and nasal polyps, which might require surgical removal. Answer A is incorrect because it is a congenital condition in which there is a bony obstruction between the nares and the pharynx. Answers C and D are not specific to the child with cystic fibrosis; therefore, they are incorrect.

128. **Answer D is correct.** Lipid-lowering agents are contraindicated in the client with active liver disease. Answers A, B, and C are incorrect because they are not contraindicated in the client with active liver disease.

129. **Answer C is correct.** Oatmeal is low in sodium and high in fiber. Limiting sodium intake and increasing fiber helps to lower cholesterol levels, which reduce blood pressure. Answer A is incorrect because cornflakes and whole milk are higher in sodium and are poor sources of fiber. Answers B and D are incorrect choices because they contain animal proteins that are high in both cholesterol and sodium.

130. **Answer A is correct.** After hypospadias repair, the child will need to avoid straddle toys, such as a rocking horse, until allowed by the surgeon. Swimming and rough play should also be avoided. Answers B, C, and D do not relate to the post-operative care of the child with hypospadias; therefore, they are incorrect.

131. **Answer A is correct.** Symptoms of morning sickness might be alleviated by eating a carbohydrate source such as dry crackers or toast before arising. Answer B is incorrect because the additional fat might increase the client's nausea. Answer C is incorrect because the client does not need to skip meals. Answer D is the treatment of hypoglycemia, not morning sickness; therefore, it is incorrect.

132. **Answer A is correct.** The stethoscope should be left in the client's room for future use. The stethoscope should not be returned to the exam room or the nurse's station; therefore, answers B and D are incorrect. The stethoscope should not be used to assess other clients; therefore, answer C is incorrect.

133. **Answer B is correct.** The medication will be needed throughout the child's lifetime. Answers A, C, and D contain inaccurate statements; therefore, they are incorrect.

134. **Answer B is correct.** Glucotrol XL is given once a day with breakfast. Answer A is incorrect because the client would develop hypoglycemia while sleeping. Answers C and D are incorrect choices because the client would develop hypoglycemia later in the day or evening.

135. **Answer D is correct.** The client with myasthenia develops progressive weakness that worsens during the day. Answer A is incorrect because it refers to symptoms of multiple sclerosis. Answer B is incorrect because it refers to symptoms of Guillain Barre syndrome. Answer C is incorrect because it refers to Parkinson's disease.

136. **Answer B is correct.** To prevent fractures, the parents should lift the infant by the buttocks rather than the ankles when diapering. Answer A is incorrect because infants with osteogenesis imperfecta have normal calcium and phosphorus levels. Answer C is incorrect because the condition is not temporary. Answer D is incorrect because the teeth and the sclera are also affected.

137. Answer A is correct. Placing the client on strict NPO status will stop the inflammatory process by reducing the secretion of pancreatic enzymes. The use of low, intermittent suction prevents release of secretion in the duodenum. Answer B is incorrect because the client requires exogenous insulin. Answer C is incorrect because it does not prevent the secretion of gastric acid. Answer D is incorrect because it does not eliminate the need for analgesia.

138. Answer B is correct. A rigid or boardlike abdomen is suggestive of peritonitis, which is a complication of diverticulitis. Answers A, C, and D are common findings in diverticulitis; therefore, they are incorrect.

139. Answer A is correct. Prostigmin is used to treat clients with myasthenia gravis. Answer B is incorrect because atropine sulfate is used in the management of the client with cholinergic crisis. Answer C is incorrect because the drug is unrelated to the treatment of myasthenia gravis. Answer D is incorrect because it is the test for myasthenia gravis.

140. Answer D is correct. The suggested diet for the client with AIDS is one that is high calorie, high protein, and low fat. Clients with AIDS have a reduced tolerance to fat because of the disease as well as side effects from some antiviral medications; therefore, answers A and C are incorrect. Answer B is incorrect because the client needs a high-protein diet.

141. Answer B is correct. The nurse can help ready the child with cerebral palsy for speech therapy by providing activities that help the child develop tongue control. Most children with cerebral palsy have visual and auditory difficulties that require glasses or hearing devices rather than rehabilitative training; therefore, answers A and C are incorrect. Answer D is incorrect because video games are not appropriate for the age or developmental level of the child with cerebral palsy.

142. Answer C is correct. Most infants begin nocturnal sleep lasting 9–11 hours by 3–4 months of age. Answers A and B are incorrect because the infant is still waking for nighttime feedings. Answer D is incorrect because it does not answer the question.

143. Answer A is correct. The child with myelomenigocele is at greatest risk for the development of latex allergy because of repeated exposure to latex products during surgery and from numerous urinary catheterizations. Answers B, C, and D are much less likely to be exposed to latex; therefore, they are incorrect.

144. Answer D is correct. The nurse or parent should use a cupped hand when performing chest percussion. Answer A is incorrect because the hand should be cupped. Answer B is incorrect because the child's position should be changed every 5–10 minutes and the whole session should be limited to 20 minutes. Answer C is incorrect because chest percussion should be done before meals.

145. Answer A is correct. No more than 1mL should be given in the vastus lateralis of the infant. Answers B, C, and D are incorrect because the dorsogluteal and ventrogluteal muscles are not used for injections in the infant.

146. Answer C is correct. Depot injections of Haldol are administered every 4 weeks. Answers A and B are incorrect because the medication is still in the client's system. Answer D is incorrect because the medication has been eliminated from the client's system, which allows the symptoms of schizophrenia to return.

147. **Answer D is correct.** Tucking a disposable diaper at the perineal opening will help prevent soiling of the cast by urine and stool. Answer A is incorrect because the head of the bed should be elevated. Answer B is incorrect because the child can place the crayons beneath the cast, causing pressure areas to develop. Answer C is incorrect because the child does not need high-calorie foods that would cause weight gain while she is immobilized by the cast.

148. **Answer B is correct.** Coolness and discoloration of the reimplanted digits indicates compromised circulation, which should be reported immediately to the physician. The temperature should be monitored, but the client would receive antibiotics to prevent infection; therefore, answer A is incorrect. Answers C and D are expected following amputation and reimplantation; therefore, they are incorrect.

149. **Answer A is correct.** Following extracorporeal lithotripsy, the urine will appear cherry red in color but will gradually change to clear urine. Answer B is incorrect because the urine will be red, not orange. Answer C is incorrect because the urine will be not be dark red or cloudy in appearance. Answer D is incorrect because it describes the urinary output of the client with acute glomerulonephritis.

150. **Answer B is correct.** An adverse reaction to Cognex (tacrine) is drug-induced hepatitis. The nurse should monitor the client for signs of jaundice. Answers A, C, and D are incorrect because they are not associated with the use of Cognex (tacrine).

151. **Answer C is correct.** Apricots are low in potassium; therefore, it is a suitable snack of the client on a potassium-restricted diet. Raisins, oranges, and bananas are all good sources of potassium; therefore, answers A, B, and C are incorrect choices.

152. **Answer B is correct.** No special preparation is needed for the blood test for *H. pylori.* Answer A is incorrect because the client is not NPO before the test. Answer C is incorrect because it refers to preparation for the breath test. Answer D is incorrect because glucose is not administered before the test.

153. **Answer B is correct.** Oral potassium supplements should be given in at least 4oz. of juice or other liquid, to prevent gastric upset and to disguise the unpleasant taste. Answers A, C, and D are incorrect because they cause gastric upset.

154. **Answer D is correct.** Fresh specimens are essential for accurate diagnosis of CMV. Answer A is incorrect because cultures of urine, sputum, and oral swab are preferred. Answer B is incorrect because pregnant caregivers should not be assigned to care for clients with suspected or known infection with CMV. Answer C is incorrect because a convalescent culture is obtained 2–4 weeks after diagnosis.

155. **Answer D is correct.** The client should receive pain medication 30 minutes before the application of Sulfamylon. Answer A is incorrect because it refers to silver nitrate. Answer B is incorrect because it refers to Silvadene. Answer C is incorrect because it refers to Betadine.

156. **Answer D is correct.** Gingival hyperplasia is a side effect of Dilantin; therefore, the nurse should provide oral hygiene and gum care every shift. Answers A, B, and C do not apply to the medication; therefore, they are incorrect.

157. **Answer C is correct.** Zofran is given before chemotherapy to prevent nausea. Answers A, B, and D are not associated with the medication; therefore, they are incorrect.

158. **Answer A is correct.** When administering ear drops to a child under 3 years of age, the nurse should pull the ear down and back to straighten the ear canal. Answers B and D are incorrect positions for administering ear drops. Answer C is used for administering ear drops to an adult client.

159. **Answer C is correct.** The nurse should carefully monitor the client taking Thorazine for signs of infection that can quickly become overwhelming. Answers A, B, and D are incorrect because they are expected side effects of the medication.

160. **Answer A is correct.** Iron is better absorbed when taken with ascorbic acid. Orange juice is an excellent source of ascorbic acid. Answer B is incorrect because the medication should be taken with orange juice or tomato juice. Answer C is incorrect because iron should not be taken with milk because it interferes with absorption. Answer D is incorrect because apple juice does not contain high amounts of ascorbic acid.

161. **Answer B is correct.** Burn injury of the arm (9%), chest (9%), and head (9%) accounts for burns covering 27% of the total body surface area. Answers A, C, and D are incorrect percentages.

162. **Answer B is correct.** With standing orders, the nurse can administer oxygen at 6L per minute via mask. Answer A is incorrect because the amount is too low to help the client with chest pain and shortness of breath. Answers C and D have oxygen levels requiring a doctor's order.

163. **Answer A is correct.** Stool from the ileostomy contains digestive enzymes that can cause severe skin breakdown. Answer B contains contradictory information; therefore, it is incorrect. Answers C and D contain inaccurate statements; therefore, they are incorrect.

164. **Answer C is correct.** Tinnitus is a sign of aspirin toxicity. Answers A, B, and D are not related to aspirin toxicity; therefore, they are incorrect.

165. **Answer B is correct.** The client with delirium tremens has an increased risk for seizures; therefore, the nurse should provide seizure precautions. Answer A is not a priority in the client's care; therefore, it is incorrect. Answer C is incorrect because the client should be kept in a dimly lit, not dark, room. Answer D is incorrect because thiamine and multivitamins are given to prevent Wernicke's encephalopathy, not delirium tremens.

166. **Answer D is correct.** Steak, baked potato, and tossed salad are lower in purine than the other choices. Liver, crab, and chicken are high in purine; therefore, answers A, B, and C are incorrect.

167. **Answer C is correct.** Placing the newborn in a side-lying position helps the urine to drain from the exposed bladder. Answer A is incorrect because it would position the child on the exposed bladder. Answers B and D are incorrect choices because they would allow the urine to pool.

168. **Answer D is correct.** Burping the baby frequently throughout the feeding will help prevent gastric distention that contributes to esophageal reflux. Answers A and B are incorrect because they allow air to collect in the baby's stomach, which contributes to reflux. Answer C is incorrect because the baby should be placed side-lying with the head elevated, to prevent aspiration.

169. **Answer B is correct.** Growth plates located in the epiphysis can be damaged by epiphyseal fractures. Answers A, C, and D are untrue statements; therefore, they are incorrect.

170. **Answer A is correct.** The nurse should replace the aspirate and administer the feeding because the amount aspirated was less than 50mL. Answers B and C are incorrect choices because the aspirate should not be discarded. Answer D is incorrect because the feeding should not be withheld.

171. **Answer B is correct.** The nurse should administer two capsules. Answers A, C, and D contain inaccurate amounts; therefore, they are incorrect.

172. **Answer B is correct.** The normal specific gravity is 1.010 to 1.025. Answers A, C, and D are inaccurate statements; therefore, they are incorrect.

173. **Answer A is correct.** To prevent spasms of the sphincter of Oddi, the client with acute pancreatitis should receive non-opiate analgesics for pain. Answer B is incorrect because the client with acute pancreatitis might be prone to bleed; therefore, Toradol is not a drug of choice for pain control. Morphine and codeine, opiate analgesics, are contraindicated for the client with acute pancreatitis; therefore, answers C and D are incorrect.

174. **Answer D is correct.** Overuse of magnesium-containing antacids results in diarrhea. Antacids containing calcium and aluminum cause constipation; therefore, answer A is incorrect. Answers B and C are not associated with the use of magnesium antacids; therefore, they are incorrect.

175. **Answer B is correct.** The head circumference of the normal newborn is approximately 33 cm, while the chest circumference is 31cm. Answer A is incorrect because the head and chest are not the same circumference. Answer C is incorrect because the head is larger in circumference than the chest. Answer D is incorrect because the difference in head circumference and chest circumference is too great.

176. **Answer D is correct.** Protamine sulfate is given to counteract the effects of enoxaprin as well as heparin. Calcium gluconate is given to counteract the effects of magnesium sulfate; therefore, answer A is incorrect. Answer B is incorrect because aquamephyton is given to counteract the effects of sodium warfarin. Answer C is incorrect because methergine is given to increase uterine contractions following delivery.

177. **Answer A is correct.** Participating in reality orientation is the most appropriate activity for the client who is confused. Answers B, C, and D are incorrect because they are not suitable activities for a client who is confused.

178. **Answer B is correct.** The nurse should recommend acetaminophen for the child's joint discomfort because it will have no effect on the bleeding time. Answers A, C, and D are all nonsteroidal anti-inflammatory medications that can prolong bleeding time; therefore, they are not suitable for the child with hemophilia.

179. **Answer D is correct.** Applying a paste of baking soda and water soothes the itching and helps to dry the vesicles. The use of baby powder is not recommended because inhalation of the powder is detrimental to the client; therefore, answer A is incorrect. Answers B and C are incorrect choices because hydrogen peroxide and saline will not relieve the itching and will prevent the vesicles from crusting.

180. **Answer A is correct.** Hypospadias results when the urinary meatus is located on the underside of the penis rather than the tip. Answer B is incorrect because it refers to ureteral reflux. Answer C is incorrect because it refers to epispadias. Answer D is incorrect because it refers to exstrophy of the bladder.

181. **Answer D is correct.** Tagamet (cimetidine) should be administered in one dose at bedtime. Answers A, B, and C have incorrect times for dosing.

182. **Answer A is correct.** Pain associated with angina is relieved by rest. Answer B is incorrect because it is not a true statement. Answer C is incorrect because pain associated with angina can be referred to the jaw, the left arm, and the back. Answer D is incorrect because pain from a myocardial infarction can be referred to areas other than the left arm.

183. **Answer A is correct.** It would not be helpful to limit the fluid intake of a client during bowel retraining. Answers B, C, and D would help the client; therefore, they are incorrect answers.

184. **Answer B is correct.** The client with Meniere's disease should limit the intake of foods that contain sodium. Answers A, C, and D have no relationship to the symptoms of Meniere's disease; therefore, they are incorrect.

185. **Answer A is correct.** The nurse should pay close attention to swelling in the client with preeclampsia. Facial swelling indicates that the client's condition is worsening and blood pressure will be increased. Answer B is not related to the question; therefore, it is incorrect. Answer C is incorrect because ankle edema is expected in pregnancy. Diminished reflexes are associated with the use of magnesium sulfate, which is the treatment of preeclampsia; therefore, answer D is incorrect.

186. **Answer D is correct.** Verbalizing feelings of anger and sadness to a staff member is an appropriate therapeutic goal for the client with a risk of self-directed violence. Answers A and C place the client in an isolated situation to deal with her feelings alone; therefore, they are incorrect. Answer B is incorrect because it does not allow the client to ventilate her feelings.

187. **Answer C is correct.** The nurse should remove any remaining ointment before applying the medication again. Answer A is incorrect because it interferes with absorption. Answer B does not apply to the question of how to administer the medication; therefore, it is incorrect. Answer D is incorrect because the medication's action is more immediate.

188. **Answer D is correct.** Telling the client what happened and where he is helps with reorientation. Answer A does not explain what happened to the client; therefore, it is incorrect. Answer B is not helpful because the client regaining consciousness will not know where he is; therefore, the answer is incorrect. The nurse should not offer false reassurances, such as "everything will be alright"; therefore, answer C is incorrect.

189. **Answer B is correct.** Following a generalized seizure, the client frequently experiences drowsiness and postictal sleep. Answer A is incorrect because the client is able to move the extremities. Answer C is incorrect because the client can remember events before the seizure. Answer D is incorrect because the blood pressure is elevated.

190. **Answer A is correct.** The client with oxylate renal calculi should limit sources of oxylate, which include strawberries, rhubarb, and spinach. Answers B, C, and D are incorrect because they are not sources of oxylate.

191. **Answer D is correct.** The child with Legg-Calve Perthes disease should be prevented from bearing weight on the affected extremity until revascularization has occurred. Answer A is incorrect because it does not relate to the condition. Answers B and C are incorrect choices because the condition does not involve the muscles or the joints.

192. **Answer B is correct.** The infant with Hirschsprung's disease will have infrequent bowel movements. Answers A, C, and D do not apply to the condition; therefore, they are incorrect.

193. **Answer B is correct.** Iron supplements should be taken with a source of vitamin C to promote absorption. Answer A is incorrect because iron should not be taken with milk. Answer C is incorrect because high-fiber sources prevent the absorption of iron. Answer D is an inaccurate statement; therefore, it is incorrect.

194. **Answer A is correct.** The client does not need to drastically reduce her caloric intake during pregnancy. Doing so would not provide adequate nourishment for proper development of the fetus. Answers B, C, and D indicate that the client understands the nurse's dietary teaching regarding obesity and hypertension; therefore, they are incorrect.

195. **Answer B is correct.** Confusion, disorientation, behavioral changes, and alterations in judgment are early signs of dementia. Answers A, C, and D do not relate to the question; therefore, they are incorrect.

196. **Answer C is correct.** In the left occipital posterior position, the heart sounds will be heard loudest through the fetal back. Answers A, B, and D are incorrect locations.

197. **Answer B is correct.** Benzodiazepines such as Ativan (lorazepam) and Klonopin (clonazepam) are given to the client withdrawing from alcohol. Answer A is incorrect because methodone is given to the client withdrawing from opiates. Answer C is incorrect because naloxone is an antidote for narcotic overdose. Answer D is incorrect because disufiram is used in aversive therapy for alcohol addiction.

198. **Answer C is correct.** The client's breakfast should be served within 30 minutes to coincide with the onset of the client's regular insulin.

199. **Answer C is correct.** The nurse should administer .07mL of the medication. Answers A, B, and D are incorrect because the dosage is incorrect.

200. **Answer A is correct.** Tetracycline is contraindicated for use in infants and young children because it stains the teeth and arrests bone development. Answers B, C, and D are incorrect because they can be used to treat infections in infants and children.

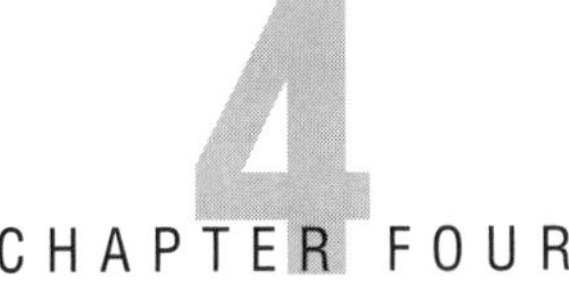

CHAPTER FOUR

Practice Exam 4 and Rationales

Quick Check

1. A client with AIDS asks the nurse why he can't have a pitcher of water at his bedside so he can drink whenever he likes. The nurse should tell the client that:

   - ❍ **A.** It would be best for him to drink tap water.
   - ❍ **B.** He should drink less water and more juice.
   - ❍ **C.** Leaving a glass of water makes it easier to calculate his intake.
   - ❍ **D.** He shouldn't drink water that has been sitting longer than 15 minutes.

Quick Answers: **251**
Detailed Answer: **254**

2. The mother of a male child with cystic fibrosis tells the nurse that she hopes her son's children won't have the disease. The nurse is aware that:

   - ❍ **A.** There is a 25% chance that his children would have cystic fibrosis.
   - ❍ **B.** Most of the males with cystic fibrosis are sterile.
   - ❍ **C.** There is a 50% chance that his children would be carriers.
   - ❍ **D.** Most males with cystic fibrosis are capable of having children, so genetic counseling is advised.

Quick Answers: **251**
Detailed Answer: **254**

3. An infant is hospitalized for treatment of botulism. Which factor is associated with botulism in the infant?

   - ❍ **A.** The infant sucks on his fingers and toes.
   - ❍ **B.** The mother sweetens the infant's cereal with honey.
   - ❍ **C.** The infant was switched to soy-based formula.
   - ❍ **D.** The infant's older sibling has an aquarium.

Quick Answers: **251**
Detailed Answer: **254**

Quick Check

4. A nurse is assessing a client hospitalized with peptic ulcer disease. Which finding should be reported to the charge nurse immediately?

Quick Answers: 251
Detailed Answer: 254

- ❍ **A.** BP 82/60, pulse 120
- ❍ **B.** Pulse 68, respirations 24
- ❍ **C.** BP 110/88, pulse 56
- ❍ **D.** Pulse 82, respirations 16

5. The nurse is teaching the client with AIDS regarding proper food preparation. Which statement indicates that the client needs further teaching?

Quick Answers: 251
Detailed Answer: 254

- ❍ **A.** "I should avoid adding pepper to food after it is cooked."
- ❍ **B.** "I can still have an occasional medium-rare steak."
- ❍ **C.** "Eating cheese and yogurt won't help prevent AIDS-related diarrhea."
- ❍ **D.** "I should eat fruits and vegetables that can be peeled."

6. A client taking Laniazid (isoniazid) asks the nurse how long she must take the medication before her sputum cultures will return to normal. The nurse recognizes that the client should have a negative sputum culture within:

Quick Answers: 251
Detailed Answer: 254

- ❍ **A.** 2 weeks
- ❍ **B.** 6 weeks
- ❍ **C.** 2 months
- ❍ **D.** 3 months

7. Which person is at greatest risk for developing Lyme's disease?

Quick Answers: 251
Detailed Answer: 254

- ❍ **A.** Computer technician
- ❍ **B.** Middle-school teacher
- ❍ **C.** Dog trainer
- ❍ **D.** Forestry worker

8. Following eruption of the primary teeth, the mother can promote chewing by giving the toddler:

Quick Answers: 251
Detailed Answer: 254

- ❍ **A.** Pieces of hot dog
- ❍ **B.** Celery sticks
- ❍ **C.** Melba toast
- ❍ **D.** Grapes

Quick Check

9. A client scheduled for an exploratory laparotomy tells the nurse that she takes kava-kava (piper methysticum)for sleep. The nurse should notify the doctor because kava-kava:

Quick Answers: 251
Detailed Answer: 254

- ❍ **A.** Increases the effects of anesthesia and post-operative analgesia
- ❍ **B.** Eliminates the need for antimicrobial therapy following surgery
- ❍ **C.** Increases urinary output, so a urinary catheter will be needed post-operatively
- ❍ **D.** Depresses the immune system, so infection is more of a problem

10. The nurse is teaching circumcision care to the mother of a newborn. Which statement indicates that the mother needs further teaching?

Quick Answers: 251
Detailed Answer: 254

- ❍ **A.** "I will apply a petroleum gauze to the area once a day."
- ❍ **B.** "I will clean the area carefully with each diaper change."
- ❍ **C.** "I can place a heat lamp next to the area to speed up the healing process."
- ❍ **D.** "I should carefully observe the area for signs of infection."

11. The chart of a client hospitalized with a fractured femur reveals that the client is colonized with MRSA. The nurse knows that the client:

Quick Answers: 251
Detailed Answer: 254

- ❍ **A.** Will not display symptoms of infection
- ❍ **B.** Is less likely to have an infection
- ❍ **C.** Can be placed in the room with others
- ❍ **D.** Cannot colonize others with MRSA

12. A client is admitted with *Clostridium difficile*. The nurse would expect the client to have:

Quick Answers: 251
Detailed Answer: 255

- ❍ **A.** Diarrhea containing blood and mucus
- ❍ **B.** Cough, fever, and shortness of breath
- ❍ **C.** Anorexia, weight loss, and fever
- ❍ **D.** Development of deep leg ulcers

Quick Check

13. An elderly client asks the nurse how often he will need to receive immunizations against pneumonia. The nurse should tell the client that she will need an immunization against pneumonia:

- ❍ **A.** Every year
- ❍ **B.** Every 2 years
- ❍ **C.** Every 5 years
- ❍ **D.** Every 10 years

Quick Answers: **251**
Detailed Answer: **255**

14. The nurse is caring for a client following a right nephrolithotomy. Post-operatively, the client should be positioned:

- ❍ **A.** On the right side
- ❍ **B.** Supine
- ❍ **C.** On the left side
- ❍ **D.** Prone

Quick Answers: **251**
Detailed Answer: **255**

15. A nursing assistant is referred to the employee health office with symptoms of latex allergy. The first symptom usually noticed by those with latex allergy is:

- ❍ **A.** Oral itching after eating bananas
- ❍ **B.** Swelling of the eyes and mouth
- ❍ **C.** Difficulty breathing
- ❍ **D.** Swelling and itching of the hands

Quick Answers: **251**
Detailed Answer: **255**

16. Acticoat (silver nitrate) dressings are applied to the arms and chest of a client with full-thickness burns. The nurse should:

- ❍ **A.** Change the dressings once per shift
- ❍ **B.** Moisten the dressings with sterile water
- ❍ **C.** Change the dressings only when they become soiled
- ❍ **D.** Moisten the dressings with normal saline

Quick Answers: **251**
Detailed Answer: **255**

17. A client is diagnosed with stage III Hodgkin's lymphoma. The nurse recognizes that the client has involvement:

- ❍ **A.** In a single lymph node or single site
- ❍ **B.** In more than one node or single organ on the same side of the diaphragm
- ❍ **C.** In lymph nodes on both sides of the diaphragm
- ❍ **D.** In disseminated organs and tissues

Quick Answers: **251**
Detailed Answer: **255**

Quick Check

18. A client has been receiving Rheumatrex (methotrexate) for severe rheumatoid arthritis. The nurse should tell the client to avoid taking:

Quick Answers: **251**
Detailed Answer: **255**

- ❍ **A.** Aspirin
- ❍ **B.** Multivitamins
- ❍ **C.** Omega 3 and omega 6 fish oils
- ❍ **D.** Acetaminophen

19. A suitable diet for a client with cirrhosis and abdominal ascites is one that is:

Quick Answers: **251**
Detailed Answer: **255**

- ❍ **A.** High in sodium, low in calories
- ❍ **B.** Low in potassium, high in calories
- ❍ **C.** High in protein, high in calories
- ❍ **D.** Low in calcium, low in calories

20. A client with gallstones in the gall bladder is scheduled for lithotripsy. For the procedure, the client will be placed:

Quick Answers: **251**
Detailed Answer: **255**

- ❍ **A.** In a prone position
- ❍ **B.** In a supine position
- ❍ **C.** In a side-lying position
- ❍ **D.** In a recumbent position

21. A client with rheumatoid arthritis is being treated with daily steroid medication. Which food should the client avoid?

Quick Answers: **251**
Detailed Answer: **255**

- ❍ **A.** Raw oysters
- ❍ **B.** Cottage cheese
- ❍ **C.** Baked chicken
- ❍ **D.** Green beans

22. A client tells the nurse that she takes St. John's wort (hypericum perforatum) three times a day for mild depression. The nurse should tell the client that:

Quick Answers: **251**
Detailed Answer: **256**

- ❍ **A.** St. John's wort seldom relieves depression.
- ❍ **B.** She should avoid eating cold cuts and aged cheese.
- ❍ **C.** Skin reactions increase with the use of sunscreens.
- ❍ **D.** St. John's wort will increase the amount of medication needed.

Quick Check

23. The physician has instructed the client with gout to avoid protein sources of purine. Which protein source is high in purine?

Quick Answers: **251**
Detailed Answer: **256**

❍ **A.** Dried beans
❍ **B.** Nuts
❍ **C.** Cheese
❍ **D.** Eggs

24. The nurse is caring for a client with a long history of bulimia. The nurse would expect the client to have:

Quick Answers: **251**
Detailed Answer: **256**

❍ **A.** Extreme weight loss
❍ **B.** Dental caries
❍ **C.** Hair loss
❍ **D.** Lanugo

25. A client with paranoid schizophrenia has an order for Thorazine (chlorpromazine) 400mg orally twice daily. Which of the following symptoms should be reported to the physician immediately?

Quick Answers: **251**
Detailed Answer: **256**

❍ **A.** Muscle spasms of the neck, difficulty in swallowing
❍ **B.** Dry mouth, constipation, blurred vision
❍ **C.** Lethargy, slurred speech, thirst
❍ **D.** Fatigue, drowsiness, photosensitivity

26. The nurse is applying a Transderm Nitro (nitrogycerin) patch to a client with angina. When applying the patch, the nurse should:

Quick Answers: **251**
Detailed Answer: **256**

❍ **A.** Shave the area before applying a new patch
❍ **B.** Remove the old patch and clean the skin with alcohol
❍ **C.** Cover the patch with plastic wrap and tape it in place
❍ **D.** Avoid cutting the patch because it will alter the dose

27. A client with myasthenia gravis is admitted with a diagnosis of cholinergic crisis. The nurse can expect the client to have:

Quick Answers: **251**
Detailed Answer: **256**

❍ **A.** Decreased blood pressure and pupillary meiosis
❍ **B.** Increased heart rate and increased respirations
❍ **C.** Increased respirations and increased blood pressure
❍ **D.** Anoxia and absence of the cough reflex

Quick Check

28. The nurse is providing dietary teaching regarding low-sodium diets for a client with hypertension. Which food should be avoided by the client on a low-sodium diet?

Quick Answers: **251**
Detailed Answer: **256**

- ❍ **A.** Dried beans
- ❍ **B.** Swiss cheese
- ❍ **C.** Peanut butter
- ❍ **D.** American cheese

29. A client is admitted to the emergency room with partial-thickness burns of his head and both arms. According to the Rule of Nines, the nurse calculates that the TBSA (total body surface area) involved is:

Quick Answers: **251**
Detailed Answer: **256**

- ❍ **A.** 20%
- ❍ **B.** 27%
- ❍ **C.** 35%
- ❍ **D.** 50%

30. The physician has ordered a paracentesis for a client with severe ascites. Before the procedure, the nurse should:

Quick Answers: **251**
Detailed Answer: **256**

- ❍ **A.** Instruct the client to void
- ❍ **B.** Shave the abdomen
- ❍ **C.** Encourage extra fluids
- ❍ **D.** Request an abdominal x-ray

31. The mother of a child with chickenpox wants to know if there is a medication that will shorten the course of the illness. Which medication is sometimes used to speed healing of the lesions and shorten the duration of fever and itching?

Quick Answers: **251**
Detailed Answer: **256**

- ❍ **A.** Zovirax (acyclovir)
- ❍ **B.** Varivax (varicella vaccine)
- ❍ **C.** VZIG (varicella-zoster immune globulin)
- ❍ **D.** Periactin (cyproheptadine)

32. Which of the following clients is most likely to be a victim of elder abuse?

Quick Answers: **251**
Detailed Answer: **257**

- ❍ **A.** A 62-year-old female with diverticulitis
- ❍ **B.** A 76-year-old female with right-sided hemiplegia
- ❍ **C.** A 65-year-old male with a hip replacement
- ❍ **D.** A 72-year-old male with diabetes mellitus

Quick Check

33. A hospitalized client with severe anemia is to receive a unit of blood. Which facet of care is most appropriate for the newly licensed practical nurse?

Quick Answers: **251**
Detailed Answer: **257**

- ❍ **A.** Initiating the IV of normal saline
- ❍ **B.** Monitoring the client's vital signs
- ❍ **C.** Initiating the blood transfusion
- ❍ **D.** Notifying the physician of a reaction

34. To reduce the possibility of having a baby with a neural tube defect, the client should be told to increase her intake of folic acid. Dietary sources of folic acid include:

Quick Answers: **251**
Detailed Answer: **257**

- ❍ **A.** Meat, liver, eggs
- ❍ **B.** Pork, fish, chicken
- ❍ **C.** Oranges, cabbage, cantaloupe
- ❍ **D.** Dried beans, sweet potatoes, Brussels sprouts

35. A client is admitted for suspected bladder cancer. Which one of the following factors is most significant in the client's diagnosis?

Quick Answers: **251**
Detailed Answer: **257**

- ❍ **A.** Smoking a pack of cigarettes a day for 30 years
- ❍ **B.** Taking hormone-replacement therapy
- ❍ **C.** Eating foods with preservatives
- ❍ **D.** Past employment involving asbestos

36. The physician has prescribed nitroglycerin buccal tablets as needed for a client with angina. The nurse should tell the client to take the tablets:

Quick Answers: **251**
Detailed Answer: **257**

- ❍ **A.** After engaging in strenuous activity
- ❍ **B.** Every 4 hours to prevent chest pain
- ❍ **C.** When he first feels chest discomfort
- ❍ **D.** At bedtime to prevent nocturnal angina

37. The nurse is caring for an infant who is on strict intake and output. The used diaper weighs 90.5 grams. The diaper's dry weight was 62 grams. The infant's urine output was:

Quick Answers: **251**
Detailed Answer: **257**

- ❍ **A.** 10mL
- ❍ **B.** 28.5mL
- ❍ **C.** 10 grams
- ❍ **D.** 152.5 grams

Quick Check

38. The nurse is teaching the parents of an infant with osteogenesis imperfecta. The nurse should explain the need for:

Quick Answers: **251**
Detailed Answer: **257**

❍ **A.** Additional calcium in the infant's diet

❍ **B.** Careful handling to prevent fractures

❍ **C.** Providing extra sensorimotor stimulation

❍ **D.** Frequent testing of visual function

39. The nurse is preparing a client with gastroesophageal reflux disease (GERD) for discharge. The nurse should tell the client to:

Quick Answers: **251**
Detailed Answer: **257**

❍ **A.** Eat a small snack before bedtime

❍ **B.** Sleep on his right side

❍ **C.** Avoid colas, tea, and coffee

❍ **D.** Increase his intake of citrus fruits

40. The nurse is administering Dilantin (phenytoin) via nasogastric (NG) tube. When giving the medication, the nurse should:

Quick Answers: **251**
Detailed Answer: **258**

❍ **A.** Flush the NG tube with 2–4mL of water before giving the medication

❍ **B.** Administer the medication, flush with 5mL of water, and clamp the NG tube

❍ **C.** Flush the NG tube with 5mL of normal saline and administer the medication

❍ **D.** Flush the NG tube with 2–4oz. of water before and after giving the medication

41. The nurse is caring for a 3-year-old in a wet hip spica cast made from plaster of Paris. When turning the 3-year-old with a wet cast, the nurse should:

Quick Answers: **251**
Detailed Answer: **258**

❍ **A.** Grasp the cast by the hand

❍ **B.** Use an assistive sling

❍ **C.** Use the palms of the hands

❍ **D.** Obtain a lifting device

42. A client has a diagnosis of discoid lupus. The primary difference in discoid lupus and systemic lupus is that discoid lupus:

Quick Answers: **251**
Detailed Answer: **258**

❍ **A.** Produces changes in the kidneys

❍ **B.** Is confined to the skin

❍ **C.** Results in damage to the heart and lungs

❍ **D.** Affects both joints and muscles

Quick Check

43. The nurse is preparing to walk the post-operative client for the first time since surgery. Before walking the client, the nurse should:

Quick Answers: **251**
Detailed Answer: **258**

- ❍ **A.** Give the client pain medication
- ❍ **B.** Assist the client in dangling his legs
- ❍ **C.** Have the client breathe deeply
- ❍ **D.** Provide the client with additional fluids

44. While performing a neurological assessment on a client with a closed head injury, the licensed practical nurse notes a positive Babinski reflex. The nurse should:

Quick Answers: **251**
Detailed Answer: **258**

- ❍ **A.** Recognize that the client's condition is improving
- ❍ **B.** Reposition the client and check reflexes again
- ❍ **C.** Do nothing because the finding is an expected one
- ❍ **D.** Notify the charge nurse of the finding

45. The physician has prescribed Gantrisin (sulfasoxazole) 1 gram in divided doses for a client with a urinary tract infection. The nurse should administer the medication:

Quick Answers: **251**
Detailed Answer: **258**

- ❍ **A.** With meals or a snack
- ❍ **B.** 30 minutes before meals
- ❍ **C.** 30 minutes after meals
- ❍ **D.** At bedtime

46. A client hospitalized with renal calculi complains of severe pain in the right flank. In addition to complaints of pain, the nurse can expect to see changes in the client's vital signs, which include:

Quick Answers: **251**
Detailed Answer: **258**

- ❍ **A.** Decreased pulse rate
- ❍ **B.** Increased blood pressure
- ❍ **C.** Decreased respiratory rate
- ❍ **D.** Increased temperature

47. A 3-year-old is diagnosed with diarrhea caused by an infection with salmonella. Which of the following most likely contributed to the child's illness?

Quick Answers: **251**
Detailed Answer: **258**

- ❍ **A.** Brushing the family dog
- ❍ **B.** Playing with a pet turtle
- ❍ **C.** Taking a pony ride
- ❍ **D.** Feeding the family cat

Quick Check

48. The nurse is administering Pyridium (phenazopyridine) to a client with cystitis. The nurse should tell the client that:

Quick Answers: **251**
Detailed Answer: **258**

❍ **A.** The urine will have a strong odor of ammonia.

❍ **B.** The urinary output will increase in amount.

❍ **C.** The urine will have a red–orange color.

❍ **D.** The urinary output will decrease in amount.

49. The nurse is caring for an infant with atopic dermatitis. An important part of the infant's care will be:

Quick Answers: **251**
Detailed Answer: **258**

❍ **A.** Keeping the infant warm

❍ **B.** Trimming the fingernails

❍ **C.** Using soap for bathing

❍ **D.** Applying peroxide to dry areas

50. The nurse is providing care for a 10-month-old infant diagnosed with a Wilms tumor. Most parents report feeling a mass when:

Quick Answers: **251**
Detailed Answer: **259**

❍ **A.** The infant is diapered or bathed

❍ **B.** The infant raises his arms

❍ C The infant has finished a bottle

❍ **D.** The infant tries to sit

51. The LPN is assigned to care for a client with a fractured femur. Which of the following should be reported to the charge nurse immediately?

Quick Answers: **251**
Detailed Answer: **259**

❍ **A.** The client complains of chest pain and feelings of apprehension

❍ **B.** Ecchymosis is noted on the side of the injured leg

❍ **C.** The client's oral temperature of 99.2°F

❍ **D.** The client complains of Level 2 pain on a scale of 1 to 5

Quick Check

52. The Joint Commission for Accreditation of Hospital Organizations (JCAHO) specifies that two client identifiers are to be used before medication administration. Which method is best for identifying patients using two patient identifiers?

Quick Answers: **251**
Detailed Answer: **259**

❍ **A.** Take the medication administration record (MAR) to the room and compare it with the name and medical number recorded on the armband

❍ **B.** Compare the medication administration record (MAR) with the client's room number and name on the armband

❍ **C.** Request that a family member identify the client, and then ask the client to state his name

❍ **D.** Ask the client to state his full name and then to write his full name

53. A nurse finds her neighbor lying unconscious in the doorway of her bathroom. After determining that the victim is unresponsive, the nurse should:

Quick Answers: **251**
Detailed Answer: **259**

❍ **A.** Start cardiac compression

❍ **B.** Give two slow deep breaths

❍ **C.** Open the airway using the head-tilt chin-lift maneuver

❍ **D.** Call for help

54. A client with AIDS-related cytomegalovirus has been started on Cytovene (ganciclovir). The client asks the nurse how long he will have to take the medication. The nurse should tell the client that the medication will be needed:

Quick Answers: **251**
Detailed Answer: **259**

❍ **A.** Until the infection clears

❍ **B.** For 6 months to a year

❍ **C.** Until the cultures are normal

❍ **D.** For the remainder of life

55. The nurse is caring for a client with a basal cell epithelioma. The nurse recognizes that the risk factors for basal cell carcinoma include having fair skin and:

Quick Answers: **251**
Detailed Answer: **259**

❍ **A.** Sun exposure

❍ **B.** Smoking

❍ **C.** Ingesting alcohol

❍ **D.** Ingesting food preservatives

Quick Check

56. While caring for a client following a Whipple procedure, the LPN notices that the drainage has become bile tinged and has increased over the past hour. The LPN should:

Quick Answers: 251
Detailed Answer: 259

- ❍ **A.** Document the finding and continue to monitor the client
- ❍ **B.** Irrigate the drainage tube with 10mL of normal saline
- ❍ **C.** Decrease the amount of intermittent suction
- ❍ **D.** Notify the RN regarding changes in the drainage

57. A client with AIDS tells the nurse that he regularly takes Echinacea to boost his immune system. The nurse should tell the client that:

Quick Answers: 251
Detailed Answer: 259

- ❍ **A.** Herbals can interfere with the action of antiviral medication.
- ❍ **B.** Supplements have proven effective in prolonging life.
- ❍ **C.** Herbals have been shown to decrease the viral load.
- ❍ **D.** Supplements appear to prevent replication of the virus.

58. A client receiving chemotherapy has Sjogren's syndrome. The nurse can help relieve the discomfort caused by Sjogren's syndrome by:

Quick Answers: 251
Detailed Answer: 259

- ❍ **A.** Providing cool, noncarbonated beverages
- ❍ **B.** Instilling eyedrops
- ❍ **C.** Administering prescribed antiemetics
- ❍ **D.** Providing small, frequent meals

59. Which one of the following symptoms is common in the client with duodenal ulcers?

Quick Answers: 251
Detailed Answer: 260

- ❍ **A.** Vomiting shortly after eating
- ❍ **B.** Epigastric pain following meals
- ❍ **C.** Frequent bouts of diarrhea
- ❍ **D.** Presence of blood in the stools

60. The physician has prescribed a Flovent (fluticasone) inhaler two puffs twice a day for a client with chronic obstructive pulmonary disease. The nurse should tell the client to report:

Quick Answers: 251
Detailed Answer: 260

- ❍ **A.** Increased weight
- ❍ **B.** A sore throat
- ❍ **C.** Difficulty in sleeping
- ❍ **D.** Changes in mood

Quick Check

61. A client treated for depression is admitted with a diagnosis of serotonin syndrome. The nurse recognizes that serotonin syndrome can be caused by:

Quick Answers: **251**
Detailed Answer: **260**

- ❍ **A.** Concurrent use of two SSRIs
- ❍ **B.** Eating foods that are high in tyramine
- ❍ **C.** Drastic decrease in dopamine levels
- ❍ **D.** Use of medications containing pseudoephedrine

62. A client is admitted with suspected pernicious anemia. Which finding is common in the client with pernicious anemia?

Quick Answers: **251**
Detailed Answer: **260**

- ❍ **A.** Complaints of feeling tired and listless
- ❍ **B.** Waxy, pale skin
- ❍ **C.** Loss of coordination and position sense
- ❍ **D.** Rapid pulse rate and heart murmur

63. Which finding is associated with secondary syphilis?

Quick Answers: **251**
Detailed Answer: **260**

- ❍ **A.** Painless, popular lesions on the perineum, fingers, and eyelids
- ❍ **B.** Absence of lesions
- ❍ **C.** Deep asymmetrical granulomatous lesions
- ❍ **D.** Well-defined generalized lesions on the palms, soles, and perineum

64. The physician has ordered an injection of morphine for a client with post-operative pain. Before administering the medication, it is essential that the nurse assess the client's:

Quick Answers: **251**
Detailed Answer: **260**

- ❍ **A.** Heart rate
- ❍ **B.** Respirations
- ❍ **C.** Temperature
- ❍ **D.** Blood pressure

65. The nurse is assessing a client following a subtotal thyroidectomy. Part of the assessment is asking the client to state her name. The primary reason for asking the client to state her name is to check for:

Quick Answers: **251**
Detailed Answer: **260**

- ❍ **A.** Post-operative bleeding
- ❍ **B.** Decreased calcium
- ❍ **C.** Laryngeal stridor
- ❍ **D.** Laryngeal nerve damage

Quick Check

66. A client is admitted for treatment of essential hypertension. Essential hypertension exists when the client maintains a blood pressure reading at or above:

Quick Answers: **251**
Detailed Answer: **260**

- ❍ **A.** 140/90
- ❍ **B.** 136/72
- ❍ **C.** 130/70
- ❍ **D.** 128/68

67. The nurse is applying karaya powder to the skin surrounding the client's ilestomy. The purpose of the karaya powder is to:

Quick Answers: **251**
Detailed Answer: **260**

- ❍ **A.** Prevent the formation of odor
- ❍ **B.** Help form a seal that will protect the skin
- ❍ **C.** Prevent the loss of electrolytes
- ❍ **D.** Increase the time between bag evacuations

68. The nurse is caring for a 9-month-old with suspected celiac disease. Which diet is appropriate?

Quick Answers: **251**
Detailed Answer: **261**

- ❍ **A.** Whole milk and oatmeal
- ❍ **B.** Breast milk and mixed cereal
- ❍ **C.** Formula and barley cereal
- ❍ **D.** Breast milk and rice cereal

69. Which lab finding would the nurse expect to find in the client with diverticulitis?

Quick Answers: **251**
Detailed Answer: **261**

- ❍ **A.** Elevated red cell count
- ❍ **B.** Decreased serum creatinine
- ❍ **C.** Elevated white cell count
- ❍ **D.** Decreased alkaline phosphatase

70. A gravida two para one has just delivered a full-term infant. Which finding indicates separation of the placenta?

Quick Answers: **251**
Detailed Answer: **261**

- ❍ **A.** Wavelike relaxation of the abdomen
- ❍ **B.** Increased length of the cord
- ❍ **C.** Decreased vaginal bleeding
- ❍ **D.** Inability to palpate the uterus

Quick Check

71. The physician has ordered a daily dose of Tagamet (cimetidine) for a client with gastric ulcers. The nurse should administer the medication:

- ❍ **A.** Before breakfast
- ❍ **B.** After breakfast
- ❍ **C.** At bedtime
- ❍ **D.** At noon

Quick Answers: **251**
Detailed Answer: **261**

72. A client admitted for treatment of a duodenal ulcer complains of sudden sharp midepigastric pain. Further assessment reveals that the client has a rigid, boardlike abdomen. The nurse recognizes that the client's symptoms most likely indicate:

- ❍ **A.** Ulcer perforation
- ❍ **B.** Increased ulcer formation
- ❍ **C.** Esophageal inflammation
- ❍ **D.** Intestinal obstruction

Quick Answers: **251**
Detailed Answer: **261**

73. Which snack is best for the child following a tonsillectomy?

- ❍ **A.** Banana popsicle
- ❍ **B.** Chocolate milk
- ❍ **C.** Fruit punch
- ❍ **D.** Cola

Quick Answers: **251**
Detailed Answer: **261**

74. The physician has prescribed Xanax (alprazolam) for a client with acute anxiety. The nurse should teach the client to avoid:

- ❍ **A.** Sun exposure
- ❍ **B.** Drinking beer
- ❍ **C.** Eating cheese
- ❍ **D.** Taking aspirin

Quick Answers: **251**
Detailed Answer: **261**

75. The nurse is instructing a post-operative client on the use of an incentive spirometer. The nurse knows that the correct use of the incentive spirometer is directly related to:

- ❍ **A.** Promoting the client's circulation
- ❍ **B.** Preparing the client for amubulation
- ❍ **C.** Strengthening the client's muscles
- ❍ **D.** Increasing the client's respiratory effort

Quick Answers: **251**
Detailed Answer: **261**

Quick Check

76. The nurse is assisting the physician with the insertion of an esophageal tamponade. Before insertion, the nurse should:

Quick Answers: **251**
Detailed Answer: **261**

❍ **A.** Inflate and deflate the gastric and esophageal balloons
❍ **B.** Measure from the tip of the client's nose to the xiphoid process
❍ **C.** Explain to the client that the tube will remain in place for 5–7 days
❍ **D.** Insert a nasogastric tube for gastric suction

77. The physician has ordered Cephulac (lactulose) for a client with increased serum ammonia. The nurse knows the medication is having its desired effect if the client experiences:

Quick Answers: **251**
Detailed Answer: **262**

❍ **A.** Increased urination
❍ **B.** Diarrhea
❍ **C.** Increased appetite
❍ **D.** Decreased weight

78. The nurse is assessing a client immediately following delivery. The nurse notes that the client's fundus is boggy. The nurse's next action should be to:

Quick Answers: **251**
Detailed Answer: **262**

❍ **A.** Assess for bladder distention
❍ **B.** Notify the physician
❍ **C.** Gently massage the fundus
❍ **D.** Administer pain medication

79. Which breakfast selection is suitable for the client on a high-fiber diet?

Quick Answers: **251**
Detailed Answer: **262**

❍ **A.** Danish pastry, tomato juice, coffee, and milk
❍ **B.** Oatmeal, grapefruit wedges, coffee, and milk
❍ **C.** Cornflakes, toast and jam, and milk
❍ **D.** Scrambled eggs, bacon, toast, and coffee

80. A male client is admitted with a tentative diagnosis of Hodgkin's lymphoma. The client with Hodgkin's lymphoma commonly reports:

Quick Answers: **251**
Detailed Answer: **262**

❍ **A.** Finding enlarged nodes in the neck while shaving
❍ **B.** Projectile vomiting upon arising
❍ **C.** Petechiae and easy bruising
❍ **D.** Frequent, painless hematuria

Quick Check

81. A client with acquired immunodeficiency syndrome has begun treatment with Pentam (pentamidine). The nurse recognizes that the medication will help to prevent:

Quick Answers: 251
Detailed Answer: 262

❍ **A.** Candida albicans

❍ **B.** Pneumocystis carinii

❍ **C.** Cryptosporidiosis

❍ **D.** Cytomegaloretinitis

82. During a well baby visit, the mother asks the nurse when the "soft spot" on the front of her baby's head will close. The nurse should tell the mother that the anterior fontanel normally closes by the time the baby is:

Quick Answers: 251
Detailed Answer: 262

❍ **A.** 4–6 months of age

❍ **B.** 7–9 months of age

❍ **C.** 10–12 months of age

❍ **D.** 12–18 months of age

83. An elderly client with anemia has a positive Schilling test. The nurse knows that the client's anemia is due to:

Quick Answers: 251
Detailed Answer: 262

❍ **A.** Chronically low iron store

❍ **B.** Abnormal shape of the red blood cells

❍ **C.** Lack of intrinsic factor

❍ **D.** Shortened lifespan of the red blood cells

84. The nurse is cleaning up a blood spill that occurred during removal of a chest tube. The nurse should clean the blood spill using:

Quick Answers: 251
Detailed Answer: 262

❍ **A.** Hydrogen peroxide

❍ **B.** Weak solution of bleach

❍ **C.** Isoprophyl alcohol

❍ **D.** Soap and water

85. A 5-month-old admitted with gastroenteritis is managed with IV fluids and is to be NPO. Which nursing intervention will provide the most comfort for the 5-month-old who is NPO?

Quick Answers: 251
Detailed Answer: 262

❍ **A.** Offering a pacifier

❍ **B.** Sitting next to the crib

❍ **C.** Providing a mobile

❍ **D.** Singing a lullaby

Quick Check

86. During the admission assessment, the nurse discovers that the client has brought her medications from home. The nurse should:

Quick Answers: **251**
Detailed Answer: **262**

- ❍ **A.** Tell the client that she can keep her medicines as long as she does not take them
- ❍ **B.** Make a list of the medications and ask a family member to take the medications home
- ❍ **C.** Allow the client to keep over-the-counter medications and herbal supplements
- ❍ **D.** Use the client's home medications because they have already been purchased

87. The nurse is reviewing the preoperative checklist for a client scheduled for a cholecystectomy. Which item is not required on the client's preoperative checklist?

Quick Answers: **251**
Detailed Answer: **262**

- ❍ **A.** History of allergies
- ❍ **B.** Most recent vital signs
- ❍ **C.** Physician's signature
- ❍ **D.** Preoperative medications

88. The nursing staff has planned a picnic for a small group of clients from the psychiatric unit. All of the clients are taking Thorazine (chlorpromazine). The nursing staff should take extra measures to:

Quick Answers: **252**
Detailed Answer: **263**

- ❍ **A.** Protect the clients from sun exposure
- ❍ **B.** Eliminate aged cheese from the menu
- ❍ **C.** Limit the amount of fluid intake by the clients
- ❍ **D.** Avoid chocolate desserts and treats on the menu

89. The nurse is caring for a client following a pneumonectomy. Which nursing intervention will help prevent an embolus?

Quick Answers: **252**
Detailed Answer: **263**

- ❍ **A.** Encouraging the client to use an incentive spirometer
- ❍ **B.** Administering thrombolytic medication as ordered
- ❍ **C.** Telling the client to turn, cough, and breathe deeply
- ❍ **D.** Ambulating the client as soon as possible

Quick Check

90. The physician has ordered B & O (belladonna and opium) suppositories for a client following a prostatectomy. The nurse recognizes that the medication will:

- ❍ **A.** Help relieve pain due to bladder spasms
- ❍ **B.** Improve the urinary output
- ❍ **C.** Reduce post-operative swelling
- ❍ **D.** Treat nausea and vomiting

Quick Answers: **252**
Detailed Answer: **263**

91. Post-operative orders have been left for a client with an above-the-knee amputation. The orders include wrapping the stump with an elastic bandage. The nurse knows that the primary reason for wrapping the stump with an elastic bandage is to:

- ❍ **A.** Decrease bleeding
- ❍ **B.** Shrink the stump
- ❍ **C.** Prevent phantom pain
- ❍ **D.** Prevent seeing the area

Quick Answers: **252**
Detailed Answer: **263**

92. A client with polycythemia vera is admitted for a phlebotomy. Assessment of the client with polycythemia vera reveals:

- ❍ **A.** Red, sore tongue; fatigue; and paresthesia
- ❍ **B.** Ruddy complexion, dyspnea, and pruritis
- ❍ **C.** Pallor; thin, spoon-shape fingernails; and pica
- ❍ **D.** Nocturnal dyspnea, rales, and weight gain

Quick Answers: **252**
Detailed Answer: **263**

93. The nurse is assisting a client with a total hip replacement to a chair. Which type of chair is appropriate for the client following a total hip replacement?

- ❍ **A.** A recliner
- ❍ **B.** A rocking chair
- ❍ **C.** A straight chair
- ❍ **D.** A sofa chair

Quick Answers: **252**
Detailed Answer: **263**

94. The physician has ordered Cotazyme (pancrelipase) for a child with cystic fibrosis. The nurse knows that the medication is given to:

- ❍ **A.** Replace the fat-soluble vitamins A, D, E, and K
- ❍ **B.** Decrease carbohydrate metabolism
- ❍ **C.** Aid in the digestion and absorption of fats, carbohydrates, and protein
- ❍ **D.** Facilitate sodium and chloride excretion

Quick Answers: **252**
Detailed Answer: **263**

Quick Check

95. The nurse at a local daycare center observes a group of preschool-age children playing. The children are playing in an unorganized fashion, with no obvious rules to the play activity. The type of play that is typical of preschool-age children is known as:

Quick Answers: 252
Detailed Answer: 263

❍ **A.** Solitary play
❍ **B.** Parallel play
❍ **C.** Associative play
❍ **D.** Cooperative play

96. Which of the following is not a part of routine cord care of the newborn?

Quick Answers: 252
Detailed Answer: 264

❍ **A.** Placing a petroleum gauze on the cord
❍ **B.** Applying an antibiotic to the cord
❍ **C.** Cleaning the cord with alcohol
❍ **D.** Folding diapers below the cord

97. A client is hospitalized with a diagnosis of antisocial personality disorder. According to Freud's psychoanalytic theory, antisocial personality disorder arises from faulty development of the:

Quick Answers: 252
Detailed Answer: 264

❍ **A.** Id
❍ **B.** Ego
❍ **C.** Superego
❍ **D.** Preconscious

98. The nurse is monitoring a client admitted with an overdose of Phenobarbital (phenobarbital). The nurse should carefully observe the client for signs of:

Quick Answers: 252
Detailed Answer: 264

❍ **A.** Hyperthermia
❍ **B.** Decreased respirations
❍ **C.** Increased blood pressure
❍ **D.** Dysuria

99. An elderly client is admitted with a fractured left hip. Which type of traction will be used to immobilize the client's left extremity?

Quick Answers: 252
Detailed Answer: 264

❍ **A.** 90–90 traction
❍ **B.** Buck's traction
❍ **C.** Bryant's traction
❍ **D.** Dunlop's traction

Quick Check

100. The physician has prescribed Zoloft (sertraline) for a client who has been taking Nardil (phenelzine). The recommended length of time between discontinuing a monoamine oxidase inhibitor and beginning therapy with a selective serotonin reuptake inhibitor is:

Quick Answers: **252**
Detailed Answer: **264**

- ❍ **A.** 2 days
- ❍ **B.** 7 days
- ❍ **C.** 10 days
- ❍ **D.** 14 days

101. A post-operative client has called the nurse's station with complaints of pain. The first action by the nurse should be to:

Quick Answers: **252**
Detailed Answer: **264**

- ❍ **A.** Check to see when the client received pain medication
- ❍ **B.** Administer the prescribed pain medication
- ❍ **C.** Notify the charge nurse of the client's complaints
- ❍ **D.** Assess the location and character of the client's pain

102. The nurse is observing a developmental assessment of an infant. Which of the following is an example of cephalocaudal development?

Quick Answers: **252**
Detailed Answer: **264**

- ❍ **A.** The infant is able to make rudimentary vocalizations before using language.
- ❍ **B.** The infant can control arm movements before she can control finger movements.
- ❍ **C.** The infant is able to raise her head before sitting.
- ❍ **D.** The infant responds to pain with her whole body before she can localize pain.

103. The physician has ordered a straight catheterization for a female client. When performing a straight catheterization on a female client, the nurse should:

Quick Answers: **252**
Detailed Answer: **264**

- ❍ **A.** Use medical asepsis when doing the catheterization
- ❍ **B.** Insert the catheter 4–6 inches
- ❍ **C.** Inflate and deflate the balloon before insertion
- ❍ **D.** Hold the catheter in place while the bladder empties

104. Before moving a client up in bed, the nurse lowers the head of the bed. The purpose of lowering the head of the bed is:

Quick Answers: **252**
Detailed Answer: **264**

- ❍ **A.** To avoid working against gravity as the client is moved
- ❍ **B.** To prevent getting wrinkles in the client's linen
- ❍ **C.** To eliminate needing additional help to move the client
- ❍ **D.** To relieve pressure on the client's sacrum

Quick Check

105. A client has returned from having an arteriogram. The nurse should give priority to:

Quick Answers: **252**
Detailed Answer: **265**

❍ **A.** Checking the radial pulse

❍ **B.** Assessing the site for bleeding

❍ **C.** Offering fluids

❍ **D.** Administering pain medication

106. The physician has ordered Dolophine (methadone) for a client withdrawing from opiates. Which finding is associated with acute methodone toxicity?

Quick Answers: **252**
Detailed Answer: **265**

❍ **A.** Fever

❍ **B.** Oliguria

❍ **C.** Nasal congestion

❍ **D.** Respiratory depression

107. A client scheduled for surgery has a preoperative order for atropine on call. The nurse should tell the client that the medication will:

Quick Answers: **252**
Detailed Answer: **265**

❍ **A.** Make him drowsy

❍ **B.** Make his mouth dry

❍ **C.** Help him to relax

❍ **D.** Prevent infection

108. The nurse is assessing a primgravida 12 hours after a Caesarean section. The nurse notes that the client's fundus is at the umbilicus and is firm. The nurse should:

Quick Answers: **252**
Detailed Answer: **265**

❍ **A.** Prepare to catheterize the client

❍ **B.** Obtain an order for an oxytocic

❍ **C.** Chart the finding

❍ **D.** Tell the client to remain in bed

109. Which of the following observations in a 4-year-old suggests the possibility of child abuse?

Quick Answers: **252**
Detailed Answer: **265**

❍ **A.** The presence of "rainbow" bruises

❍ **B.** Sucking the thumb when going to sleep

❍ **C.** Crying during painful procedures

❍ **D.** Eagerness to talk to strangers

Quick Check

110. A client with a history of alcoholism cannot remember the events of the past week even though he has receipts from various places of business. The client's inability to recall events is known as:

Quick Answers: **252**
Detailed Answer: **265**

- ❍ **A.** Alcoholic hallucinosis
- ❍ **B.** A hangover
- ❍ **C.** A blackout
- ❍ **D.** Sunday morning paralysis

111. The nurse is caring for a client with degenerative joint disease. Which finding is associated with degenerative joint disease?

Quick Answers: **252**
Detailed Answer: **265**

- ❍ **A.** Joint pain that intensifies with activity and diminishes with rest
- ❍ **B.** Bilateral and symmetric joint involvement
- ❍ **C.** Involvement of the fingers and hands
- ❍ **D.** Complaints of early-morning stiffness

112. The physician has ordered an injection of Demerol (meperidine) for a client with pancreatitis. The nurse should:

Quick Answers: **252**
Detailed Answer: **265**

- ❍ **A.** Administer the injection using the Z track method
- ❍ **B.** Hold pressure on the injection site for 3–5 minutes
- ❍ **C.** Administer the medication subcutaneously in the arm
- ❍ **D.** Prep the skin using a betadine wipe

113. The nurse is preparing a client with Addison's disease for discharge. The nurse should explain that the client can help prevent complications by:

Quick Answers: **252**
Detailed Answer: **265**

- ❍ **A.** Avoiding dietary sources of sodium
- ❍ **B.** Dressing in lightweight clothing
- ❍ **C.** Restricting foods rich in potassium
- ❍ **D.** Staying out of crowds

114. A 10-year-old received an injury to his face and mouth in a bicycle accident. Examination reveals that a permanent tooth has been evulsed. Emergency care following evulsion of a permanent tooth includes:

Quick Answers: **252**
Detailed Answer: **265**

- ❍ **A.** Rinsing the tooth in milk before reimplantation
- ❍ **B.** Wiping the tooth with gauze before reimplantation
- ❍ **C.** Holding the tooth by the root as it is rinsed
- ❍ **D.** Putting the tooth underneath the child's tongue

Quick Check

115. A 6-year-old is admitted with a diagnosis of leukemia. The most frequent presenting symptoms of leukemia include:

Quick Answers: **252**
Detailed Answer: **266**

❍ **A.** Headache, nausea, and vomiting

❍ **B.** Pallor, easy bruising, and joint pain

❍ **C.** Delayed growth, anorexia, and alopecia

❍ **D.** Poor wound healing, polyuria, and fever

116. The LPN is assigning tasks to the nursing assistant. Which task is beyond the scope of practice for the nursing assistant?

Quick Answers: **252**
Detailed Answer: **266**

❍ **A.** Collecting a stool specimen for occult blood

❍ B Obtaining a urine specimen for a routine urinalysis

❍ **C.** Performing a tape test for pinworms

❍ **D.** Aspirating nasogatric secretions for occult blood

117. The nurse is caring for a client following an exploratory laparotomy. Which of the following assessment findings requires intervention?

Quick Answers: **252**
Detailed Answer: **266**

❍ **A.** The abdominal dressing is clean, dry, and intact.

❍ **B.** The hourly urinary output of 20mL is dark amber in color.

❍ **C.** The nasogastric tube output of 15mL is bile colored.

❍ **D.** The IV is infusing with no signs of infiltration.

118. The nurse is caring for a client following a colonoscopy in which conscious sedation was used. Initial assessment of the client reveals the following: BP 128/72, temperature 97, pulse 64, respirations 14, oxygen saturation 90%, and Glascow score of 13. An IV of normal saline is infusing at 20 drops per minute. Which nursing intervention should receive priority?

Quick Answers: **252**
Detailed Answer: **266**

❍ **A.** Administering an analgesic

❍ **B.** Administering oxygen per standing order

❍ **C.** Covering the client with a blanket

❍ **D.** Discontinuing the IV fluid

119. The physician has prescribed Phenergan (promethazine) with codeine for a client with pleurisy. The nurse recognizes that the medication was ordered for its:

Quick Answers: **252**
Detailed Answer: **266**

❍ **A.** Expectorant effects

❍ **B.** Anti-inflammatory properties

❍ **C.** Antitussive effects

❍ **D.** Ability to relieve pain

Quick Check

120. The primary cause of anemia in clients with chronic renal failure is:

- ❍ **A.** The urinary loss of red blood cells
- ❍ **B.** The lack of erythropoietin
- ❍ **C.** Alterations in the shape of red blood cells
- ❍ **D.** The decrease in iron stores

Quick Answers: **252**
Detailed Answer: **266**

121. The nurse is about to administer the client's medication when the client states that the medication "looks different" than what she took before. The safest action for the nurse to take is to:

- ❍ **A.** Tell the client that the medication is the same
- ❍ **B.** Reassure the client that the doctor has prescribed correctly
- ❍ **C.** Explain that pharmacies make generic substitutions
- ❍ **D.** Recheck the MAR (medication administration record) to validate the medication's correctness

Quick Answers: **252**
Detailed Answer: **266**

122. The physician has prescribed Laradopa (levodopa) for a client with Parkinson's disease. The nurse should:

- ❍ **A.** Tell the client that the medication will not be absorbed if it is taken with food
- ❍ **B.** Explain that monthly lab work will be needed while the client is taking the medication
- ❍ **C.** Tell the client that the medication will be needed only until the symptoms disappear
- ❍ **D.** Instruct the client to rise slowly from a sitting position

Quick Answers: **252**
Detailed Answer: **266**

123. Dietary management of the client with congestive heart failure includes the restriction of:

- ❍ **A.** Sodium
- ❍ **B.** Calcium
- ❍ **C.** Potassium
- ❍ **D.** Magnesium

Quick Answers: **252**
Detailed Answer: **266**

124. The physician has ordered diuretic therapy and fluid restrictions for a client admitted with a stroke. The nurse knows that diuretic therapy and fluid restrictions are ordered during the acute phase of a stroke to:

- ❍ **A.** Reduce cardiac output
- ❍ **B.** Prevent an embolus
- ❍ **C.** Reduce cerebral edema
- ❍ **D.** Minimize incontinence

Quick Answers: **252**
Detailed Answer: **267**

Quick Check

125. The nurse is caring for a client with esophageal cancer. The client's history will likely reveal:

- ❍ **A.** A diet high in fiber
- ❍ **B.** Presence of gastroesophageal reflux
- ❍ **C.** Occasional use of alcohol
- ❍ **D.** A diet low in fat

Quick Answers: **252**
Detailed Answer: **267**

126. Which food is the best source of calcium and potassium?

- ❍ **A.** Broccoli
- ❍ **B.** Sweet potato
- ❍ **C.** Spinach
- ❍ **D.** Avocado

Quick Answers: **252**
Detailed Answer: **267**

127. The physician has ordered a PSA and acid phosphatase for a client admitted with complaints of dysuria. The nurse knows that a PSA and acid phosphatase are screening tests for:

- ❍ **A.** Cancer of the bladder
- ❍ **B.** Cancer of the prostate
- ❍ **C.** Cancer of the vas deferens
- ❍ **D.** Cancer of the testes

Quick Answers: **252**
Detailed Answer: **267**

128. The client's morning lithium level is 1.2mEq/L. The nurse recognizes that:

- ❍ **A.** The level is too low to be therapeutic.
- ❍ **B.** The client can be expected to have signs of toxicity.
- ❍ **C.** The level is within the therapeutic range.
- ❍ **D.** The client needs to eat more sodium-rich foods.

Quick Answers: **252**
Detailed Answer: **267**

129. Which emergency treatment is appropriate for the client who suddenly develops ventricular fibrillations?

- ❍ **A.** Cardioversion
- ❍ **B.** Intubation
- ❍ **C.** Defibrillation
- ❍ **D.** Anticonvulsant medication

Quick Answers: **252**
Detailed Answer: **267**

Quick Check

130. The nurse is caring for a client following a stroke that left him with apraxia. The nurse knows that the client will:

Quick Answers: **252**
Detailed Answer: **267**

- ❍ **A.** Be unable to communicate through speech
- ❍ **B.** Have difficulty swallowing
- ❍ **C.** Have difficulty with voluntary movements
- ❍ **D.** Be unable to perform previously learned skills

131. The nurse is positioning a client with right hemiplegia. To prevent subluxation of the client's right shoulder, the nurse should:

Quick Answers: **252**
Detailed Answer: **267**

- ❍ **A.** Use a pillow to support the client's arm when she is sitting in a chair
- ❍ **B.** Elevate the arm and hand above chest level when she is lying in bed
- ❍ **C.** Place a pillow under the axilla to elevate the elbow when she is lying in bed
- ❍ **D.** Use a pillow to support the client's hand when she is sitting in a chair

132. A client with thrombophlebitis is receiving Lovenox (enoxaparin). Which method is recommended for administering Lovenox?

Quick Answers: **252**
Detailed Answer: **267**

- ❍ **A.** Z track in the dorsogluteal muscle
- ❍ **B.** Intramuscularly in the deltoid muscle
- ❍ **C.** Subcutaneously in the abdominal tissue
- ❍ **D.** Orally after breakfast

133. A client with angina is to be discharged with a prescription for nitroglycerin tablets. The client should be instructed to:

Quick Answers: **252**
Detailed Answer: **267**

- ❍ **A.** Take one tablet daily with a glass of water
- ❍ **B.** Leave the medication in a dark-brown bottle
- ❍ **C.** Replenish the medication supply every year
- ❍ **D.** Leave the cotton in the bottle to protect the tablets

134. The physician has ordered Parnate (tranylcypromine) for a client with depression. The nurse should tell the client to avoid foods containing tryamine because it can result in:

Quick Answers: **252**
Detailed Answer: **268**

- ❍ **A.** Elevations in blood pressure
- ❍ **B.** Decreased libido
- ❍ **C.** Elevations in temperature
- ❍ **D.** Increased depression

Quick Check

135. A client is receiving external radiation for cancer of the larynx. As a result of the treatment, the client will most likely complain of:

Quick Answers: **252**
Detailed Answer: **268**

- ❍ **A.** Generalized pruritis
- ❍ **B.** Dyspnea
- ❍ **C.** Sore throat
- ❍ **D.** Bone pain

136. The nurse is caring for a client with a T4 spinal cord injury when he begins to have symptoms of autonomic dysreflexia. After placing the client in high Fowler's position, the nurse should:

Quick Answers: **252**
Detailed Answer: **268**

- ❍ **A.** Administer a prescribed analgesic
- ❍ **B.** Check for patency of the catheter
- ❍ **C.** Tell the client to breathe slowly
- ❍ **D.** Check the temperature

137. Hospital policy recommends that all children under the age of 3 years be placed in a crib. When providing care for a child in a crib, the nurse should give priority to:

Quick Answers: **252**
Detailed Answer: **268**

- ❍ **A.** Keeping the side rails locked at the halfway point
- ❍ **B.** Maintaining one hand on the child whenever side rails are down
- ❍ **C.** Positioning the child farther away from the lowered side rail
- ❍ **D.** Telling the parent that the side rails can stay down as long as someone is in the room

138. An infant with respiratory synctial virus has been started on Virazole (ribavirin). When caring for the infant receiving Virazole, the nurse should:

Quick Answers: **252**
Detailed Answer: **268**

- ❍ **A.** Discontinue isolation precautions while the medication is being administered
- ❍ **B.** Use contact precautions only when opening the mist tent
- ❍ **C.** Temporarily stop administration of the medication when the mist tent needs to be opened
- ❍ **D.** Increase the rate of medication administration when the mist tent needs to be opened

Quick Check

139. Although children can develop allergies to a variety of foods, the most common food allergens are:

Quick Answers: **252**
Detailed Answer: **268**

- ❍ **A.** Fruit, eggs, and corn
- ❍ **B.** Wheat, oats, and grain
- ❍ **C.** Cow's milk, rice, and tomatoes
- ❍ **D.** Eggs, cow's milk, and peanuts

140. A 9-month-old is admitted with a diagnosis of eczema. The nurse would expect the 9-month-old to have eczematous lesions over:

Quick Answers: **252**
Detailed Answer: **268**

- ❍ **A.** The abdomen, cheeks, and scalp
- ❍ **B.** The buttocks, abdomen, and back
- ❍ **C.** The back and flexor surfaces of the arms and legs
- ❍ **D.** The cheeks and extensor surfaces of arms and legs

141. Which one of the following factors has the greatest influence on the recovery and sobriety of a client with a chemical addiction?

Quick Answers: **252**
Detailed Answer: **268**

- ❍ **A.** The family's understanding of the client's addiction
- ❍ **B.** The quality of the treatment program and follow-up
- ❍ **C.** The client's own desire to become drug-free
- ❍ **D.** The nursing staff's attitude toward addiction

142. Which symptom differentiates chronic otitis media from acute otitis media?

Quick Answers: **252**
Detailed Answer: **268**

- ❍ **A.** Elevated temperature
- ❍ **B.** Pain in the affected ear
- ❍ **C.** Nausea and vomiting
- ❍ **D.** Feelings of fullness in the ear

143. A 6-year-old is admitted with suspected rheumatic fever. Which finding is associated with rheumatic fever?

Quick Answers: **252**
Detailed Answer: **269**

- ❍ **A.** A history of low birth weight
- ❍ **B.** A case of strep throat several weeks ago
- ❍ **C.** Presence of sickle cell trait
- ❍ **D.** Inability to digest certain grains

Quick Check

144. Which of the following signs is characteristic of the child with Duchenne's muscular dystrophy?

Quick Answers: **252**
Detailed Answer: **269**

- ❍ **A.** The use of Gower's maneuver to rise to a standing position
- ❍ **B.** Bilateral knee pain located at the tibial tubercle
- ❍ **C.** Concave curvature of the lumbar spine
- ❍ **D.** Aseptic necrosis of the head of the femur

145. An obstetrical client is admitted in active labor. When the membranes rupture, the nurse would expect to find:

Quick Answers: **252**
Detailed Answer: **269**

- ❍ **A.** A large amount of bright-red discharge
- ❍ **B.** A moderate amount of straw-colored discharge
- ❍ **C.** A small amount of green-colored discharge
- ❍ **D.** A scant amount of dark-brown discharge

146. Fetal heart tones can be heard using a fetoscope as early as:

Quick Answers: **252**
Detailed Answer: **269**

- ❍ **A.** 5 weeks gestation
- ❍ **B.** 10 weeks gestation
- ❍ **C.** 15 weeks gestation
- ❍ **D.** 18 weeks gestation

147. The nurse is teaching the pregnant client ways to prevent heartburn. The nurse should tell the client to:

Quick Answers: **252**
Detailed Answer: **269**

- ❍ **A.** Sleep on her right side
- ❍ **B.** Eat dry crackers at bedtime
- ❍ **C.** Sleep on a small pillow
- ❍ **D.** Avoid caffeinated beverages

148. A child with cystic fibrosis takes pancreatic enzymes with each of his meals and between meal snacks. Which finding indicates that the prescribed amount of pancreatic replacement is adequate?

Quick Answers: **252**
Detailed Answer: **269**

- ❍ **A.** Improved respiratory function
- ❍ **B.** Decreased sodium excretion
- ❍ **C.** Increased weight
- ❍ **D.** Decreased chloride excretion

Quick Check

149. The mother of a child with impetigo asks the nurse when her child will be able to return to school. The nurse's response is based on the knowledge that the lesions of impetigo resolve in:

- ❍ **A.** 24 hours
- ❍ **B.** 5 days
- ❍ **C.** 1 week
- ❍ **D.** 2 weeks

Quick Answers: **252**
Detailed Answer: **269**

150. Infants born to diabetic mothers are often described as large for gestational age. The primary reason for the infant's large size is:

- ❍ **A.** Overstimulation of the thyroid
- ❍ **B.** Maternal hyperglycemia
- ❍ **C.** Improved maternal nutrition
- ❍ **D.** Increased production of the pituitary

Quick Answers: **252**
Detailed Answer: **269**

151. The physician has ordered a Guthrie test for a newborn. The nurse recognizes that the test is ordered to detect:

- ❍ **A.** Cystic fibrosis
- ❍ **B.** Phenylketonuria
- ❍ **C.** Hypothyroidism
- ❍ **D.** Sickle cell anemia

Quick Answers: **252**
Detailed Answer: **269**

152. A client with emphysema has an order for Elixophyllin (theophylline). The desired action of theophylline for a client with emphysema is:

- ❍ **A.** Reduction of bronchial secretions
- ❍ **B.** Decreased alveolar spasms
- ❍ **C.** Restoration of bronchial compliance
- ❍ **D.** Relaxation of bronchial smooth muscle

Quick Answers: **252**
Detailed Answer: **269**

153. The physician has ordered a low-calorie, low-fat, low-sodium diet for a client with hypertension. Which menu selection is appropriate for the client?

- ❍ **A.** Mixed green salad, blue cheese dressing, crackers, tea
- ❍ **B.** Frankfurter and roll, baked beans, celery and carrots, cola
- ❍ **C.** Taco salad, tortilla chips, sour cream, tea
- ❍ **D.** Baked chicken, apple, angel food cake, 1% milk

Quick Answers: **252**
Detailed Answer: **269**

Quick Check

154. A postpartal client wants to know how the nutrient value of breast milk differs from that of cow's milk. The nurse should tell the client that breast milk is:

Quick Answers: **252**
Detailed Answer: **270**

- ❍ **A.** Higher in fat
- ❍ **B.** Higher in iron
- ❍ **C.** Higher in calcium
- ❍ **D.** Higher in sodium

155. The nurse is administering medication to a client with paranoid schizophrenia. The client accepts the medication but does not place it in his mouth. The nurse should:

Quick Answers: **252**
Detailed Answer: **270**

- ❍ **A.** Tell the client that if he does not take the medication, he will have to get an injection
- ❍ **B.** Tell the client to put the medicine in his mouth and swallow it with the water
- ❍ **C.** Tell a nursing assistant to remain with the client until he takes the medication
- ❍ **D.** Tell the client he will have to take his medication or he cannot go with the others to recreation

156. A client with Crohn's disease has been started on Entocort EC (budesonide) 9mg daily. The nurse should tell the client to take the medication:

Quick Answers: **252**
Detailed Answer: **270**

- ❍ **A.** With grapefruit juice
- ❍ **B.** On an empty stomach
- ❍ **C.** Between meals
- ❍ **D.** With meals or a snack

157. The nurse is teaching an obstetrical client regarding the appearance of edema in the last trimester. Which statement by the client indicates a need for further teaching?

Quick Answers: **252**
Detailed Answer: **270**

- ❍ **A.** "I need to drink six to eight glasses of water a day."
- ❍ **B.** "I can expect to have edema of my feet and ankles."
- ❍ **C.** "Edema of my face and hands is a normal occurrence."
- ❍ **D.** "It's important for me to avoid prolonged standing."

Quick Check

158. While reviewing the client's lab report, the nurse notes that the client has a potassium level of 3.0 mEq/L. What is the best source of potassium?

Quick Answers: **252**
Detailed Answer: **270**

❍ **A.** One cup of apple juice

❍ **B.** One cup of orange juice

❍ **C.** One cup of cranberry juice

❍ **D.** One cup of prune juice

159. A client admitted with renal calculi is experiencing severe pain in the right flank and nausea. The immediate nursing intervention is to:

Quick Answers: **252**
Detailed Answer: **270**

❍ **A.** Administer pain medication as ordered

❍ **B.** Encourage oral fluids

❍ **C.** Administer an antiemetic as ordered

❍ **D.** Evaluate the hydration status

160. The physician has ordered a sterile urine specimen from a client with an in-dwelling catheter. The nurse should:

Quick Answers: **252**
Detailed Answer: **270**

❍ **A.** Open the spout on the urine bag and allow urine to flow into a sterile specimen cup

❍ **B.** Disconnect the drainage tube from the collection bag and allow urine to drain into a sterile specimen cup

❍ **C.** Disconnect the drainage tube from the catheter and allow urine to drain from the bag into a sterile specimen cup

❍ **D.** Use a sterile syringe and needle to remove urine from the port nearest the client and place the urine into a sterile specimen cup

161. Otitis media occurs more frequently in infants and young children because of the unique anatomic features of the:

Quick Answers: **252**
Detailed Answer: **270**

❍ **A.** Nasopharynx

❍ **B.** External ear canals

❍ **C.** Eustachian tubes

❍ **D.** Tympanic membranes

162. The nurse is admitting a newborn to the nursery. Which finding is expected in the full-term newborn?

Quick Answers: **252**
Detailed Answer: **270**

❍ **A.** Absence of sucking pads

❍ **B.** Presence of vernix caseosa

❍ **C.** Presence of the scarf sign

❍ **D.** Absence of solar creases

Quick Check

163. A client who was admitted with a closed head injury is asked to tell the nurse today's date. The nurse is assessing the client's orientation to:

Quick Answers: 252
Detailed Answer: 270

- ❍ **A.** Person
- ❍ **B.** Place
- ❍ **C.** Time
- ❍ **D.** Objects

164. Which of the following tasks is within the developmental norm for the 22-month-old child?

Quick Answers: 252
Detailed Answer: 270

- ❍ **A.** Feeds herself with a spoon
- ❍ **B.** Dresses and undresses without help
- ❍ **C.** Shares her toys with others
- ❍ **D.** Speaks in 8- to 10-word sentences

165. A pediatric client is admitted with Munchausen's syndrome by proxy. The nurse would expect the child to have:

Quick Answers: 252
Detailed Answer: 271

- ❍ **A.** Extreme tooth decay
- ❍ **B.** Unexplained illness
- ❍ **C.** Dermatitis of the lips and tongue
- ❍ **D.** Inability to sweat

166. A client refuses to take the medication prescribed for her. Which action should the nurse take first?

Quick Answers: 252
Detailed Answer: 271

- ❍ **A.** Encourage the client to take the medication
- ❍ **B.** Ask the client her reasons for refusing the medication
- ❍ **C.** Document that the client refused her medication
- ❍ **D.** Report the client's refusal to take the medication to the charge nurse

167. A nurse complains that a client is noncompliant because she prefers to take herbs prescribed by her herbalist rather than taking "real medicine." The nurse's statement is an example of:

Quick Answers: 252
Detailed Answer: 271

- ❍ **A.** Ethnicity
- ❍ **B.** Cultural sensitivity
- ❍ **C.** Ethnocentrism
- ❍ **D.** Cultural tolerance

Quick Check

168. The nurse is checking the fetal heart rates of a client in labor. The normal range for fetal heart rates is:

Quick Answers: **252**
Detailed Answer: **271**

- ❍ **A.** 90–110 beats per minute
- ❍ **B.** 110–160 beats per minute
- ❍ **C.** 160–200 beats per minute
- ❍ **D.** 200–250 beats per minute

169. Which one of the following measures decreases abdominal discomfort when the post-operative client is asked to cough?

Quick Answers: **252**
Detailed Answer: **271**

- ❍ **A.** Exhaling forcefully between coughs
- ❍ **B.** Splinting the incision with a pillow
- ❍ **C.** Maintaining muscle tension in the operative site
- ❍ **D.** Taking panting respirations between coughs

170. The nurse is caring for a client with arteriosclerotic heart disease. The nurse recognizes that a nonmodifiable risk factor in the development of arteriosclerotic heart disease is:

Quick Answers: **252**
Detailed Answer: **271**

- ❍ **A.** Family history
- ❍ **B.** Hypertension
- ❍ **C.** Diet
- ❍ **D.** Exercise

171. The physician has ordered Nardil (phenelzine), an MAO inhibitor for a client who is currently taking Paxil (paroxetine). The nurse should:

Quick Answers: **252**
Detailed Answer: **271**

- ❍ **A.** Give the medications together as ordered
- ❍ **B.** Clarify the orders with the physician
- ❍ **C.** Request an order for anti-Parkinsonian medication
- ❍ **D.** Administer the medications at different times

172. Which technique should the nurse use to prevent air from entering the stomach during a nasogastric tube feeding?

Quick Answers: **252**
Detailed Answer: **271**

- ❍ **A.** Pour all the formula into the syringe barrel before opening the clamp
- ❍ **B.** Open the clamp and pour the formula in a continuous flow down the side of the syringe barrel
- ❍ **C.** Release the clamp before pouring all the formula into the syringe barrel
- ❍ **D.** Open the clamp and allow a small amount of formula to enter the stomach before adding more formula

Quick Check

173. The nurse is assessing a client who has undergone a right lobectomy. Which assessment should alert the nurse to the possibility of internal bleeding?

Quick Answers: 252
Detailed Answer: 271

- ❍ **A.** Urinary output of 200mL during the past 3 hours
- ❍ **B.** Sanguineous chest tube drainage at a rate of 50mL per hour for the past 3 hours
- ❍ **C.** Restless and shortness of breath
- ❍ **D.** Decreased pulse rate and decreased respirations

174. A client with congestive heart failure loses 4.1kg while hospitalized. The client's weight loss is approximately:

Quick Answers: 252
Detailed Answer: 271

- ❍ **A.** 2 pounds
- ❍ **B.** 4 pounds
- ❍ **C.** 7 pounds
- ❍ **D.** 9 pounds

175. A 40-year-old client with a myocardial infarction tells the nurse, "My father died with a heart attack when he was in his forties, and I guess I will, too." Which response by the nurse is most appropriate?

Quick Answers: 252
Detailed Answer: 272

- ❍ **A.** "Tell me more about what you are feeling."
- ❍ **B.** "Are you thinking you won't recover from this?"
- ❍ **C.** "You have an excellent doctor, so I'm sure everything will be fine."
- ❍ **D.** "I would think that's unlikely because we have much better treatment now."

176. Which nursing action is most appropriate immediately following the removal of a nasogastric tube?

Quick Answers: 252
Detailed Answer: 272

- ❍ **A.** Providing mouth care
- ❍ **B.** Auscultating bowel sounds
- ❍ **C.** Offering fluids
- ❍ **D.** Checking for abdominal distention

Quick Check

177. An elderly client injured in a fall is admitted with fractures of the ribs and a closed right pneumothorax. The nurse should position the client:

Quick Answers: **252**
Detailed Answer: **272**

❍ **A.** In modified Trendelenburg position with the lower extremities elevated

❍ **B.** In semi-Fowler's position tilted toward the right side

❍ **C.** In dorsal recumbent position with the lower extremities flat

❍ **D.** In semi-Fowler's position tilted toward the left side

178. A client develops cravings while withdrawing from alcohol. Which measure will best help the client maintain sobriety?

Quick Answers: **252**
Detailed Answer: **272**

❍ **A.** Placing the client in seclusion for 24 hours

❍ **B.** Restricting visits from family and friends

❍ **C.** Gaining support from other recovering alcoholics

❍ **D.** Assigning a staff member to stay until the cravings pass

179. A client with Addison's disease has a diagnosis of fluid volume deficit related to inadequate adrenal hormone secretion. Which fluids are most appropriate for the client with Addison's disease?

Quick Answers: **252**
Detailed Answer: **272**

❍ **A.** Milk and diet soda

❍ **B.** Water and tea

❍ **C.** Bouillon and juice

❍ **D.** Coffee and juice

180. The nurse is preparing to administer a DTP, Hib, and hepatitis B immunizations to an infant. The nurse should:

Quick Answers: **252**
Detailed Answer: **272**

❍ **A.** Administer all the immunizations in one site

❍ **B.** Administer the DTP in one leg, and the Hib and the hepatitis B in the other leg

❍ **C.** Administer the DTP in the leg, the Hib in the other leg, and the hepatitis B in the arm

❍ **D.** Administer the DTP and Hib in one leg, and the hepatitis B in the arm

Quick Check

181. Lab results indicate that a client receiving heparin has a prolonged bleeding time. Which medication is the antidote for heparin?

Quick Answers: **252**
Detailed Answer: **272**

- ❍ **A.** Aquamephyton (phytonadione)
- ❍ **B.** Ticlid (ticlopidine)
- ❍ **C.** Protamine sulfate (protamine sulfate)
- ❍ **D.** Amicar (aminocaproic acid)

182. A newborn of 32 weeks gestation is diagnosed with respiratory distress syndrome 3 hours after birth. An assessment finding in the newborn with respiratory distress syndrome is:

Quick Answers: **252**
Detailed Answer: **272**

- ❍ **A.** Feeding difficulties
- ❍ **B.** Nasal flaring
- ❍ **C.** Increased blood pressure
- ❍ **D.** Temperature instability

183. To reduce the risk of SIDS (sudden infant death syndrome), the nurse should tell parents to place the infant:

Quick Answers: **252**
Detailed Answer: **272**

- ❍ **A.** Prone while he is sleeping
- ❍ **B.** Side-lying while he is awake
- ❍ **C.** On his back while he is sleeping
- ❍ **D.** Prone while he is awake

184. Which of the following play activities is most developmentally appropriate for the toddler?

Quick Answers: **253**
Detailed Answer: **272**

- ❍ **A.** Watching cartoons
- ❍ **B.** Pulling a toy wagon
- ❍ **C.** Watching a mobile
- ❍ **D.** Coloring with crayons in a coloring book

185. The physician has discharged a client with diverticulitis with a prescription for Metamucil (psyllium). When teaching the client how to prepare the medication, the nurse should tell the client to:

Quick Answers: **253**
Detailed Answer: **273**

- ❍ **A.** Dissolve the medication in gelatin or applesauce
- ❍ **B.** Mix the medication with water and drink it immediately
- ❍ **C.** Sprinkle the medication on ice cream or sherbet
- ❍ **D.** Take the medication with an ounce of antacid

Quick Check

186. Young children living in housing that was built before the 1970s are at risk for:

- ❍ **A.** Lead poisoning
- ❍ **B.** Pernicious anemia
- ❍ **C.** Iron poisoning
- ❍ **D.** Sprue

Quick Answers: **253**
Detailed Answer: **273**

187. Which of the following findings is associated with fluid overload in the child with renal disease?

- ❍ **A.** Sluggish capillary refill and slow heart rate
- ❍ **B.** Distention of the jugular veins and pitting edema
- ❍ **C.** Decreased blood pressure and increased heart rate
- ❍ **D.** Increased blood pressure and bilateral wheezes

Quick Answers: **253**
Detailed Answer: **273**

188. A client with allergic dermatitis has a prescription for a Medrol (methylprenisolone) dose pack. The client asks why the number of pills decreases each day. The nurse's response is based on the knowledge that a gradual decreasing of the daily dose is necessary to prevent:

- ❍ **A.** Cushing's syndrome
- ❍ **B.** Thyroid storm
- ❍ **C.** Cholinergic crisis
- ❍ **D.** Addisonian crisis

Quick Answers: **253**
Detailed Answer: **273**

189. A child with beta thalassemia has developed hemosiderosis. To prevent organ damage, the child will receive chelation therapy with:

- ❍ **A.** Chemet (succimer)
- ❍ **B.** Versenate (calcium disodium versenate)
- ❍ **C.** Desferal (deferoxamine)
- ❍ **D.** EDTA (calcium disodium edetate)

Quick Answers: **253**
Detailed Answer: **273**

190. The nurse is caring for a client 1 week post-burn injury. The nurse should expect the client to benefit from a diet that is:

- ❍ **A.** High in protein, low in sodium, and low in carbohydrates
- ❍ **B.** Low in fat, low in sodium, and high in calories
- ❍ **C.** High in protein, high in carbohydrates, and high in calories
- ❍ **D.** High in protein, high in fat, and low in calories

Quick Answers: **253**
Detailed Answer: **273**

Quick Check

191. Which of the following describes a nosocomial infection?

Quick Answers: **253**
Detailed Answer: **273**

❍ **A.** A client develops MRSA while hospitalized for treatment of a fractured hip.

❍ **B.** A client develops a kidney infection from an extended bladder infection.

❍ **C.** A client develops hepatitis A after eating in a local restaurant.

❍ **D.** A client develops pneumonia after attending a sporting event.

192. An 8-month-old infant has been diagnosed with iron deficiency anemia. What food should be added to the infant's diet?

Quick Answers: **253**
Detailed Answer: **273**

❍ **A.** Orange juice

❍ **B.** Fortified rice cereal

❍ **C.** Whole milk

❍ **D.** Strained meat

193. The American Cancer Society's current recommendation is that women should have a baseline mammogram done between the ages of:

Quick Answers: **253**
Detailed Answer: **273**

❍ **A.** 25 and 30

❍ **B.** 30 and 35

❍ **C.** 35 and 40

❍ **D.** 40 and 45

194. The nurse is caring for a 6-year-old following revision of a ventriculoperitoneal shunt. An expected nursing intervention is:

Quick Answers: **253**
Detailed Answer: **273**

❍ **A.** Request for an x-ray to evaluate shunt placement

❍ **B.** Daily measurement of head circumference

❍ **C.** Frequent palpation of the fontanels

❍ **D.** Maintaining the child in a prone position

195. Stranger anxiety is defined as the distress that occurs when the infant is separated from the parents or caregivers. Stranger anxiety first peaks at:

Quick Answers: **253**
Detailed Answer: **274**

❍ **A.** 1–3 months of age

❍ **B.** 3–6 months of age

❍ **C.** 7–9 months of age

❍ **D.** 12–15 months of age

Quick Check

196. The nurse is assessing an infant with coarctation of the aorta. The nurse can expect to find:

- ❍ **A.** Deep cyanosis
- ❍ **B.** Clubbing of the fingers and toes
- ❍ **C.** Loud cardiac murmur
- ❍ **D.** Diminished femoral pulses

Quick Answers: **253**
Detailed Answer: **274**

197. Which client is most likely to be affected with Cooley's anemia?

- ❍ **A.** A child of Mediterranean descent
- ❍ **B.** A child of Asian descent
- ❍ **C.** A child of African descent
- ❍ **D.** A child of European descent

Quick Answers: **253**
Detailed Answer: **274**

198. The primary nursing consideration when working with a newly admitted adolescent with anorexia nervosa is:

- ❍ **A.** Identifying stressors that contributed to the disorder
- ❍ **B.** Including family members in the client's care
- ❍ **C.** Establishing a trusting relationship
- ❍ **D.** Restoring the client's nutritional status

Quick Answers: **253**
Detailed Answer: **274**

199. The nurse is palpating the fontanels of a 2-month-old. The fontanels should feel:

- ❍ **A.** Tense and bulging
- ❍ **B.** Soft and sunken
- ❍ **C.** Flat and firm
- ❍ **D.** Flat and tense

Quick Answers: **253**
Detailed Answer: **274**

200. An infant born at 25 weeks gestation was treated with prolonged oxygen therapy. Prolonged oxygen therapy places the infant at risk for:

- ❍ **A.** Cerebral palsy
- ❍ **B.** Retinitis pigmentosa
- ❍ **C.** Hydrocephalus
- ❍ **D.** Retinopathy of prematurity

Quick Answers: **253**
Detailed Answer: **274**

Quick Check Answer Key

1. D
2. B
3. B
4. A
5. B
6. D
7. D
8. C
9. A
10. C
11. A
12. A
13. C
14. C
15. D
16. B
17. C
18. B
19. C
20. A
21. A
22. B
23. A
24. B
25. A
26. D
27. A
28. D
29. B
30. A
31. A
32. B
33. B
34. C
35. A
36. C
37. B
38. B
39. C
40. D
41. C
42. B
43. B
44. D
45. B
46. B
47. B
48. C
49. B
50. A
51. A
52. A
53. D
54. D
55. A
56. D
57. A
58. B
59. D
60. B
61. A
62. C
63. D
64. B
65. D
66. A
67. B
68. D
69. C
70. B
71. C
72. A
73. A
74. B
75. D
76. A
77. B
78. C
79. B
80. A
81. B
82. D
83. C
84. B
85. A
86. B
87. C

88. A
89. D
90. A
91. B
92. B
93. A
94. C
95. C
96. A
97. A
98. B
99. B
100. D
101. D
102. C
103. D
104. A
105. B
106. D
107. B
108. C
109. A
110. C
111. A
112. B
113. D
114. A
115. B
116. D
117. B
118. B
119. C
120. B
121. D
122. D
123. A
124. C
125. B
126. C
127. B
128. C
129. C
130. D
131. A
132. C
133. B
134. A
135. C
136. B
137. B
138. C
139. D
140. D
141. C
142. A
143. B
144. A
145. B
146. D
147. D
148. C
149. D
150. B
151. B
152. D
153. D
154. A
155. B
156. D
157. C
158. D
159. A
160. D
161. C
162. B
163. C
164. A
165. B
166. B
167. C
168. B
169. B
170. A
171. B
172. A
173. C
174. D
175. A
176. A
177. B
178. C
179. C
180. B
181. C
182. B
183. C

184. B

185. B

186. A

187. B

188. D

189. C

190. C

191. A

192. B

193. C

194. B

195. C

196. D

197. A

198. D

199. C

200. D

Answers and Rationales

1. **Answer D is correct.** The client with AIDS should not drink water that has been sitting longer than 15 minutes because of bacterial contamination. Answer A is incorrect because tap water is not better for the client. Answer B is incorrect because juices should not replace water intake. Answer C is not an accurate statement; therefore, it is incorrect.

2. **Answer B is correct.** Approximately 99% of males with cystic fibrosis are sterile because of obstruction of the vas deferens. Answers A, C, and D are incorrect because most males with cystic fibrosis are incapable of reproduction.

3. **Answer B is correct.** Infants under the age of 2 years should not be fed honey because of the danger of infection with *Clostridium botulinum*. Answers A, C, and D have no relationship to the situation; therefore, they are incorrect.

4. **Answer A is correct.** Decreased blood pressure and increased pulse rate are signs of bleeding. Answers B, C, and D are within normal limits; therefore, they are incorrect.

5. **Answer B is correct.** Undercooked meat is a source of toxoplasmosis cysts. Toxoplasmosis is a major cause of encephalitis in clients with AIDS. Answers A, C, and D are accurate statements reflecting the client's understanding of the nurse's teaching; therefore, they are incorrect.

6. **Answer D is correct.** The client taking isoniazid should have a negative sputum culture within 3 months. Answers A, B, and C are incorrect because there has not been sufficient time for the medication to be effective.

7. **Answer D is correct.** Lyme's disease is transmitted by ticks found on deer and mice in wooded areas. Answers A and B have little risk for the disease. Dog trainers are exposed to dog ticks that carry Rocky Mountain Spotted Fever but not Lyme's disease; therefore, answer C is incorrect.

8. **Answer C is correct.** Melba toast promotes chewing and is easily managed by the toddler. Pieces of hot dog, celery sticks, and grapes are unsuitable for the toddler because of the risk of aspiration.

9. **Answer A is correct.** Kava-kava increases the effects of central nervous system depressants. Answers B, C, and D are not related to the use of kava-kava; therefore, they are incorrect.

10. **Answer C is correct.** The mother does not need to place an external heat source near the infant. It will not promote healing, and there is a chance that the newborn could be burned; therefore, the mother needs further teaching. Answers A, B, and D indicate correct care of the newborn who has been circumcised; therefore, they are incorrect.

11. **Answer A is correct.** The client who is colonized with MRSA will have no symptoms associated with infection. Answer B is incorrect because the client is more likely to develop an infection with MRSA following invasive procedures. Answer C is incorrect because the client should not be placed in the room with others. Answer D is incorrect because the client can colonize others, including healthcare workers, with MRSA.

12. **Answer A is correct.** Pseudomembranous colitis results from infection with *Clostridium difficile.* Symptoms of pseudomembranous colitis include diarrhea containing blood, mucus, and white blood cells. Answers B, C, and D are incorrect because they are not symptoms of infection with *Clostridium difficile.*

13. **Answer C is correct.** Immunization against pneumonia is recommended every 5 years for persons over age 65, as well as for those with a chronic illness. Answers A and B are incorrect because the client still has immunity from the vaccine. Answer D is incorrect because the client should have received the booster immunization much sooner.

14. **Answer C is correct.** Following a nephrolithotomy, the client should be positioned on the unoperative side. Answers A, B, and D are incorrect positions for the client following a nephrolithotomy.

15. **Answer D is correct.** The first sign of a latex allergy is usually contact dermatitis, which includes swelling and itching of the hands. Answers A, B, and C can also occur but are not the first signs of latex allergy; therefore, they are incorrect.

16. **Answer B is correct.** The dressings should be moistened with sterile water. Answer A is incorrect because Acticoat dressings remain in place up to 5 days. Answer C is incorrect because the dressings should be changed every 4 or 5 days. Answer D is incorrect because normal saline should not be used to moisten the dressing.

17. **Answer C is correct.** Stage III Hodgkin's lymphoma is characterized by lymph node involvement on both sides of the diaphragm. Answer A refers to stage I Hodgkin's lymphoma; therefore, it is incorrect. Answer B refers to stage II Hodgkin's lymphoma; therefore, it is incorrect. Answer D refers to stage IV Hodgkin's lymphoma; therefore, it is incorrect.

18. **Answer B is correct.** The client taking methotrexate should avoid multivitamins because they contain folic acid. Folic acid is the antidote for methotrexate. Answers A and D are incorrect because aspirin and acetaminophen are given to relieve pain and inflammation associated with rheumatoid arthritis. Answer C is incorrect because omega 3 and omega 6 fish oils have proven beneficial for the client with rheumatoid arthritis.

19. **Answer C is correct.** The client with ascites requires additional protein and calories unless the client's condition deteriorates because of renal involvement. In that case, protein intake is restricted. Answer A is incorrect because the client needs a low-sodium diet. Answer B is incorrect because the client does not need to decrease his intake of potassium. Answer D is incorrect because the client needs adequate amounts of calcium-rich foods that are also excellent sources of protein.

20. **Answer A is correct** because it is the position used for lithotripsy for the client with gallstones in the gall bladder. Answer B is incorrect because it is the position used for lithotripsy for the client with gallstones in the common bile duct. Answers C and D are incorrect because side-lying and recumbent positions do not allow the maximum effect of therapy.

21. **Answer A is correct.** Persons receiving steroids should eat only cooked or processed foods. Raw oysters carry hepatitis A as well as *E. coli.* Answers B, C, and D are all suitable foods for the client taking steroid medication; therefore, they are incorrect.

22. **Answer B is correct.** St. John's wort has properties similar to those of monoamine oxidase inhibitors (MAOI). Eating foods high in tryramine (aged cheese, chocolate, salami, liver, and so on) can result in a hypertensive crisis. Answer A is incorrect because it can relieve mild to moderate depression. Answer C is incorrect because use of a sunscreen prevents skin reactions to sun exposure. Answer D is incorrect because the use of St. John's wort decreases the amount of medication needed.

23. **Answer A is correct.** Foods high in purine include dried beans, peas, spinach, oatmeal, poultry, fish, liver, lobster, and oysters. Answers B, C, and D are incorrect because they are low in purine. Other sources low in purine include most vegetables, milk, and gelatin.

24. **Answer B is correct.** The client with bulimia is prone to dental caries due to erosion of the tooth enamel from frequent bouts of self-induced vomiting. Answers A, C, and D are findings associated with anorexia nervosa, not bulimia; therefore, they are incorrect.

25. **Answer A is correct.** Adverse reactions to Thorazine include dystonia. Spasms of the neck and difficulty swallowing can lead to airway compromise. Answers B, C, and D are expected side effects that occur with the use of Thorazine. They do not require that the physician be notified immediately; therefore, they are incorrect.

26. **Answer D is correct.** Transderm Nitro is a reservoir patch that releases the medication via a semipermeable membrane. Cutting the patch allows too much of the drug to be released. Answer A is incorrect because the area should not be shaved because it can cause skin irritation. Answer B is incorrect because the skin is cleaned with soap and water. Answer C is incorrect because the patch is not covered with plastic wrap.

27. **Answer A is correct.** Cholinergic crisis is the result of overmedication with anticholinesterase inhibitors. Clients with cholinergic crisis have the following symptoms: nausea, vomiting, diarrhea, blurred vision, pallor, decreased blood pressure, and pupillary meiosis. Myasthenia crisis is the result of under medication with cholinesterase inhibitors. Answers B, C, and D are incorrect because they are symptoms of myasthenia crisis.

28. **Answer D is correct.** The client should avoid eating American and processed cheeses such as Colby and Cheddar because they are high in sodium. Dried beans, peanut butter, and Swiss cheese are low in sodium; therefore, answers A, B, and C are incorrect.

29. **Answer B is correct.** According to the Rule of Nines, the arms (18%) + the head (9%) = 27% TBSA burn injury. Answers A, B, and D are inaccurate percentages for the TBSA; therefore, they are incorrect.

30. **Answer A is correct.** The client should void before the paracentesis to prevent accidental trauma to the bladder. Answer B is incorrect because the abdomen is not shaved. Answer C is incorrect because the client does not need extra fluids, which would cause bladder distention. Answer D is incorrect because the physician, not the nurse, would request an x-ray, if needed.

31. **Answer A is correct.** Acyclovir shortens the course of chickenpox, but the American Academy of Pediatrics does not recommend it for healthy children because of the cost. Answer B is incorrect because it is the vaccine used to prevent chickenpox. Answer C is incorrect because it is the immune globulin given to those who have been

exposed to chickenpox. Answer D is incorrect because it is an antihistamine used to control itching associated with chickenpox.

32. **Answer B is correct.** Females with chronic debilitating conditions who are dependent on others for most or all of their care are most likely to be the victims of elder abuse. Answers A, C, and D are incorrect because the clients are less likely to be dependent on others for their care; therefore, they are less likely to be victims of elder abuse. Although they might also be victims, men are less likely to report abuse than women.

33. **Answer B is correct.** The most appropriate facet of care for the newly licensed practical nurse is the monitoring of the client's vital signs. Answers A and C are incorrect because initiation of IV fluids and administration of blood is the responsibility of the registered nurse. Answer D is incorrect because in the hospital setting, the registered nurse would be responsible for notifying the physician of a reaction.

34. **Answer C is correct.** Dark-green, leafy vegetables; the cabbage family; beets; kidney beans; cantaloupe; and oranges are good sources of folic acid (B9). Meat, liver, eggs, dried beans, sweet potatoes, and Brussels sprouts are good sources of B12; therefore, answers A and D are incorrect. Pork, fish, and chicken are good sources of B6; therefore, answer B is incorrect.

35. **Answer A is correct.** Cigarette smoking is the number one cause of bladder cancer. Answer B is incorrect because it is associated with breast cancer, not bladder cancer. Answer C is wrong because it is a primary cause of gastric cancer. Answer D is incorrect because it is a cause of certain types of lung cancer.

36. **Answer C is correct.** Nitrogycerin tablets should be used as soon as the client first notices chest pain or discomfort. Answer A is incorrect because the medication should be used before engaging in activity. Strenuous activity should be avoided. Answer B is incorrect because the medication should be used when pain occurs, not on a regular schedule. Answer D is incorrect because the medication will not prevent nocturnal angina.

37. **Answer B is correct.** To obtain the urine output, the weight of the dry diaper (62 grams) is subtracted from the weight of the used diaper (90.5 grams), for a urine output of 28.5 grams, or 28.5mL (1 gram = 1mL). Answer A is an inaccurate amount; therefore, it is incorrect. Output is measured in milliliters, not grams; therefore, answers C and D are incorrect.

38. **Answer B is correct.** The infant with osteogenesis imperfecta (ribbon bones) should be handled with care to prevent fractures. Adding calcium to the infant's diet will not improve the condition; therefore, answer A is incorrect. Answers C and D are not related to the disorder; therefore, they are incorrect.

39. **Answer C is correct.** The client with gastroesophageal reflux disease (GERD) should avoid beverages containing caffeine because they increase the production of hydrochloric acid, which erodes the esophagus. Answer A is incorrect because the client should not eat for 3–4 hours before going to bed. The client should sleep on his left side, not his right side; therefore, answer B is incorrect. Citrus juices are acidic, which can contribute to reflux and esophageal erosion; therefore, answer D is incorrect.

40. **Answer D is correct.** The nurse should flush the NG tube with 2–4oz. of water before

and after giving the medication. Answers A and B are incorrect because they do not use sufficient amounts of water. Answer C is incorrect because water, not normal saline, is used to flush the NG tube.

41. **Answer C is correct.** The nurse should handle the cast using the palms of the hands, to prevent indentations in the cast. Answer A is incorrect because grasping the cast with the hands will produce indentations that cause pressure points. Answers B and D are incorrect choices because assistive slings and lifting devices would frighten the 3-year-old and are not needed.

42. **Answer B is correct.** Discoid lupus is confined to the skin, producing "coinlike" lesions on the skin. Answers A, C, and D refer to systemic lupus; therefore, they are incorrect.

43. **Answer B is correct.** Before walking the client for the first time since surgery, the nurse should ask the client to sit on the side of the bed and dangle his legs, to prevent postural hypotension. Pain medication should not be given before walking; therefore, answer A is incorrect. Answers C and D have no relationship to walking the client; therefore, they are incorrect.

44. **Answer D is correct.** A positive Babinski reflex in adults should be reported to the charge nurse because it indicates an abnormal finding. Answer A is incorrect because a positive Babinski sign in the adult is abnormal, therefore it does not indicate that the client's condition is improving. Answer B is incorrect because changing the position will not alter the finding. Answer C is incorrect because a positive Babinski reflex is an expected finding in the infant but not in adults.

45. **Answer B is correct.** Gantrisin and other sulfa drugs should be given 30 minutes before meals to enhance absorption. Answer A is incorrect because the medication should be given before eating. Answer C is incorrect because the medication should be given on an empty stomach. Answer D is incorrect because the medication is to be given in divided doses throughout the day.

46. **Answer B is correct.** The client in pain usually has an increased blood pressure. Answers A and C are incorrect because the client in pain will have an increase in the pulse rate and respirations. Temperature is not affected by pain; therefore, answer D is incorrect.

47. **Answer B is correct.** Salmonella infection is commonly associated with turtles. Answers A, C, and D are incorrect because they are not sources of salmonella infection.

48. **Answer C is correct.** The medication will cause the urine to become red-orange in color. Answers A, B, and D are not associated with the use of Pyridium; therefore, they are incorrect.

49. **Answer B is correct.** The infant's fingernails should be kept short to prevent scratching the skin. Keeping the infant warm will increase itching; therefore, answer A is incorrect. Soap should not be used because it dries the skin; therefore, answer C is incorrect. Peroxide is damaging to the tissues; therefore, answer D is incorrect.

50. **Answer A is correct.** A Wilms tumor is found by most parents when the infant is being diapered or bathed. Answers B, C, and D are not associated with a Wilms tumor; therefore, they are incorrect.

51. **Answer A is correct.** Complaints of chest pain and feelings of apprehension are associated with pulmonary emboli, which can occur after the fracture of long bones. These findings should be reported immediately so that interventions can begin. Answer B is incorrect because ecchymosis is common following fractures. Answer C is incorrect because a low-grade temperature is expected because of the inflammatory response. Answer D is incorrect because Level 2 pain is expected in the client with a recent fracture.

52. **Answer A is correct.** JCAHO guidelines state that at least two client identifiers should be used whenever administering medications or blood products, whenever samples or specimens are taken, and when providing treatments. Neither of the identifiers is to be the client's room number. Answer B is incorrect because the client's room number is not used as an identifier. Answer C and D are incorrect because the best identifiers according to JCAHO are the client's armband, medical record number, and/or date of birth.

53. **Answer D is correct.** According to the American Heart Association, the nurse should call for help before instituting CPR. Answer A is incorrect because the nurse would first call for help. The nurse would not start cardiac compressions before evaluating the client's carotid pulse. Answer B is incorrect because the nurse would first call for help. The nurse would not administer rescue breathing until she established that the client was not breathing on her own. Answer C is incorrect because the nurse would open the airway after calling for help.

54. **Answer D is correct.** The medication must be taken for the remainder of the client's life to prevent the reoccurrence of CMV infection. Answers A, B, and C are inaccurate statements; therefore, they are incorrect.

55. **Answer A is correct.** Basal cell epithelioma, skin cancer, is related to sun exposure. Answers B, C, and D are incorrect because they are not associated with the development of basal cell epithelioma.

56. **Answer D is correct.** The appearance of increased drainage that is clear, colorless, or bile tinged indicates disruption or leakage at one of the anastamosis sites, which requires immediate attention. Answer A is incorrect because the client's condition will worsen without prompt intervention. Answers B and C are incorrect choices because they cannot be performed without a physician's order.

57. **Answer A is correct.** Herbals such as Echinacea can interfere with the action of antiviral medications; therefore, the client should discuss the use of herbals with his physician. Answer B is incorrect because supplements have not been shown to prolong life. Answer C is incorrect because herbals have not been shown to be effective in decreasing the viral load. Answer D is incorrect because supplements do not prevent replication of the virus.

58. **Answer B is correct.** The client with Sjogren's syndrome complains of dryness of the eyes. The nurse can help relieve the client's discomfort by instilling eyedrops. Answers A, B, and C do not relieve the symptoms of Sjogren's syndrome; therefore, they are incorrect.

59. **Answer D is correct.** Melena, or blood in the stool, is common in the client with duodenal ulcers. Answers A and B are symptoms of gastric ulcers; therefore, they are incorrect. Diarrhea is not a symptom of duodenal ulcers; therefore, answer C is incorrect.

60. **Answer B is correct.** Clients who use steroid medications, such as fluticasone, can develop adverse side effects, including oral infections with candida albicans. Symptoms of candida albicans include sore throat and white patches on the oral mucosa. Increased weight, difficulty in sleeping, and changes in mood are expected side effects; therefore, answers A, C, and D are incorrect.

61. **Answer A is correct.** Concurrent use of two SSRIs can result in serotonin syndrome, a potentially lethal condition. Answer B is incorrect because it refers to the "Parnate-cheese" reaction or hypertension that results when the client taking an MAO inhibitor ingests sources of tyramine. Answer C in incorrect because it refers to neuroleptic malignant syndrome or elevations in temperature caused by antipsychotic medication. Answer D is incorrect because it refers to the hypertension that results when MAO inhibitors are used with cold and hayfever medications containing pseudoephedrine.

62. **Answer C is correct.** Pernicious anemia is characterized by changes in neurological function such as loss of coordination and loss of position sense. Answers A, B, and D are applicable to all types of anemia; therefore, they are incorrect.

63. **Answer D is correct.** Secondary syphilis is characterized by well-defined generalized lesions on the palms, soles, and perineum. Lesions can enlarge and erode, leaving highly contagious pink or grayish white lesions. Answer A describes the chancre associated with primary syphilis; therefore, it is incorrect. Answer B describes the latent stage of syphilis; therefore, it is incorrect. Answer C describes late syphilis; therefore, it is incorrect.

64. **Answer B is correct.** Morphine can severely depress the client's respirations. Answer A is incorrect because the assessment of heart rate, a part of pain assessment, is not an essential assessment for administering morphine. Answer C is incorrect because temperature is not affected by the administration of morphine. Answer D is incorrect because assessment of blood pressure, a part of pain assessment, is not an essential assessment for administering morphine.

65. **Answer D is correct.** Hoarseness and weak voice are signs of laryngeal nerve damage. These would be evident when the client states her name. Answer A is incorrect because it is not assessed by having the client state her name. The nurse would check the client's dressing and check behind the neck for signs of post-operative bleeding. Answer B is incorrect because it is not assessed by having the client state her name. Signs of decreased calcium include tingling around the mouth and muscle twitching. Answer C is incorrect because it is not assessed by having the client state her name. Signs of laryngeal stridor include harsh, high-pitched respirations.

66. **Answer A is correct.** Essential hypertension is defined as maintenance of a blood pressure reading at or above 140/90. Answers B, C, and D are incorrect because the blood pressures are lower than 140/90.

67. **Answer B is correct.** Karaya powder is applied to help form a seal that will protect the skin from the liquid stool. Answer A is incorrect because karaya powder will not

prevent the formation of odor. Answer C is incorrect because karaya powder will not prevent the loss of electrolytes from the ileostomy. Answer D is incorrect because karaya powder will not increase the time between bag evaluations.

68. **Answer D is correct.** The appropriate diet for the 9-month-old with suspected celiac disease is breast milk and rice cereal. Answer A is incorrect because the 9-month-old is too young to have whole milk, and oats contain gluten, which is associated with celiac disease. Both mixed cereal and barley cereal contain gluten, which is associated with celiac disease; therefore, answers B and C are incorrect.

69. **Answer C is correct.** An elevated white cell count is expected in inflammatory conditions such as diverticulitis. Answers A, B, and D are not associated with inflammation; therefore, they are incorrect.

70. **Answer B is correct.** Increased length of the cord is a sign that the placenta has separated. Answers A, C, and D are not associated with separation of the placenta; therefore, they are incorrect.

71. **Answer C is correct.** It is recommended that a daily dose of cimetadine be given at bedtime. Answers A, B, and D are inaccurate times; therefore, they are incorrect.

72. **Answer A is correct.** Perforation of a duodenal ulcer is characterized by sudden sharp midepigastric pain caused by the emptying of duodenal contents into the peritoneum. The abdomen is tender, rigid, and boardlike. Answer B is not associated with the client's sudden onset of symptoms; therefore, it is incorrect. Answer C is incorrect because the client would complain of heartburn or reflux. Answer D is incorrect because the client would have increased abdominal distention, visible peristaltic waves, and high-pitched bowel sounds.

73. **Answer A is correct.** The banana popsicle is best for the child following a tonsillectomy because it is cold and the yellow color does not allow it to be confused with any bleeding that the child might have. Answer B is incorrect because milk products form a film on the operative area and thicken saliva. Answer C is incorrect because fruit punch contains fruit juices that might cause a burning sensation in the throat following a tonsillectomy. Answer D is incorrect because the carbonation from cola causes a burning sensation in the throat following a tonsillectomy.

74. **Answer B is correct.** The client taking alprazolam should not use alcohol, which includes beer, because alcohol potentiates the effect of the medication. Answers A and D are not associated with the use of alprazolam; therefore, they are incorrect. Answer C is associated with the use of MAO inhibitors; therefore, it is incorrect.

75. **Answer D is correct.** The correct use of the incentive spirometer will increase the client's respiratory effort and effectiveness. Answers A and B are indirectly affected by the correct use of the incentive spirometer; therefore, they are incorrect. Answer C is not affected by the use of an incentive spiromenter; therefore, it is incorrect.

76. **Answer A is correct.** Unless the manufacturer recommends otherwise, the nurse should inflate and deflate the gastric and esophageal balloons to make sure they are not defective. Answer B refers to the insertion of a standard nasogastric tube; therefore, it is incorrect. Answer C is incorrect because the esophageal tamponade is usually removed after 48 hours. Answer D is incorrect because the esophageal tamponade has a port for gastric suction.

77. **Answer B is correct.** Lactulose is given to produce diarrhea, which lowers the client's serum ammonia levels. Answers A, C, and D are not associated with the use of lactulose; therefore, they are incorrect.

78. **Answer C is correct.** Gently massaging the fundus immediately following delivery will help it to contract. Answer A is incorrect because the uterus would be displaced to one side if the bladder was distended. Answer B is incorrect. The nurse should first massage the fundus before notifying the doctor. Answer D is incorrect because uterine relaxation is not associated with pain.

79. **Answer B is correct.** Oatmeal and grapefruit wedges are high in fiber. Answers A, C, and D are incorrect because they contain less fiber.

80. **Answer A is correct.** Many clients with Hodgkin's lymphoma report finding enlarged nodes in the neck when shaving. Answer B is associated with brain tumors; therefore, it is incorrect. Answer C is associated with leukemia; therefore, it is incorrect. Answer D is associated with renal cancer; therefore, it is incorrect.

81. **Answer B is correct.** Pentamidine is used to prevent pneumocystis carinni pneumonia (PCP). Answers A, C, and D are not associated with the use of pentamidine; therefore, they are incorrect.

82. **Answer D is correct.** The anterior fontanel usually closes by the time the baby is 12–18 months of age. Answers A, B and C are incorrect because the baby is too young for the anterior fontanel to be closed.

83. **Answer C is correct.** A positive Schilling test indicates that the client has pernicious anemia, which is due to the lack of intrinsic factor. Answer A describes iron-deficiency anemia; therefore, it is incorrect. Answer B describes sickle cell anemia; therefore, it is incorrect. Answer D describes Cooley's anemia; therefore, it is incorrect.

84. **Answer B is correct.** According to universal precautions, blood spills should be cleaned up immediately using a weak solution of bleach (1 part bleach to 10 parts water). Answers A, C, and D are not recommended for cleaning up accidental blood spills; therefore, they are incorrect.

85. **Answer A is correct.** Providing a pacifier will provide the most comfort for the 5-month-old by providing oral gratification. Answers B, C, and D will comfort the infant, but not as much as the pacifier while he is NPO.

86. **Answer B is correct.** The nurse should make a list of the medications and ask a family member to take the medications home. If no family member is available, the medication should remain locked in the medication room until the client is discharged home. Answer A is incorrect because the client might take the medication without the nurse's knowledge, which might result in overmedication. Answer C is incorrect because over-the-counter medications and herbal supplements can interact with medications the physician might order. Answer D is incorrect because only medications supplied by the hospital pharmacy should be used while the client is hospitalized unless the physician writes an order allowing the nurse to administer medication previously purchased by the client.

87. **Answer C is correct.** The physician's signature is not included on the preoperative checklist because it is a check sheet for the assessment and preparation of the client

for surgery. The physician's signature is required on the preoperative orders and the consent form for surgery. Answers A, B, and D are incorrect because they are required on the client's preoperative checklist.

88. **Answer A is correct.** Thorazine (chlorpromazine) causes an increase in sun sensitivity; therefore, the nursing staff should take extra measures to protect the clients from sun exposure. Aged cheese and chocolate are eliminated from the diet of a client taking an MAO inhibitor; therefore, answers B and D are incorrect. Answer C is incorrect because the client taking Thorazine needs extra fluid because the anticholinergic effects of the medication cause dry mouth.

89. **Answer D is correct.** Ambulating the client as soon as possible prevents venous stasis and helps to prevent embolus formation. Answers A and C are measures to increase the effectiveness of respirations and help to prevent pneumonia; therefore, they are incorrect. Answer B is a treatment to break up an existing embolus; therefore, it is incorrect.

90. **Answer A is correct.** B & O suppositories relieve pain following a prostatectomy by reducing bladder spasms. The medication does not improve urinary output, does not reduce post-operative swelling, and does not treat nausea and vomiting; therefore, answers B, C, and D are incorrect.

91. **Answer B is correct.** The primary reason for wrapping the stump with an elastic bandage is to shrink the stump and get it ready for application of a prosthetic device. Answer A is incorrect because the application of an elastic bandage will not decrease bleeding. Answer C is incorrect because the application of an elastic bandage will not prevent phantom pain. Application of an elastic bandage will prevent the client from seeing the area, but this is not the primary reason for its use; therefore, answer D is incorrect.

92. **Answer B is correct.** Symptoms associated with polycythemia include ruddy complexion, spleenomegaly, headache, fatigue, dyspena, angina, and pruritis. Answer A is incorrect because it is associated with pernicious anemia. Answer C is incorrect because it is associated with anemia. Answer D is incorrect because the symptoms are associated with left-sided heart failure.

93. **Answer A is correct.** Following a total hip replacement, the nurse should assist the client to sit in a recliner, which limits the amount of hip flexion to 60° or less. Answers B, C, and D are incorrect because they allow the hip to be flexed more than 90°, which might dislocate the hip prosthesis.

94. **Answer C is correct.** Cotazyme (pancrelipase) increases the digestion and absorption of fats, carbohydrates, and proteins in the GI tract. Deficiencies in the fat-soluble vitamins (A, D, E, K) are corrected by administering the water-soluble forms of those vitamins; therefore, answer A is incorrect. Answer B is incorrect because Cotazyme increases carbohydrate metabolism. Answer D is incorrect because Cotazyme has no effect on sodium and chloride excretion.

95. **Answer C is correct.** The typical play of preschool-age children is described as associative play. In associative play, children of the same sex play together with no obvious rules for play activity and without leaders. Answer A is incorrect because it is the typical play activity of the infant. Answer B is incorrect because it is the typical play

activity of the toddler. Answer D is incorrect because it is the typical play activity of the school-age child.

96. **Answer A is correct.** Petroleum gauze should not be applied to the cord, which separates by a process of drying. Answers B, C, and D are all parts of routine cord care; therefore, they are incorrect.

97. **Answer A is correct.** According to Freud's psychoanalytic theory, antisocial personality disorder arises from faulty development of the id. Answers B, C, and D are incorrect because they are not related to the development of antisocial personality disorder.

98. **Answer B is correct.** Phenobarbital is a central nervous system depressant that is capable of producing decreased respirations and apnea. Answer A is associated with an overdose of aspirin; therefore, it is incorrect. Answer C is incorrect because the blood pressure would be decreased. Answer D is not associated with an overdose of Phenobarbital; therefore, it is incorrect.

99. **Answer B is correct.** Buck's traction is a skin traction used for short-time immobilization of hip fractures before surgical correction. Answer A is incorrect because 90-90 traction is a skeletal traction used to immobilize fractures of the femur. Answer C is incorrect because Bryant's traction is used only for children who weigh less than 30 pounds. Answer D is incorrect because Dunlop's traction is used to treat fractures of the humerus.

100. **Answer D is correct.** Concurrent use of an SSRI and an MAO inhibitor can produce serotonin syndrome; therefore, the client should discontinue the MAO inhibitor 14 days before beginning therapy with an SSRI. Answers A, B, and C are incorrect because the time is too brief between the use of the MAO inhibitor and the beginning of therapy with an SSRI.

101. **Answer D is correct.** The nurse should first assess the client to determine the location and character of the pain. Answers A, B, and C are incorrect because they are not the first action that the nurse should take.

102. **Answer C is correct.** Cephalocaudal development refers to head-to-tail (toe) development; therefore, the infant can raise her head before she can sit. Answer A is an example of simple-to-complex development; therefore, it is incorrect. Answer B is an example of proximodistal development; therefore, it is incorrect. Answer D is an example of general-to-specific development; therefore, it is incorrect.

103. **Answer D is correct.** When performing a straight catheterization, the nurse should hold the catheter in place as the bladder empties to prevent it from slipping out. Answer A is incorrect because surgical, not medical, asepsis is used when performing a catheterization. Answer B is incorrect because the catheter should be inserted 2–3 inches. Answer C is incorrect because the straight catheter does not have a balloon for inflation.

104. **Answer A is correct.** Moving the client up in the bed is easier with the head of the bed lowered because the nurse does not have to work against the force of gravity. Answer B is incorrect because lowering the head of the bed will not prevent wrinkles in the linen. Answer C is incorrect because lowering the head of the bed will not eliminate the need for additional help to move the client. Answer D is incorrect because lowering the head of the bed will not relieve pressure on the client's sacrum.

105. Answer B is correct. During an arteriogram, contrast media is injected directly into the artery. The nurse should give priority to assessing the site for bleeding. Answers A, C, and D are incorrect because they do not take priority over assessing the site for bleeding.

106. Answer D is correct. Methodone is an opiod agonist; therefore, it is capable of producing respiratory depression.

107. Answer B is correct. Atropine is given to dry secretions and lessens the likelihood of aspiration. Answers A, C, and D are inaccurate statements; therefore, they are incorrect.

108. Answer C is correct. The client's assessment findings are within normal 12 hours after a Caesarean section; therefore, the nurse should chart the finding. Answer A is incorrect because the assessment does not reveal the presence of bladder distention. Answer B is incorrect because the assessment does not reveal uterine atony. Answer D is incorrect because the client needs to ambulate.

109. Answer A is correct. "Rainbow" bruises refer to bruises in various stages of healing. Although they are not conclusive proof of physical abuse, they do suggest the possibility. Answer B is incorrect because the 4-year-old might still suck the thumb when going to sleep. The victim of child abuse usually endures painful procedures with little expression of emotion; therefore, answer C is incorrect. Victims of child abuse are usually reluctant to talk to strangers; therefore, answer D is incorrect.

110. Answer C is correct. An alcoholic blackout refers to the inability to remember what occurred before or after a period of alcohol intake. Answer A is incorrect because it occurs after a period of heavy drinking or when the usual alcohol intake is reduced. Alcoholic hallucinosis is characterized by hallucinations. Answer B is incorrect because it refers to the headache and gastrointestinal symptoms experienced after drinking alcohol. Sunday morning paralysis refers to radial nerve palsy commonly observed when a stuporous person lies with his arm pressed over a projecting surface; therefore, answer D is incorrect.

111. Answer A is correct. Degenerative joint disease (osteoarthritis) is characterized by joint pain that intensifies with activity and diminishes with rest. Answers B, C, and D are typical findings in the client with rheumatoid arthritis; therefore, they are incorrect.

112. Answer B is correct. The client with pancreatitis has decreased levels of vitamin K, making him more likely to have prolonged bleeding with injections; therefore, the nurse should hold pressure on the injection site for 3–5 minutes. Answer A is incorrect because the medication is not administered using the Z track method. Answer C is incorrect because the medication is not administered subcutaneously. Answer D is incorrect because alcohol, not betadine, is used to prep the skin.

113. Answer D is correct. The client with Addison's disease is treated with corticosteroid therapy that reduces the client's immunity. The client needs to stay out of crowds to prevent complications posed by infection. Answers A and C are incorrect because the client needs additional sources of sodium and potassium in the diet. Answer B is incorrect because the client with Addison's disease should dress in warm clothing to prevent easy chilling.

114. Answer A is correct. The evulsed tooth should be rinsed in milk, in saline solution, or under running water before reimplantation. Answer B is incorrect because it will disturb the adhering periodontal membrane. Answer C is incorrect because the tooth should be held by the crown, not the root. Answer D is incorrect because the child might swallow or aspirate the tooth.

115. **Answer B is correct.** Presenting symptoms of leukemia include pallor, fatigue, anorexia, petechiae, and bone or joint pain. Answers A, C, and D are incorrect because they are not associated with leukemia.

116. **Answer D is correct.** The skill of aspirating nasogastric secretions is beyond the scope of practice of the nursing assistant. Answers A, B, and C are incorrect because they are within the scope of practice of the nursing assistant.

117. **Answer B is correct.** The hourly urinary output should be maintained between 30mL and 50mL per hour. The fact that the urine is dark amber indicates that the client is not receiving adequate fluids to prevent dehydration. Answers A, C, and D do not call for any interventions; therefore, they are incorrect.

118. **Answer B is correct.** The client's oxygen saturation is low; therefore, the nurse should give priority to administering oxygen per standing order. Answer A is incorrect because there is nothing that indicates that the client needs an analgesic. Answer C is incorrect because the client's temperature is satisfactory. Answer D is incorrect because the Glascow score of 13 indicates that the client is not fully recovered from the effects of conscious sedation; therefore, the IV should not be discontinued.

119. **Answer C is correct.** Phenergan with codeine is an antitussive that relieves coughing and affords the client an opportunity to rest. Answers A and B are not properties of the medication; therefore, they are incorrect. Answer D is incorrect because the amount of codeine in the medication is not sufficient to relieve pain.

120. **Answer B is correct.** The primary cause of anemia in the client with chronic renal failure is the lack of erythropoietin. Answer A is incorrect because it is not the primary cause of anemia in the client with chronic renal failure. Answer C is incorrect because it refers to sickle cell anemia. Answer D is incorrect because it refers to iron-deficiency anemia.

121. **Answer D is correct.** The nurse should recheck the MAR to make sure the medication she is about to give is correct. Answers A and B are incorrect because they do not provide for the client's safety. Answer C is incorrect because the pharmacist might or might not have made a substitution. The nurse needs to validate generic substitution before administering the medication.

122. **Answer D is correct.** A side effect of Laradopa (levodopa) is orthostatic hypotension; therefore, the nurse should tell the client to rise slowly from a sitting position. Answer A is incorrect because the medication can be given with a snack to prevent gastric irritation. Answer B is incorrect because the client does not need monthly lab work. Answer C is incorrect because the medication only controls the symptoms of Parkinson's disease; it does not cure the disease. Therefore, the medication will be taken indefinitely.

123. **Answer A is correct.** Dietary management of the client with congestive heart failure includes a sodium-restricted diet. Answers B, C, and D are incorrect because they are not restricted in the client with congestive heart failure.

124. **Answer C is correct.** Diuretic therapy and restriction of fluids are ordered during the acute phase of a stroke to reduce cerebral edema. Answer A is incorrect because the orders are not intended to reduce cardiac output. Answer B is incorrect because the measures will not prevent an embolus. Answer D is incorrect because the measures are not intended to minimize incontinence.

125. **Answer B is correct.** Long-term exposure to gastric contents such as that caused by gastroesophageal reflux plays a role in the development of esophageal cancer. Answers A and D are incorrect because they are not associated with esophageal cancer. A history of prolonged use of alcohol and tobacco is associated with esophageal cancer; therefore, answer C is incorrect.

126. **Answer C is correct.** Spinach is an excellent source of both calcium and potassium. Broccoli is a good source of calcium but not potassium; therefore, answer A is incorrect. Sweet potato and avocado are good sources of potassium but not calcium; therefore, answers B and D are incorrect.

127. **Answer B is correct.** The PSA (prostate specific antigen) and acid phosphatase are valuable screening tests for cancer of the prostate. The PSA is not a screening test for cancers of the bladder, vas deferens, or testes; therefore, answers A, C, and D are incorrect.

128. **Answer C is correct.** The client's lithium level is within the therapeutic range. Answer A is incorrect because the lithium level is not too low to be therapeutic. Answer B is incorrect because the client is not within the range of toxicity. Answer D is incorrect because eating more sodium-rich foods will reduce the lithium level.

129. **Answer C is correct.** The treatment for ventricular fibrillations (V-fib) is defibrillation (D-fib). Answers A, B, and D are not emergency treatments for the client who suddenly develops ventricular fibrillations.

130. **Answer D is correct.** The client with apraxia is unable to recognize the purpose of familiar objects; therefore, he is unable to perform previously learned skills such as combing his hair. Answer A is incorrect because it refers to aphasia. Answer B is incorrect because it refers to dysphagia. Answer C is incorrect because it refers to ataxia.

131. **Answer A is correct.** Using a pillow or sling to support the client's arm while she is sitting will help prevent subluxation of the affected shoulder. Answers B, C, and D are incorrect because they do not prevent subluxation of the client's affected shoulder.

132. **Answer C is correct.** The recommended way of administering Lovenox (enoxaparin) is subcutaneously in the abdominal tissue. Answers A and B are not recommended ways of administering Lovenox (enoxaparin); therefore, they are incorrect. Answer D is incorrect because Lovenox (enoxaprin) is not available in an oral form.

133. **Answer B is correct.** Nitroglycerin should be kept in a dark-brown bottle to protect it from light, which causes deterioration of the medication. Answer A is incorrect because the medication is placed beneath the tongue when needed, not taken daily. Answer C is incorrect because the medication supply should be replenished every 6 months, not every year. Answer D is incorrect because the cotton should be removed from the bottle because it absorbs the medication.

134. **Answer A is correct.** Ingestion of foods containing tyramine by the client taking Parnate, an MAO inhibitor, can result in elevations in blood pressure. Answers B, C, and D are not associated with the interaction of Parnate or other MAO inhibitors; therefore, they are incorrect.

135. **Answer C is correct.** Because of the location, the client receiving external radiation for cancer of the larynx will most likely complain of a sore throat. Generalized pruritis, dyspnea, and bone pain are not associated with external radiation for cancer of the larynx; therefore, answers A, B, and D are incorrect.

136. **Answer B is correct.** Symptoms of autonomic dysreflexia are often triggered by bladder distention or fecal impaction; therefore, after raising the client's head, the nurse should check for patency of the catheter. Answer A is incorrect because administering a prescribed analgesic will not alleviate the symptoms of autonomic dysreflexia. Answer C is incorrect because breathing slowly does not alleviate autonomic dysreflexia. Answer D is incorrect because the changes in the client's temperature are not associated with autonomic dysreflexia.

137. **Answer B is correct.** The nurse or parent should maintain one hand on the child whenever the side rails are down to prevent the child falling from the crib. Answer A is incorrect because the child can fall over rails that are locked at the halfway point. Positioning the child farther away from the lowered side rail will not prevent falls because the child can quickly move to the other side so that falls can result; therefore, answer C is incorrect. Answer D is incorrect because the child can fall from the crib.

138. **Answer C is correct.** The nurse should temporarily stop the administration of the Virazole when the mist tent needs to be opened to allow the medication particles to settle. Answer A is incorrect because contact precautions should be used even though the infant is receiving Virazole. Answer B is incorrect because contact precautions are used whether the mist tent is opened or closed. Answer D is incorrect because increasing or decreasing the rate of medication administration is not a nursing function.

139. **Answer D is correct.** The most common food allergens are proteins such as those contained in eggs, cow's milk, and peanuts. Answers A, B, and C are incorrect because they are not the most common food allergens.

140. **Answer D is correct.** Eczematous lesions are more common on the cheeks and extensor surfaces of the arms and legs. Answer A is incorrect because the abdomen is not a common site of eczematous lesions. Answer B is incorrect because the buttocks, abdomen, and back are not common sites of eczematous lesions. Answer C is incorrect because the back and flexor surfaces of the arms and legs are not common sites of eczematous lesions.

141. **Answer C is correct.** The client's own desire to become drug-free has the most influence on recovery and sobriety. Answers A, B, and D are important factors, but they do not have the greatest influence on the client's recovery; therefore, they are incorrect.

142. **Answer A is correct.** Acute otitis media is characterized by elevations in temperature as high as 104°F. Pain in the affected ear, nausea and vomiting, and feelings of fullness characterize both chronic otitis media and acute otitis media; therefore, answers B, C, and D are incorrect.

143. Answer B is correct. Rheumatic fever is associated with a history of a sequella to strep throat. Answers A, C, and D are not associated with rheumatic fever; therefore, they are incorrect.

144. Answer A is correct. The child with Duchenne's muscular dystrophy must use Gower's maneuver to rise to a standing position. The child puts his hands on his knees and moves the hands up the legs until he is standing. Answer B is incorrect because it refers to the child with Osgood-Schlatter disease. Answer C is incorrect because it refers to the child with lordosis. Answer D is incorrect because it refers to the child with Legg-Calve-Perthes disease.

145. Answer B is correct. Amniotic fluid is straw colored in appearance. Answer A is incorrect because it indicates active bleeding. Answer C is incorrect because it indicates the passage of meconium, which is associated with fetal distress. Answer D is incorrect because the discharge should be straw colored, not dark brown in appearance.

146. Answer D is correct. Fetal heart tones can be heard using a fetoscope as early as 18 weeks gestation. Answers A, B, and C are incorrect because fetal heart tones cannot be heard using a fetoscope before 18 weeks gestation.

147. Answer D is correct. The client can help prevent heartburn by avoiding caffeinated beverages. Answers A and C are incorrect because the client should sleep on her left side with her head elevated on several pillows. Answer B is incorrect because eating dry crackers at bedtime can increase problems with heartburn.

148. Answer C is correct. Pancreatic enzyme replacement is given to facilitate the digestion of fats, proteins, and carbohydrates. Therefore, if the amount of pancreatic enzyme is adequate, the client will have an increase in weight. Answer A is incorrect because pancreatic enzyme replacement has no effect on respiratory function. Answer B is incorrect because pancreatic enzyme replacement does not decrease sodium excretion. Answer D is incorrect because pancreatic enzyme replacement does not decrease chloride excretion.

149. Answer D is correct. The lesions of impetigo resolve in 2 weeks, and it will be safe for the child to return to school. Answers A, B, and C are incorrect because the lesions will still be present and the child will be contagious.

150. Answer B is correct. Infants born to diabetic mothers have microsomia or large bodies because of maternal hyperglycemia. Answers A, C, and D do not relate specifically to infants of diabetic mothers; therefore, they are incorrect.

151. Answer B is correct. The Guthrie test is a screening test for newborns to detect phenylketonuria. Cystic fibrosis is confirmed by a sweat test; therefore, answer A is incorrect . Hypothyroidsim is confirmed by a T3 and T4; therefore, answer C is incorrect. Sickle cell is confirmed by the Sickledex; therefore, answer D is incorrect.

152. Answer D is correct. Elixophylline (theophylline) is a bronchodilator that acts to relax bronchial smooth muscle. Answers A, B, and C are incorrect because they are not actions of theophylline.

153. Answer D is correct. A meal of baked chicken, apple, angel food cake, and 1% milk is low in calories, low in fat, and low in sodium. Answer A is incorrect because blue cheese dressing and crackers are high in sodium. Answer B is incorrect because frankfurters are high in calories, fat, and sodium. Answer C is incorrect because taco seasoning, meat, chips, and sour cream are high in calories, fat, and sodium.

154. Answer A is correct. Breast milk is higher in fat than cow's milk. Answers B, C, and D are inaccurate statements regarding breast milk; therefore, they are incorrect.

155. Answer B is correct. The nurse should direct the client to put the medicine in his mouth and swallow it with some water. Answer A is incorrect because it is threatening to the client. Answer C is incorrect because medication administration and supervision is a responsibility of the nurse, not the nursing assistant. Answer D is incorrect because the nurse is threatening the client.

156. Answer D is correct. Entocort EC (budesonide) is a long-acting corticosteroid that should be taken with meals or a snack to prevent gastric upset. Answer A is incorrect because the medication should not be taken with grapefruit juice. Entocort EC (budesonide) should be taken with food; therefore, answers B and C are incorrect.

157. Answer C is correct. Edema of the face and hands is not a normal occurrence in pregnancy; therefore, the client needs further teaching. Answers A, B, and D indicate that the client understands the nurse's teaching; therefore, they are incorrect.

158. Answer D is correct. One cup of prune juice provides 707mg of potassium. Answers A, B, and C are incorrect because they provide less potassium than prune juice. (One cup of apple juice provides 295mg of potassium, one cup of orange juice provides 496mg of potassium, and one cup of cranberry juice provides 152mg of potassium.)

159. Answer A is correct. The immediate nursing intervention is the administration of pain medication. Answers B, C, and D will be done later; therefore, they are incorrect.

160. Answer D is correct. The urine should be removed using a sterile syringe and needle. Removing the urine from the port nearest the client ensures that the urine is more sterile. Answer A is incorrect because urine in the bag is not sterile. Answer B is incorrect because urine in the drainage tube is not sterile. Answer C is incorrect because urine in the bag is not sterile.

161. Answer C is correct. In infants and young children, the Eustachian tube is shorter, straighter, and wider, making it more vulnerable to otitis media. Answers A, B, and D are incorrect because they are not related to the occurrence of otitis media.

162. Answer B is correct. Vernix caseosa covers the body of the full-term infant. Absence of sucking pads, presence of the scarf sign, and the absence of solar creases are expected findings in the preterm infant; therefore, answers A, C, and D are incorrect.

163. Answer C is correct. The nurse can assess the client's orientation to time by asking the date, the month, the year, or the season. Asking the client to state his name or to identify family members or friends is a way of assessing the client's orientation to person; therefore, answer A is incorrect. Answer B is incorrect because it elicits information regarding where the client is at the present time. Answer D is incorrect because it elicits information regarding the client's recognition of familiar objects.

164. Answer A is correct. The 22-month-old child can be expected to feed herself with a spoon. Answers B, C, and D are developmental tasks of the older child; therefore, they are incorrect.

165. **Answer B is correct.** Munchausen's syndrome by proxy is characterized by unexplained illness brought on by another person, usually the mother, for the purpose of gaining attention. Answer A refers to nursing bottle syndrome; therefore, it is incorrect. Answer C refers to oral allergy syndrome; therefore, it is incorrect. Answer D refers to Christ-Siemen's Touraine syndrome; therefore, it is incorrect.

166. **Answer B is correct.** The nurse should first try to determine the client's reason for refusing the medication so that she can decide what action needs to be taken. The nurse should not encourage the client to do anything she does not want to do; therefore, answer A is incorrect. Answers C and D are incorrect because they are not the first action the nurse should take.

167. **Answer C is correct.** The nurse believes that her way of treating illness (real medication) is superior to the client's way of treating illness (herbals). Answer A refers to belonging to a particular ethnic group; therefore, it is incorrect. Answers B and D are incorrect choices because the nurse's statement did not reflect cultural sensitivity or cultural tolerance.

168. **Answer B is correct.** The normal range for fetal heart tones is 110–160bpm. Answer A is incorrect because the heart rate is too slow. Answers C and D are incorrect choices because the heart rate is too rapid.

169. **Answer B is correct.** The client can decrease abdominal discomfort by splinting the incision with a pillow. Answers A and C are incorrect because they increase abdominal discomfort. Answer D is incorrect because it does not decrease abdominal discomfort.

170. **Answer A is correct.** A family history of arteriosclerotic heart disease is a nonmodifiable risk factor in the development of arteriorsclerotic heart disease. Answers B, C, and D are incorrect because the risk of developing arteriosclerotic heart disease can be modified or altered by controlling hypertension, eliminating high cholesterol and high saturated fats from the diet, and enrolling in a program of regular exercise.

171. **Answer B is correct.** The concurrent use of an MAO inhibitor such as Nardil and an SSRI such as Paxil is contraindicated because it can result in serotonin syndrome. Answers A and D are incorrect because the concurrent use of the medications is contraindicated. Answer C is incorrect because anti-Parkinsonian medication is used for the client with neuroleptic malignant syndrome, not serotonin syndrome.

172. **Answer A is correct.** To prevent air from entering the stomach, the nurse should pour all the formula into the syringe barrel before opening the clamp. Answers B, C, and D are incorrect because they do not prevent air from entering the stomach during nasogastric tube feeding.

173. **Answer C is correct.** Signs of possible internal bleeding include restless and shortness of breath. Answer A is incorrect because the urinary output is within normal limits. Answer B is incorrect because the color and rate of chest tube drainage is within the expected range following a lobectomy. Answer D is incorrect because the pulse rate and respiratory rate would be increased with internal bleeding.

174. **Answer D is correct.** A weight of 2.2 pounds is equal to 1kg; therefore, 4.1kg equals 9.02kg. Answers A, B, and C are inaccurate answers; therefore, they are incorrect.

175. **Answer A is correct.** Asking the client to tell more about what he is feeling gives the client an opportunity to discuss his fears and apprehensions. Answer B is incorrect because it is a closed question. Answer C is incorrect because it minimizes the client's feelings and offers false reassurances. Answer D is incorrect because it minimizes the client's feelings.

176. **Answer A is correct.** Providing mouth care should be done immediately after the removal of a nasogastric tube. Answers B, C, and D are incorrect because they are done later.

177. **Answer B is correct.** Positioning the client in semi-Fowler's position tilted toward the right side will help to splint the fractured ribs and will allow the uninvolved left lung to fully inflate. Answers A and C are incorrect because they would make breathing more difficult. Answer D is incorrect because it would not allow the full expansion of the uninvolved lung.

178. **Answer C is correct.** An established means of dealing with cravings and maintaining sobriety is gaining support from other recovering alcoholics. Answers A and B are incorrect because they are punitive and will not help the client deal with his cravings. Answer D will help provide for the client's safety during withdrawal, but it will not help the client maintain sobriety; therefore, it is incorrect.

179. **Answer C is correct.** The client with Addison's disease needs an increased sodium intake. Bouillon and juices such as tomato juice are high in sodium. Answers A, B, and D are incorrect because they do not contain high levels of sodium.

180. **Answer B is correct.** When administering the DTP, Hib, and hepatitis B vaccines, it is recommended that the DTP be administered in one leg and the Hib and hepatitis B vaccine be administered in the other leg. Answer A is incorrect because all the immunizations are not given in one site. No immunizations are to be given in the infant's arm; therefore, answers C and D are incorrect.

181. **Answer C is correct.** Protamine sulfate is the antidote for heparin overdose. Aquamephyton is the antidote for sodium warfarin overdose; therefore, answer A is incorrect. Ticlid is used to inhibit platelet aggregation and decrease the incidence of strokes; therefore, answer B is incorrect. Amicar is used in the management of hemorrhage caused by thrombolytic agents; therefore, answer D is incorrect.

182. **Answer B is correct.** Assessment findings in the newborn with respiratory distress syndrome include nasal flaring, grunting respirations, and retractions. Answers A, C, and D are not associated with respiratory distress syndrome; therefore, they are incorrect.

183. **Answer C is correct.** Placing the infant on his back while he is sleeping helps to reduce the risk of SIDS. Answers A, B, and D are incorrect because they have not been shown to reduce the risk of SIDS.

184. **Answer B is correct.** Pulling a toy wagon is the most developmentally appropriate play activity for the toddler. Answer A is incorrect because the toddler's attention span is too short for watching cartoons. Watching a mobile is developmentally appropriate for the infant, not the toddler; therefore, answer C is incorrect. Answer D is incorrect because the toddler lacks the fine motor development needed for using a coloring book and crayons.

185. **Answer B is correct.** Metamucil should be mixed with the recommended amount of water and drunk immediately. Answers A, C, and D are improper ways of preparing the medication; therefore, they are incorrect.

186. **Answer A is correct.** Before the mid-1970s, lead-based paint was used extensively. Children living in housing built before that time are at risk for lead poisoning. Answer B is incorrect because it is due to a lack of intrinsic factor needed for the production of red blood cells. Answer C is incorrect because it is related to the overuse of iron supplements or vitamins containing iron. Answer D is incorrect because it is related to the ingestion of grains such as oats, barley, wheat, and rye.

187. **Answer B is correct.** Distention of the jugular veins and pitting edema are findings associated with fluid overload in the child with renal disease. Answers A, C, and D are not characteristics of fluid overload; therefore, they are incorrect.

188. **Answer D is correct.** Gradual decreasing of the daily dose of steroid medication is necessary to prevent an Addisonian crisis caused by adrenocortical hyposecretion. Cushing's syndrome is the result of adrenocortical hypersecretion; therefore, answer A is incorrect. Answer B is incorrect because a thyroid storm is the result of untreated hyperthyroidism. Answer C is incorrect because a cholinergic crisis is the result of overmedication with anticholinesterase drugs.

189. **Answer C is correct.** Desferal (deferoxamine) is the chelating agent used to treat the child with hemosiderosis. Succimer, Versenate, and EDTA are chelating agents used to treat the child with lead poisoning; therefore, answers A, B, and D are incorrect.

190. **Answer C is correct.** The client recovering from a burn injury should have a diet that is high in protein, high in carbohydrates, and high in calories to meet the body's requirements for tissue repair. Answer A is incorrect because the client needs additional carbohydrates. Answer B is incorrect because the client would benefit from increased fat. Answer D is incorrect because the client needs additional calories.

191. **Answer A is correct.** Nosocomial infections are infections acquired in the healthcare facility. Answer B is incorrect because the infection was not acquired in the healthcare facility. Answers C and D refer to community acquired infections; therefore, they are incorrect.

192. **Answer B is correct.** Fortified rice cereal will provide the infant with an additional source of iron. Orange juice and whole milk are poor sources of iron and should not be added to the diet until the infant is older; therefore, answers A and C are incorrect. Answer D is incorrect because strained meat should not be added until the infant is older.

193. **Answer C is correct.** According to the American Cancer Society, women should have a baseline mammogram done between the ages of 35 and 40. After age 40, women should have an annual mammogram. Answers A, B, and D are incorrect because they do not follow the recommendations of the American Cancer Society.

194. **Answer B is correct.** The nurse should measure the child's head circumference daily to determine the effectiveness of the shunt. Answer A is incorrect because it is a medical intervention. Answer C is incorrect because the fontanels would be closed. Answer D is incorrect because it is not necessary to maintain the child in a prone position.

195. Answer C is correct. Stranger anxiety first peaks when the infant is 7–9 months of age. Stranger anxiety does not peak before age 7 months; therefore, answers A and B are incorrect. Answer D is incorrect because stranger anxiety first peaks before 12 months of age.

196. Answer D is correct. Coarctation of the aorta is an acyanotic heart defect characterized by the presence of diminished femoral pulses and bounding radial and brachial pulses. Answers A, B, and C are incorrect because they describe the child with a cyanotic heart defect.

197. Answer A is correct. Cooley's anemia, also known as thalassemia major, is a genetic disease primarily affecting those of Mediterranean descent. Answers B, C, and D are incorrect because they are not likely to be affected with Cooley's anemia.

198. Answer D is correct. The primary nursing consideration is restoring the client's nutritional status. Answers A, B, and C are an important part of the client's care but are not the primary nursing considerations of the newly admitted client with anorexia nervosa; therefore, they are incorrect.

199. Answer C is correct. The fontanels of a 2-month-old should feel flat and firm to the touch. Tense, bulging fontanels indicate increased intracranial pressure; therefore, answers A and D are incorrect. Soft, sunken fontanels indicate dehydration; therefore, answer B is incorrect.

200. Answer D is correct. Retinopathy of prematurity is caused by damage to immature blood vessels in the retina, which can be the result of high levels of oxygen. Answers A, B, and C are not associated with prolonged oxygen therapy; therefore, they are incorrect.

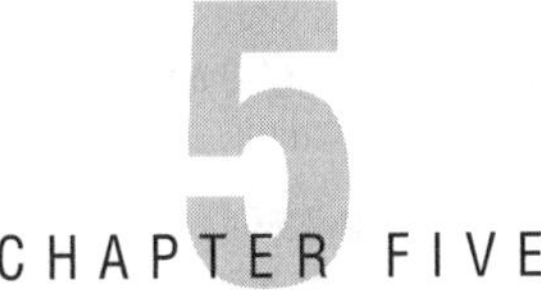

CHAPTER FIVE

Practice Exam 5 and Rationales

Quick Check

1. The nurse is in the process of administering PO medications. Which of the following drugs should not be administered at the same time?

   Quick Answers: **318**
   Detailed Answer: **321**

   - ❍ **A.** Levofloxacin (Levaquin) and Mylanta
   - ❍ **B.** Furosemide (Lasix) and Simethicone (Mylicon)
   - ❍ **C.** Cyclobenzaprine (Flexeril) and Carbidopa (Sinemet)
   - ❍ **D.** Sucralfate (Carafate) and docusate calcium (Surfak)

2. The nurse caring for a client with hyperthyroidism would expect which group of clinical manifestations to be exhibited?

   Quick Answers: **318**
   Detailed Answer: **321**

   - ❍ **A.** Confusion, weakness, and increased weight
   - ❍ **B.** Shortness of breath, dyspnea, and decreased libido
   - ❍ **C.** Restlessness, fatigue, and weight loss
   - ❍ **D.** Diuresis, hypokalemia, and tachycardia

3. Which medication would the nurse expect to be prescribed for a client exhibiting tetany after thyroid surgery?

   Quick Answers: **318**
   Detailed Answer: **321**

   - ❍ **A.** Calcium
   - ❍ **B.** Sodium
   - ❍ **C.** Potassium
   - ❍ **D.** Iodide

4. The nurse should assess a client who has a peptic ulcer for signs of bleeding. Which symptom would best indicate this complication?

   Quick Answers: **318**
   Detailed Answer: **321**

   - ❍ **A.** Melena
   - ❍ **B.** Hematuria
   - ❍ **C.** Hemoptysis
   - ❍ **D.** Ecchymosis

5. The nurse is preparing to administer insulin to a diabetic. Ten units regular and 35 units of NPH are ordered. Which of the following is the proper procedure for drawing up the medications?

   ❍ **A.** Draw up the insulin in two separate syringes, to prevent confusion

   ❍ **B.** Draw up the NPH insulin before drawing up the regular

   ❍ **C.** Inject air into the NPH vial, draw up 35 units, then inject air into the regular insulin vial and withdraw until insulin is at the 45 unit level.

   ❍ **D.** Inject 35 units of air into the NPH, inject 10 units of air into the regular, withdraw 10 units of regular, and then withdraw 35 units of NPH

Quick Check

Quick Answers: **318**
Detailed Answer: **321**

6. What does the nurse recognize as the primary reason that food and fluids are withheld from clients with pancreatitis?

   ❍ **A.** Decrease blood flow to the pancreas

   ❍ **B.** Decrease stimulation of the pancreas

   ❍ **C.** Increase secretion of pancreatic enzymes

   ❍ **D.** Increase insulin production by the pancreas

Quick Answers: **318**
Detailed Answer: **321**

7. The nurse is administering digoxin (Lanoxin) to a client with congestive heart failure. What is the expected therapeutic effect of this drug?

   ❍ **A.** Increased force of heart contraction

   ❍ **B.** Increased heart rate

   ❍ **C.** Decreased perfusion of the heart muscle

   ❍ **D.** Decreased cardiac output

Quick Answers: **318**
Detailed Answer: **321**

8. A client has just returned from a bronchoscopy. Which safety measure is most important for the nurse to implement?

   ❍ **A.** Maintaining the client in the supine position

   ❍ **B.** Providing the client with saline gargles every 15 minutes for 2 hours

   ❍ **C.** Monitoring the client for return of the gag reflex before PO intake

   ❍ **D.** Splinting the abdomen when coughing

Quick Answers: **318**
Detailed Answer: **321**

Quick Check

9. A 45-year-old client returned from a colon resection 2 hours ago. Which vital signs indicate possible hemorrhagic shock?

Quick Answers: **318**
Detailed Answer: **321**

❍ **A.** BP 120/80, heart rate 88

❍ **B.** BP 170/100, heart rate 120

❍ **C.** BP 160/98, heart rate 54

❍ **D.** BP 96/60, heart rate 120

10. A client with newly diagnosed acquired immunodeficiency syndrome (AIDS) asks the nurse if it's necessary to tell co-workers about the diagnosis. The nurse's response is based on which correct understanding?

Quick Answers: **318**
Detailed Answer: **322**

❍ **A.** Transmission of AIDS doesn't occur through casual contact

❍ **B.** Employees have a right to choose with whom they will work

❍ **C.** Clients with an AIDS diagnosis should not work in public places

❍ **D.** The law requires that employers be informed of an AIDS diagnosis

11. A client is returning to the room after a thyroidectomy. Which piece of equipment should the nurse place at the bedside?

Quick Answers: **318**
Detailed Answer: **322**

❍ **A.** A tracheotomy set

❍ **B.** A hemostat

❍ **C.** A chest tube system

❍ **D.** Wire cutters

12. A client with a hip fracture is receiving heparin sub-cutaneously. Which laboratory test should the nurse monitor when administering this medication?

Quick Answers: **318**
Detailed Answer: **322**

❍ **A.** Prothrombin time

❍ **B.** Vitamin K level

❍ **C.** Activated partial thromboplastin time

❍ **D.** Fibrin split levels

13. What teaching should the nurse reinforce to a young male adult regarding when he should perform testicular self-examinations?

Quick Answers: **318**
Detailed Answer: **322**

❍ **A.** Weekly after becoming sexually active

❍ **B.** Monthly while in the shower

❍ **C.** Bimonthly after age 40

❍ **D.** Annually on his birthday

Quick Check

14. The nurse is reinforcing teaching to a client with a hiatal hernia. Which would be included in the teaching plan?

- ❍ **A.** Eat a puréed diet
- ❍ **B.** Avoid the intake of sweets
- ❍ **C.** Remain in an upright position after meals
- ❍ **D.** Limit protein to 3 oz. once a day

Quick Answers: **318**
Detailed Answer: **322**

15. A client who is in end-stage cirrhosis should restrict which of these foods?

- ❍ **A.** Apples
- ❍ **B.** Broccoli
- ❍ **C.** Beef
- ❍ **D.** Rolls

Quick Answers: **318**
Detailed Answer: **322**

16. The nurse is providing initial first aid for a client with thermal burn injury in a community setting. Which action is appropriate?

- ❍ **A.** Apply betadine ointment over the area affected
- ❍ **B.** Cover the burn with an occlusive dressing
- ❍ **C.** Flush the burned area with cool water
- ❍ **D.** Remove any adhered clothing that is on the burn area

Quick Answers: **318**
Detailed Answer: **322**

17. A client with suspected myasthenias gravis has been administered the drug edrophonium chloride (Tensilon). Which effect would the nurse expect the client to exhibit after administration?

- ❍ **A.** Decreased motor strength
- ❍ **B.** Decreased seizure activity
- ❍ **C.** Increased muscle strength
- ❍ **D.** Increased cognitive functioning

Quick Answers: **318**
Detailed Answer: **322**

18. A client is admitted with hypothyroidism. Which clinical manifestation would the nurse expect the client to exhibit?

- ❍ **A.** Diarrhea
- ❍ **B.** Intolerance to cold
- ❍ **C.** Hyperactivity
- ❍ **D.** Diaphoresis

Quick Answers: **318**
Detailed Answer: **322**

Quick Check

19. The nurse caring for a client with Alzheimer's disease should initiate which of the following when requesting an action by the client?

Quick Answers: **318**
Detailed Answer: **322**

- ❍ **A.** Provide a detailed explanation
- ❍ **B.** Give one direction at a time
- ❍ **C.** Offer two choices for each activity
- ❍ **D.** Provide all instructions at one time

20. A nurse would expect a newly diagnosed insulin-dependent diabetic to exhibit which clinical manifestations?

Quick Answers: **318**
Detailed Answer: **322**

- ❍ **A.** Decreased appetite and constipation
- ❍ **B.** Weight gain and headache
- ❍ **C.** Nausea and hand tremors
- ❍ **D.** Increased urination and thirst

21. Which medication is important to have available for clients who have received Versed?

Quick Answers: **318**
Detailed Answer: **322**

- ❍ **A.** Diazepam (Valium)
- ❍ **B.** Naloxone (Narcan)
- ❍ **C.** Flumazenil (Romazicon)
- ❍ **D.** Florinef (Fludrocortisone)

22. The nurse is caring for a client who is nauseated and in danger of aspiration. Which action would the nurse take first?

Quick Answers: **318**
Detailed Answer: **323**

- ❍ **A.** Administer an ordered antiemetic medication
- ❍ **B.** Obtain an ice bag and apply to the client's throat
- ❍ **C.** Turn the client to one side
- ❍ **D.** Notify the physician

23. What is the action of the nurse who assesses dehiscence of a clients' surgical wound?

Quick Answers: **318**
Detailed Answer: **323**

- ❍ **A.** Place the client in the prone position
- ❍ **B.** Apply a sterile saline-moistened dressing to the wound
- ❍ **C.** Administer atropine to decrease abdominal secretions
- ❍ **D.** Wrap the abdomen with an ACE bandage

Quick Check

24. A client with hepatitis C is about to undergo a liver biopsy. Which of the following would the nurse expect to reiterate to this client?

Quick Answers: **318**
Detailed Answer: **323**

❍ **A.** The client should lie on the left side after the procedure.

❍ **B.** The client will have cleansing enemas the morning of the procedure.

❍ **C.** Blood coagulation studies might be done before the biopsy.

❍ **D.** The procedure is noninvasive and causes no pain.

25. The nurse is caring for a client after a tracheostomy procedure. The client is anxious, with a respiratory rate of 32 and an oxygen saturation of 88. The nurse's first action should be to:

Quick Answers: **318**
Detailed Answer: **323**

❍ **A.** Suction the client

❍ **B.** Turn the client to the left Sim's position

❍ **C.** Notify the physician

❍ **D.** Recheck the O_2 saturation

26. The nurse has reinforced teaching to a client who is on isoniazid (INH). Which diet selection would let the nurse know that the teaching has been ineffective?

Quick Answers: **318**
Detailed Answer: **323**

❍ **A.** Tuna casserole

❍ **B.** Ham salad

❍ **C.** Baked potato

❍ **D.** Broiled beef roast

27. A nurse is working in a nursing home and evaluating temperatures that have been recorded by the nurse's assistant. A temperature of 100.4°F is noted. Which of these responses should the nurse take?

Quick Answers: **318**
Detailed Answer: **323**

❍ **A.** Record the temperature on the client's chart as the only action

❍ **B.** Retake the client's temperature in 30 minutes to assess for an increase

❍ **C.** Have the client drink a glass of water and retake the temperature

❍ **D.** Call the doctor immediately and report the client's temperature

Quick Check

28. A nurse is observing a student perform an assessment. When the student nurse asks the client to "stick out his tongue," the student is assessing the function of which of the following cranial nerves?

Quick Answers: **318**
Detailed Answer: **323**

- ❍ **A.** II optic
- ❍ **B.** I olfactory
- ❍ **C.** X vagus
- ❍ **D.** XII hypoglossal

29. Which set of vital signs would best indicate an increase in intracranial pressure in a client with a head injury?

Quick Answers: **318**
Detailed Answer: **323**

- ❍ **A.** BP 180/70, pulse 50, respirations 16, temperature 101°F
- ❍ **B.** BP 100/70, pulse 64, respirations 20, temperature 98.6°F
- ❍ **C.** BP 96/70, pulse 132, respirations 20, temperature 98.6°F
- ❍ **D.** BP 130/80, pulse 50, respirations 18, temperature 99.6°F

30. The nurse is assessing the laboratory results of a client scheduled to receive phenytoin (Dilantin). The Dilantin level, drawn 2 hours ago, is 30mcg/mL. What is the appropriate nursing action?

Quick Answers: **318**
Detailed Answer: **323**

- ❍ **A.** Administer the Dilantin as scheduled
- ❍ **B.** Hold the scheduled dose and notify the charge nurse
- ❍ **C.** Decrease the dosage of the Dilantin from 100mg to 50mg
- ❍ **D.** Increase the dosage to 200mg from 100mg

31. A client with sickle cell disease is admitted with pneumonia. Which nursing intervention would be most helpful to prevent a sickling crisis?

Quick Answers: **318**
Detailed Answer: **323**

- ❍ **A.** Obtaining blood pressures every 2 hours
- ❍ **B.** Administering pain medication every 3–4 hours as ordered
- ❍ **C.** Assessing breath sounds once a shift
- ❍ **D.** Monitoring IV fluids at ordered rate of 200mL/hr.

Quick Check

32. A client is admitted with a diagnosis of pernicious anemia. Which of the following signs or symptoms would indicate that the client has been noncompliant with ordered B12 injections?

Quick Answers: **318**
Detailed Answer: **324**

- ❍ **A.** Hyperactivity in the evening hours
- ❍ **B.** Weight gain of 5 pounds in 1 week
- ❍ **C.** Paresthesia of hands and feet
- ❍ **D.** Diarrhea stools several times a day

33. The nurse has given dietary instructions about food to be included in a low-purine diet. Which selection by the client with gout would indicate that teaching has been ineffective?

Quick Answers: **318**
Detailed Answer: **324**

- ❍ **A.** Cabbage
- ❍ **B.** An apple
- ❍ **C.** Peach cobbler
- ❍ **D.** Spinach

34. Which of these tasks would it be most appropriate to assign to a nursing assistant?

Quick Answers: **318**
Detailed Answer: **324**

- ❍ **A.** Obtaining vital signs on a client with chest pain
- ❍ **B.** Obtaining blood sugars on a newly admitted client with diabetes
- ❍ **C.** Feeding a newly admitted stroke client
- ❍ **D.** Assisting a client 2 days post-operative abdominal surgery

35. The orthopedic nurse should be particularly alert for a fat embolus in which of the following clients having the greatest risk for this complication after a fracture?

Quick Answers: **318**
Detailed Answer: **324**

- ❍ **A.** A 50-year-old with a fractured fibula
- ❍ **B.** A 20-year-old female with a wrist fracture
- ❍ **C.** A 21-year-old male with a fractured femur
- ❍ **D.** An 8-year-old with a fractured arm

36. The nurse is reinforcing teaching to a client with iron-deficiency anemia about a high-iron diet. The nurse recognizes that teaching has been effective when the client selects which meal plan?

Quick Answers: **318**
Detailed Answer: **324**

- ❍ **A.** Hamburger, French fries, orange juice
- ❍ **B.** Sliced veal, spinach salad, whole-wheat roll
- ❍ **C.** Vegetable lasagna, Caesar salad, toast
- ❍ **D.** Bacon, lettuce, and tomato sandwich; potato chips; tea

Quick Check

37. An elderly female is admitted with a fractured right femoral neck. Which clinical manifestation would the nurse expect to find?

Quick Answers: **318**
Detailed Answer: **324**

- ❍ **A.** Free movement of the right leg
- ❍ **B.** Abduction of the right leg
- ❍ **C.** Internal rotation of the right hip
- ❍ **D.** Shortening of the right leg

38. The nurse is observing a student perform the skill of intramuscular injection by the Z track method. Which technique would the student utilize to prevent tracking of the medication?

Quick Answers: **318**
Detailed Answer: **324**

- ❍ **A.** Inject the medication in the deltoid muscle when described by the patient
- ❍ **B.** Use a 22-gauge needle
- ❍ **C.** Omit aspirating for blood before injecting
- ❍ **D.** Draw up 0.2mL of air after the proper medication dose

39. Which action by the nurse would be most effective in relieving phantom limb pain on a client with an above-the-knee amputation?

Quick Answers: **318**
Detailed Answer: **324**

- ❍ **A.** Acknowledging the presence of the pain
- ❍ **B.** Elevating the stump on a pillow
- ❍ **C.** Applying ordered transcutaneous nerve stimulator (TENS) unit
- ❍ **D.** Rewrapping the stump

40. The nurse caring for a client with anemia recognizes which clinical manifestation as the one that is specific for a hemolytic type of anemia?

Quick Answers: **318**
Detailed Answer: **324**

- ❍ **A.** Jaundice
- ❍ **B.** Anorexia
- ❍ **C.** Tachycardia
- ❍ **D.** Fatigue

41. A client has been given the drug Neulasta (pegfilgastrin). Which laboratory value indicates that the drug is producing the desired effect?

Quick Answers: **318**
Detailed Answer: **324**

- ❍ **A.** Hemoglobin of 13.5g/dL
- ❍ **B.** White blood cell count of 6,000/mm
- ❍ **C.** Platelet count of 300,000/mm
- ❍ **D.** HCT 39%

Quick Check

42. The nurse is responding to questions from a client with polycythemia vera. Which would be included in the nurses explanations? The client should:

Quick Answers: **318**
Detailed Answer: **324**

- ❍ **A.** Avoid large crowds
- ❍ **B.** Keep the head of the bed elevated at night
- ❍ **C.** Wear socks and gloves when going outside
- ❍ **D.** Recognize clinical manifestations of thrombosis

43. The physician has ordered a minimal bacteria diet for a client with cancer. Which seasoning is not permitted for this client?

Quick Answers: **318**
Detailed Answer: **325**

- ❍ **A.** Salt
- ❍ **B.** Lemon juice
- ❍ **C.** Pepper
- ❍ **D.** Ketchup

44. The nurse is caring for a client with a hip fracture who is being discharged with a prescription for alendronate (Fosamax). Which statement would indicate a need for further teaching?

Quick Answers: **318**
Detailed Answer: **325**

- ❍ **A.** "I should take the medication immediately before bedtime."
- ❍ **B.** "I should remain in an upright position for 30 minutes after taking the medication."
- ❍ **C.** "The medication should be taken by mouth with water."
- ❍ **D.** "I should not have any food intake with this medication."

45. Acetaminophen (Tylenol) 240mg is ordered for an infant who weighs 12 pounds. The usual dose for an infant is 10–15mg per kilogram of body weight. A nurse should take which action?

Quick Answers: **318**
Detailed Answer: **325**

- ❍ **A.** Give the medication as ordered
- ❍ **B.** Administer two-thirds of the prescribed dose
- ❍ **C.** Weigh the infant without clothes
- ❍ **D.** Discuss the order with the physician

Quick Check

46. The nurse is caring for a client recovering from a bone fracture. Which diet selection would be best for this client?

Quick Answers: 318
Detailed Answer: 325

- ❍ **A.** Loaded baked potato, fried chicken, and tea
- ❍ **B.** Dressed cheeseburger, French fries, and Coke
- ❍ **C.** Tuna fish salad on sourdough bread, potato chips, and skim milk
- ❍ **D.** Mandarin orange salad, broiled chicken, and milk

47. The nurse recognizes that it would be contraindicated to induce vomiting if someone had ingested which of the following?

Quick Answers: 318
Detailed Answer: 325

- ❍ **A.** Ibuprofen
- ❍ **B.** Aspirin
- ❍ **C.** Vitamins
- ❍ **D.** Gasoline

48. A client with ulcerative colitis has impaired nutrition due to diarrhea. Which diet selection by the client would indicate a need for further teaching about foods that can worsen the diarrhea?

Quick Answers: 318
Detailed Answer: 325

- ❍ **A.** Tossed salad
- ❍ **B.** Baked chicken
- ❍ **C.** Broiled fish
- ❍ **D.** Steamed rice

49. The nurse has just received report from the RN. Which of the following clients should the nurse visit first?

Quick Answers: 318
Detailed Answer: 325

- ❍ **A.** A 50-year-old COPD client with a PCO_2 of 50
- ❍ **B.** A 24-year-old admitted after an MVA complaining of shortness of breath
- ❍ **C.** A client with cancer requesting pain medication
- ❍ **D.** A 1-day post-operative cholecystectomy with a temperature of 100°F

50. The nurse is performing a self-breast exam when she discovers a mass. Which characteristic of the mass would be most indicative of a malignancy?

Quick Answers: 318
Detailed Answer: 325

- ❍ **A.** Tender to touch
- ❍ **B.** Regular shape
- ❍ **C.** Moves easily
- ❍ **D.** Firm to the touch

Quick Check

51. The nurse is caring for a client after a motor vehicle accident. The client has a fractured tibia, and bone is noted protruding through the skin. Which action would be the highest priority?

Quick Answers: **318**
Detailed Answer: **325**

- ❍ **A.** Provide manual traction above and below the leg
- ❍ **B.** Cover the bone area with a sterile dressing
- ❍ **C.** Apply an ACE bandage around the entire lower limb
- ❍ **D.** Place the client in the prone position

52. A child is to receive heparin sodium 5 units per kilogram of body weight by subcutaneous route every 4 hours. The child weighs 52.8 lb. How many units should the child receive in a 24-hour period?

Quick Answers: **318**
Detailed Answer: **325**

- ❍ **A.** 300
- ❍ **B.** 480
- ❍ **C.** 720
- ❍ **D.** 960

53. Which comment made by a client with congestive heart failure should cause a need for nursing follow-up?

Quick Answers: **318**
Detailed Answer: **325**

- ❍ **A.** "My heart rate has been between 60 and 70 the past week."
- ❍ **B.** "My oral temperature was 98°F yesterday."
- ❍ **C.** "I have been urinating every 4 hours for the past 2 days."
- ❍ **D.** "I have gained 3 pounds since yesterday."

54. The nurse caring for a client diagnosed with bone cancer is exhibiting mental confusion and a BP of 150/100. Which laboratory value would correlate with the client's symptoms reflecting a common complication with this diagnosis?

Quick Answers: **318**
Detailed Answer: **326**

- ❍ **A.** Potassium 5.2mEq/L
- ❍ **B.** Calcium 13mg/dL
- ❍ **C.** Inorganic phosphorus 1.7mEq/L
- ❍ **D.** Sodium 138mEq/L

Quick Check

55. The nurse is discussing pain from cholecystitis with a client. Which statement made by the client most accurately describes the typical pain of this disorder?

Quick Answers: **318**
Detailed Answer: **326**

❍ **A.** "The pain is usually below my sternum."
❍ **B.** "Eating food makes the pain better."
❍ **C.** "The pain gets worse after I eat fatty foods."
❍ **D.** "The pain is usually related to constipation."

56. The nurse is preparing a client for cervical uterine radiation implant insertion. Which will be included in the nurse's explanations?

Quick Answers: **318**
Detailed Answer: **326**

❍ **A.** TV or telephone use will not be allowed while the implant is in place.
❍ **B.** A Foley catheter is usually inserted.
❍ **C.** A high-fiber diet is recommended.
❍ **D.** Excretions will be considered radioactive.

57. A client with end stage cirrhosis can sometimes develop mental changes. What is the most likely cause?

Quick Answers: **318**
Detailed Answer: **326**

❍ **A.** Elevated blood ammonia
❍ **B.** Decreased serum proteins
❍ **C.** Leukocytosis
❍ **D.** Hyperglycemia

58. The nurse is caring for a client after a liver biopsy. The nurse should carefully monitor the client for the development of which of the following?

Quick Answers: **318**
Detailed Answer: **326**

❍ **A.** Respiratory alkalosis
❍ **B.** Metabolic acidosis
❍ **C.** Pneumothorax
❍ **D.** Cardiac tamponade

59. The LPN/LVN is assisting a client immediately after a paracentesis. Which of the following actions is the priority?

Quick Answers: **318**
Detailed Answer: **326**

❍ **A.** Obtaining vital signs
❍ **B.** Positioning the client for comfort
❍ **C.** Detailed documentation of the procedure
❍ **D.** Reporting the amount removed to the client

Quick Check

60. A client has received platelet infusions. Which finding would indicate the most therapeutic effect from the transfusions?

- ❍ **A.** Hgb level increase from 8.9 to 10.6
- ❍ **B.** Temperature reading of 99.4°F
- ❍ **C.** White blood cell count of 11,000
- ❍ **D.** Decrease in oozing of blood from IV site

Quick Answers: **318**
Detailed Answer: **326**

61. A client is admitted with Parkinson's disease. The client has been taking Carbidopa/levodopa (Sinemet) for 1 year. Which clinical manifestation would be most important to report?

- ❍ **A.** Dryness of the mouth
- ❍ **B.** Spasmodic eye winking
- ❍ **C.** Dark urine
- ❍ **D.** Dizziness

Quick Answers: **318**
Detailed Answer: **326**

62. The nurse who is caring for a client with cancer notes a WBC of 1,000. Which intervention would be most appropriate to include when caring for this client?

- ❍ **A.** Assess temperature every 4 hours, due to risk for hypothermia
- ❍ **B.** Instruct the client to avoid large crowds and people who are sick
- ❍ **C.** Instruct in the use of a soft toothbrush
- ❍ **D.** Assess for hematuria

Quick Answers: **318**
Detailed Answer: **326**

63. A client has a subtotal thyroidectomy. The nurse is observed requesting that the client state her name frequently. The primary reason for this assessment is to monitor for which of the following?

- ❍ **A.** Laryngeal nerve damage
- ❍ **B.** Hemorrhage
- ❍ **C.** Lower airway obstruction
- ❍ **D.** Tetany

Quick Answers: **318**
Detailed Answer: **326**

64. The nurse is caring for a client with cancer of the cervix. What clinical data would the nurse expect to find in the client's history?

- ❍ **A.** Post-coital vaginal bleeding
- ❍ **B.** Nausea and vomiting
- ❍ **C.** Foul-smelling vaginal discharge
- ❍ **D.** Hyperthermia

Quick Answers: **318**
Detailed Answer: **326**

Quick Check

65. The nurse is caring for a client with hyperthyroidism. Which clinical manifestation should be reported to the physician immediately?

Quick Answers: **318**
Detailed Answer: **327**

❍ **A.** Urinary retention

❍ **B.** Heart failure

❍ **C.** Drowsiness

❍ **D.** Sedation

66. A client with suspected leukemia is about to undergo a bone marrow aspiration from the sternum. What position would the nurse assist the client into for this procedure?

Quick Answers: **318**
Detailed Answer: **327**

❍ **A.** Dorsal recumbent

❍ **B.** Supine

❍ **C.** Fowler's

❍ **D.** Lithotomy

67. The nurse is caring for a client with a head injury who has increased ICP. The physician plans to reduce the cerebral edema by constricting the cerebral blood vessels. Which of the following would accomplish this action?

Quick Answers: **318**
Detailed Answer: **327**

❍ **A.** Hyperventilation per mechanical ventilation

❍ **B.** Insertion of a ventricular shunt

❍ **C.** Furosemide (Lasix)

❍ **D.** Dexamethasone (Decadron)

68. A client with a T6 injury 6 months ago develops facial flushing and a BP of 210/106. After elevating the head of the bed, which is the most appropriate nursing action?

Quick Answers: **318**
Detailed Answer: **327**

❍ **A.** Notify the physician

❍ **B.** Assess the client for a distended bladder

❍ **C.** Apply oxygen at 3L/min

❍ **D.** Administer Procardia sublinqually

69. The nurse is reading an admission history for a client recovering from a stroke. Medication history reveals the drug clopidogrel (Plavix). Which clinical manifestation alerts the nurse to an adverse effect of this drug?

Quick Answers: **318**
Detailed Answer: **327**

❍ **A.** Epistaxis

❍ **B.** Abdominal distention

❍ **C.** Nausea

❍ **D.** Hyperactivity

Quick Check

70. The nurse caring for a client with a head injury would recognize which assessment finding as the most indicative of increased ICP?

- ❍ **A.** Nausea and vomiting
- ❍ **B.** Headache
- ❍ **C.** Dizziness
- ❍ **D.** Papilledema

Quick Answers: **318**
Detailed Answer: **327**

71. A client with Prinzmetal angina is experiencing migraine headaches. The physician has prescribed Sumatriptan succinate (Imitrex). Which nursing action is most appropriate?

- ❍ **A.** Notify the charge nurse to question the prescription order.
- ❍ **B.** Try to obtain samples for the client to take home.
- ❍ **C.** Reinforce teaching regarding this drug.
- ❍ **D.** Consult with social services about financial assistance with obtaining the drug.

Quick Answers: **318**
Detailed Answer: **327**

72. A client with COPD is in respiratory failure. Which of the following results would be the most sensitive indicator that the client will probably be placed on a mechanical ventilator?

- ❍ **A.** PCO_2 58
- ❍ **B.** SaO_2 90
- ❍ **C.** pH 7.23
- ❍ **D.** HCO_3 30

Quick Answers: **318**
Detailed Answer: **327**

73. The nurse is caring for a client with multiple rib fractures and a pulmonary contusion. Assessment findings include a respiratory rate of 40, a heart rate of 126, and restlessness. Which associated assessment finding would require immediate intervention?

- ❍ **A.** Occasional hemoptysis
- ❍ **B.** Midline trachea with wheezing on auscultation
- ❍ **C.** Subcutaneous air and absent breath sounds
- ❍ **D.** Pain while deep breathing, with rales in the upper lobes

Quick Answers: **318**
Detailed Answer: **327**

74. The nurse is caring for a client with myasthenias gravis who is having trouble breathing. Which position would assist the client to breathe best?

- ❍ **A.** Supine with no pillow, to maintain patent airway
- ❍ **B.** Side lying with back support
- ❍ **C.** Prone with head turned to one side
- ❍ **D.** Sitting or in high Fowler's

Quick Answers: **318**
Detailed Answer: **327**

Quick Check

75. The nurse has received a report from the RN on several clients with respiratory problems. Upon receiving the following client reports, which client should be seen first?

Quick Answers: 318
Detailed Answer: 327

❍ **A.** Client with emphysema expecting discharge
❍ **B.** Bronchitis client receiving IV antibiotics
❍ **C.** Bronchitis client with edema and neck vein distention
❍ **D.** COPD client with PO_2 of 85

76. A client has sustained damage to the preoccipital lobe. The nurse should remain particularly alert for which of the following problems?

Quick Answers: 318
Detailed Answer: 328

❍ **A.** Visual impairment
❍ **B.** Swallowing difficulty
❍ **C.** Impaired judgment
❍ **D.** Hearing impairment

77. Which clinical manifestation would the nurse expect if a client was experiencing right-sided congestive heart failure?

Quick Answers: 318
Detailed Answer: 328

❍ **A.** Jugular vein distention
❍ **B.** Dry, nonproductive cough
❍ **C.** Orthopnea
❍ **D.** Crackles on chest auscultation

78. A client with a subdural hematoma is receiving Mannitol and Lasix. The nurse recognizes that these two drugs are given to reverse which effect?

Quick Answers: 318
Detailed Answer: 328

❍ **A.** Energy failure
❍ **B.** Excessive intracellular calcium accumulation
❍ **C.** Cerebral edema
❍ **D.** Excessive glutamate release

79. The nurse is assessing a client after a car accident. Partial airway obstruction is suspected. Which clinical manifestation is a late sign of airway obstruction?

Quick Answers: 318
Detailed Answer: 328

❍ **A.** Rales auscultated in breath sounds
❍ **B.** Restlessness
❍ **C.** Cyanotic ear lobes
❍ **D.** Inspiratory stridor

Quick Check

80. What is the primary reason for a client with COPD to avoid smoking?

Quick Answers: **318**
Detailed Answer: **328**

- ❍ **A.** It affects peripheral blood vessels.
- ❍ **B.** It causes vasoconstriction.
- ❍ **C.** It destroys the lung parenchyma.
- ❍ **D.** It paralyzes ciliary activity.

81. A client receiving a magnetic resonance imaging procedure should have which of the following implemented?

Quick Answers: **318**
Detailed Answer: **328**

- ❍ **A.** Informed consent and atropine 0.4mg
- ❍ **B.** Injection site scrub for 15 minutes
- ❍ **C.** Removal of any jewelry and inquiry regarding metal implants
- ❍ **D.** Administration of diphenhydramine (Benadryl) 50mg by mouth

82. The LPN/LVN is caring for a client with a diagnosis of diabetes insipidus. Which of the following clinical manifestations is expected?

Quick Answers: **318**
Detailed Answer: **328**

- ❍ **A.** Polyuria
- ❍ **B.** Nose bleed
- ❍ **C.** Clot formation
- ❍ **D.** Oliguria

83. The nurse is caring for a client with an acoustic neuroma brain tumor. The location of this tumor warrants particular concern for which of the following?

Quick Answers: **318**
Detailed Answer: **328**

- ❍ **A.** Constipation
- ❍ **B.** Fluid volume
- ❍ **C.** Individual coping
- ❍ **D.** Injury from falls

84. The client is admitted with a chest injury. The nurse's assessment reveals that an area over the right clavicle is puffy and that there is a "crackling" noise with palpation. The nurse should further assess the client for which of the following problems?

Quick Answers: **318**
Detailed Answer: **328**

- ❍ **A.** Flail chest
- ❍ **B.** Subcutaneous emphysema
- ❍ **C.** Infiltrated subclavian IV
- ❍ **D.** Pneumothorax

Quick Check

85. The influenza vaccine cannot be given to clients in which age group?

Quick Answers: **318**
Detailed Answer: **328**

- ❍ **A.** Less than 6 months of age
- ❍ **B.** 6–23 months
- ❍ **C.** 18- to 35-year-olds
- ❍ **D.** Those over age 50

86. The nurse recognizes that Nimotop (Nimodipine) is given to clients with aneurysms for which of the following reasons?

Quick Answers: **318**
Detailed Answer: **328**

- ❍ **A.** Prevent the influx of calcium into cells
- ❍ **B.** Restore the client's blood pressure to a normal reading
- ❍ **C.** Prevent the inflammatory process
- ❍ **D.** Dissolve the clot that has formed

87. A client with seizures has jerking of the right arm and twitching of the face, but remains alert and aware of the seizure. This behavior is characteristic of which type of seizure?

Quick Answers: **318**
Detailed Answer: **329**

- ❍ **A.** Absence
- ❍ **B.** Complex partial
- ❍ **C.** Simple partial
- ❍ **D.** Tonic-clonic

88. It is essential that the nurse have which piece of equipment at the bedside of a client on a ventilator?

Quick Answers: **319**
Detailed Answer: **329**

- ❍ **A.** Cardiac monitor
- ❍ **B.** Intravenous controller
- ❍ **C.** Manual resuscitator
- ❍ **D.** Oxygen by nasal cannula

89. A client has returned to the surgical unit after a laryngectomy. When suctioning the tracheostomy, the nurse should not allow the suction pressure to exceed which level?

Quick Answers: **319**
Detailed Answer: **329**

- ❍ **A.** 120mmHg
- ❍ **B.** 145mmHg
- ❍ **C.** 160mmHg
- ❍ **D.** 185mmHg

Quick Check

90. The nurse has given instructions on pursed lip breathing to a client with emphysema. Which statement by the client would indicate effective teaching?

Quick Answers: **319**
Detailed Answer: **329**

❍ **A.** "I should inhale through the mouth."

❍ **B.** "I should tighten my abdominal muscles with inhalation."

❍ **C.** "I should contract my abdominal muscles with exhalation."

❍ **D.** "I should make inhalation twice as long as exhalation."

91. A client is receiving Theodur. The nurse monitors the theophylline blood level and assesses that the level is within therapeutic range when it is at what level?

Quick Answers: **319**
Detailed Answer: **329**

❍ **A.** 5ug/mL

❍ **B.** 8ug/mL

❍ **C.** 15ug/mL

❍ **D.** 25ug/mL

92. A client diagnosed with emphysema is going to the clinic for assistance with smoking cessation. Which drug would the nurse expect to be included in the treatment plan?

Quick Answers: **319**
Detailed Answer: **329**

❍ **A.** Bupropion SR (Zyban)

❍ **B.** Metoproterenol (Alupent)

❍ **C.** Oxitropuim (Oxivent)

❍ **D.** Alprazolam (Xanax)

93. A pneumonectomy is performed on a client with lung cancer. Which of the following would not be an expected prescription?

Quick Answers: **319**
Detailed Answer: **329**

❍ **A.** Closed-chest drainage

❍ **B.** Pain-control measures

❍ **C.** Supplemental oxygen

❍ **D.** Coughing and deep-breathing exercises

94. When planning the care for a client after a posterior fossa (infratentorial) craniotomy, which would be contraindicated?

Quick Answers: **319**
Detailed Answer: **329**

❍ **A.** Keeping the client's head flat

❍ **B.** Elevating the head of the bed 30°

❍ **C.** Log-rolling or turning as a unit

❍ **D.** Keeping the neck in a neutral position

Quick Check

95. The nurse is explaining a low-residue diet to a client with ulcerative colitis. Which food would need to be eliminated from this client's diet?

Quick Answers: **319**
Detailed Answer: **329**

❍ **A.** Roasted chicken

❍ **B.** Noodles

❍ **C.** Cooked broccoli

❍ **D.** Roast beef

96. The nurse is reinforcing teaching of a client with diverticulitis about appropriate foods. Which food would be avoided?

Quick Answers: **319**
Detailed Answer: **329**

❍ **A.** Bran

❍ **B.** Fresh peach

❍ **C.** Cucumber salad

❍ **D.** Dinner roll

97. A client is admitted with possible paralytic illeus. Which question during the nursing history is least helpful in obtaining information regarding this diagnosis?

Quick Answers: **319**
Detailed Answer: **329**

❍ **A.** "Tell me about your pain."

❍ **B.** "What does your vomit look like?"

❍ **C.** "Describe your usual diet."

❍ **D.** "Have you noticed an increase in abdominal size?"

98. A client is being treated with carbamazepine (Tegretol). Which laboratory value might indicate a side effect of this drug?

Quick Answers: **319**
Detailed Answer: **329**

❍ **A.** BUN 10mg/dL

❍ **B.** Hemoglobin 13.0gm/dL

❍ **C.** WBC 4,000/mm^3

❍ **D.** Platelets 200,000/mm^3

99. A client has received damage to the parietal lobe. Which symptom would be expected due to this tumor's location?

Quick Answers: **319**
Detailed Answer: **330**

❍ **A.** Hemiplegia

❍ **B.** Aphasia

❍ **C.** Paresthesia

❍ **D.** Nausea

Quick Check

100. A client weighing 120 pounds has received burns over 40% of his body at 1200 hours. Using the Parkland formula, calculate the expected amount of fluid that the client should receive by 2000 hours as fluid-replacement therapy?

Quick Answers: **319**
Detailed Answer: **330**

- ❍ **A.** 2160
- ❍ **B.** 4320
- ❍ **C.** 6480
- ❍ **D.** 8640

101. Which post-operative assessment finding on a client with a femoral popliteal graft of the right leg would require immediate charge nurse notification?

Quick Answers: **319**
Detailed Answer: **330**

- ❍ **A.** Edema of the right extremity and pain at the incision site
- ❍ **B.** A temperature of 99.6°F and redness of the incision
- ❍ **C.** Serous drainage noted at the surgical area
- ❍ **D.** A loss of posterior tibial and dorsalis pedis pulses on the right leg

102. The nurse is caring for a client with nausea and vomiting. Laboratory results reveal a potassium level of 2.9mEq. Which ECG finding would the nurse expect to find due to the client's potassium results?

Quick Answers: **319**
Detailed Answer: **330**

- ❍ **A.** Depressed ST segments
- ❍ **B.** Elevated T waves
- ❍ **C.** Absent P waves
- ❍ **D.** Flattened QRSs

103. The nurse is preparing a patient for surgery on the lower abdomen. Which position would the nurse most likely place the client in for surgery on this area?

Quick Answers: **319**
Detailed Answer: **330**

- ❍ **A.** Lithotomy
- ❍ **B.** Sims
- ❍ **C.** Prone
- ❍ **D.** Trendelenburg

Quick Check

104. The physician has prescribed a cleansing enema to a client scheduled for colon surgery. The nurse would place the client:

Quick Answers: **319**
Detailed Answer: **330**

❍ **A.** Prone
❍ **B.** Supine
❍ **C.** Left Sims
❍ **D.** Dorsal recumbent

105. The nurse is caring for a client with chest trauma. Which finding would be most indicative of a tension pneumothorax?

Quick Answers: **319**
Detailed Answer: **330**

❍ **A.** Frothy hemoptysis
❍ **B.** Trachea shift toward unaffected side of the chest
❍ **C.** Subcutaneous emphysema noted anterior chest
❍ **D.** Opening chest wound with a whistle sound emitting from the area

106. The nurse is reviewing a history on a new admission for surgery in the morning. Which long-term medication in the client's history would be most important to report to the physician?

Quick Answers: **319**
Detailed Answer: **330**

❍ **A.** Prednisone
❍ **B.** Lisinopril (Zestril)
❍ **C.** Docusate (Colace)
❍ **D.** Calcium carbonate (Oscal D)

107. The nurse is explaining about the drug zafirlukast (Accolate) to a client with asthma. Which comment by the client would indicate ineffective teaching?

Quick Answers: **319**
Detailed Answer: **330**

❍ **A.** "I should take this medication with meals."
❍ **B.** "I need to report flulike symptoms to my doctor."
❍ **C.** "My doctor might order liver tests while I'm on this drug."
❍ **D.** "If I'm already having an asthma attack, this drug will not stop it."

108. A client is 4 hours post-operative left brain cerebral aneurysm clipping. Which assessment finding would cause the nurse the most concern?

Quick Answers: **319**
Detailed Answer: **331**

❍ **A.** Temperature 99.4°F, heart rate 110, respiratory rate 24
❍ **B.** Drowsiness, urinary output of 50mL in the past hour, 1cm blood drainage noted on surgical dressing
❍ **C.** BP 120/60, lethargic, right-sided weakness
❍ **D.** Alert and oriented, BP 168/96, heart rate 70

Quick Check

109. A client with pancreatic cancer has just been given a negative prognosis by the oncologist. The nurse hears the client state, "I don't believe the doctor, and I think he has me confused with another patient." This is an example of which of Kubler-Ross' stages of dying?

Quick Answers: **319**
Detailed Answer: **331**

❍ **A.** Denial

❍ **B.** Anger

❍ **C.** Depression

❍ **D.** Bargaining

110. The nurse is discussing staff assignments. Which client assignment should be given to the nurse's assistant?

Quick Answers: **319**
Detailed Answer: **331**

❍ **A.** Emergency exploratory laparotomy with a colon resection the previous shift

❍ **B.** Client with a stroke scheduled for discharge to rehabilitation

❍ **C.** A client with terminal cancer in severe pain

❍ **D.** New admission with diverticulitis

111. A client is being discharged on Coumadin after hospitalization for atrial fibrillation. The nurse recognizes that which of the following foods would be restricted while the client is on this medication?

Quick Answers: **319**
Detailed Answer: **331**

❍ **A.** Cabbage

❍ **B.** Apples

❍ **C.** Potatoes

❍ **D.** Macaroni

112. Which assessment finding in a client with emphysema indicates to the nurse that the respiratory problem is chronic?

Quick Answers: **319**
Detailed Answer: **331**

❍ **A.** Wheezing on exhalation

❍ **B.** Productive cough

❍ **C.** Clubbing of fingers

❍ **D.** Cyanosis

113. A client who has just undergone a laparoscopic tubal ligation complains of "free air pain." What would be the nurse's best action?

Quick Answers: **319**
Detailed Answer: **331**

❍ **A.** Ambulate the client

❍ **B.** Instruct the client to breathe deeply and cough

❍ **C.** Maintain the client on bed rest with her legs elevated

❍ **D.** Insert an NG tube to low wall suction

Quick Check

114. The nurse is planning shift duties. Which is the least appropriate task for the nursing assistant?

Quick Answers: **319**
Detailed Answer: **331**

- ❍ **A.** Assisting a COPD client admitted 2 days ago to get up in the chair
- ❍ **B.** Feeding a client with bronchitis who has an old paralysis on the right side
- ❍ **C.** Accompanying a discharged emphysema client to the transportation area
- ❍ **D.** Assessing an emphysema client complaining of difficulty breathing

115. Which nursing order would the nurse anticipate for a client with pancreatitis?

Quick Answers: **319**
Detailed Answer: **331**

- ❍ **A.** Force fluids to 3,000mL/24 hours
- ❍ **B.** Insert a nasogastric tube and connect it to low intermittent suction
- ❍ **C.** Place the client in reverse Trendelenburg position
- ❍ **D.** Place the client in enteric isolation

116. Assessment findings for the client admitted with a stroke reveal an absence of the gag reflex. The nurse suspects injury to which cranial nerve?

Quick Answers: **319**
Detailed Answer: **331**

- ❍ **A.** XII (hypoglossal)
- ❍ **B.** X (vagus)
- ❍ **C.** IX (glossopharyngeal)
- ❍ **D.** VII (facial)

117. The nurse arrives at a four-wheeler accident finding the client nonresponsive, apneic, and pulseless. After calling for a spectator to help, what would be the nurse's next action?

Quick Answers: **319**
Detailed Answer: **331**

- ❍ **A.** Ventilate with a mouth-to-mask device
- ❍ **B.** Begin chest compressions
- ❍ **C.** Administer a precordial thump
- ❍ **D.** Open the airway

Quick Check

118. A client with gallstones and obstructive jaundice is experiencing severe itching. The physician has prescribed cholestyramine (Questran). The client asks, "How does this drug work?" What is the nurse's best response?

Quick Answers: **319**
Detailed Answer: **332**

❍ **A.** "It blocks histamine, reducing the allergic response."
❍ **B.** "It inhibits the enzyme responsible for bile excretion."
❍ **C.** "It decreases the amount of bile in the gallbladder."
❍ **D.** "It binds with bile acids and is excreted in bowel movements with stool."

119. A client with ulcerative colitis requires an illeostomy. The nurse would instruct the client to do which of the following measures as an essential part of caring for the stoma?

Quick Answers: **319**
Detailed Answer: **332**

❍ **A.** Perform massage of the stoma three times a day
❍ **B.** Include high-fiber foods, especially nuts, in the diet
❍ **C.** Limit fluid intake to prevent loose stools
❍ **D.** Cleanse the peristomal skin meticulously

120. Diphenoxylate hydrochloride and atropine sulfate (Lomotil) is prescribed for the client with ulcerative colitis. The nurse realizes that the medication is having a therapeutic effect when which of the following is noted?

Quick Answers: **319**
Detailed Answer: **332**

❍ **A.** There is an absence of peristalasis.
❍ **B.** The number of diarrhea stools decreases.
❍ **C.** Cramping in the abdomen has increased.
❍ **D.** Abdominal girth size increases.

121. The physician is about to remove a chest tube. Which client instruction is appropriate?

Quick Answers: **319**
Detailed Answer: **332**

❍ **A.** Take a deep breath, exhale, and bear down
❍ **B.** Hold the breath for 2 minutes and exhale slowly
❍ **C.** Exhale upon actual removal of the tube
❍ **D.** Continually breath deeply in and out during removal

122. A client with severe anxiety has been prescribed haloperidol (Haldol). What clinical manifestation suggests that the client is experiencing side effects from this medication?

Quick Answers: **319**
Detailed Answer: **332**

❍ **A.** Cough
❍ **B.** Tremors
❍ **C.** Diarrhea
❍ **D.** Pitting edema

Quick Check

123. A client with a femur fracture is exhibiting shortness of breath, pain upon deep breathing, and a cough that produces blood-tinged sputum. The nurse would determine that these clinical manifestations are indicative of which of the following?

Quick Answers: **319**
Detailed Answer: **332**

❍ **A.** Congestive heart failure

❍ **B.** Pulmonary embolus

❍ **C.** Adult respiratory distress syndrome

❍ **D.** Tension pneumothorax

124. A client with Alzheimer's disease has been prescribed donepezil (Aricept). Which information should the nurse include when explaining about Aricept?

Quick Answers: **319**
Detailed Answer: **332**

❍ **A.** "Take the medication with meals."

❍ **B.** "The medicine can cause dizziness, so rise slowly."

❍ **C.** "If a dose is skipped, take two the next time."

❍ **D.** "The pill can cause an increase in heart rate."

125. A client who had an abdominal aortic aneurysm repair is having delayed healing of the wound. Which laboratory test result would most closely correlate to this problem?

Quick Answers: **319**
Detailed Answer: **332**

❍ **A.** Decreased albumin

❍ **B.** Decreased creatinine

❍ **C.** Increased calcium

❍ **D.** Increased sodium

126. A client with diagnosed diabetes visits the clinic complaining of shakiness and tingling sensations. Which of the following questions is most important for the LPN/LVN to ask?

Quick Answers: **319**
Detailed Answer: **332**

❍ **A.** When did you last eat?

❍ **B.** Did you bring your medication with you?

❍ **C.** What was your blood glucose and when was it checked?

❍ **D.** Is there anyone available to drive you home today?

127. Which exam is most reliable in diagnosing peptic ulcer disease?

Quick Answers: **319**
Detailed Answer: **332**

❍ **A.** Upper-gastrointestinal x-ray

❍ **B.** Gastric analysis

❍ **C.** Endoscopy

❍ **D.** Barium studies

Quick Check

128. A client recovering from a thyroidectomy tells the nurse, "I feel numbness and my face is twitching." What is the nurse's best initial action?

Quick Answers: **319**
Detailed Answer: **332**

- ❍ **A.** Offer mouth care
- ❍ **B.** Loosen the neck dressing
- ❍ **C.** Notify the physician
- ❍ **D.** Document the finding as the only action

129. A client is to undergo insertion of an esophageal gastric balloon tube. Which instruction would the nurse include in teaching about the purpose of the device?

Quick Answers: **319**
Detailed Answer: **333**

- ❍ **A.** "The device applies pressure to the veins in the esophagus and stomach."
- ❍ **B.** "It is used to prevent the accumulation of ascites."
- ❍ **C.** "It will prevent bleeding of arteries in the esophagus."
- ❍ **D.** "The doctor will use the tube to inject sclerosing solution into esophageal varices."

130. A client is admitted to the chemical dependency unit for evaluation of alcoholism. Which question is part of an alcoholism-assessment tool called the CAGE questionnaire?

Quick Answers: **319**
Detailed Answer: **333**

- ❍ **A.** How often do you have a drink containing alcohol?
- ❍ **B.** Have people annoyed you by criticizing your drinking?
- ❍ **C.** Have you or someone else ever been injured as a result of your drinking?
- ❍ **D.** How many drinks containing alcohol do you have on a typical day when you are drinking?

131. A client has an order to remove the nasogastric tube. Which is the correct nursing action to remove the tube?

Quick Answers: **319**
Detailed Answer: **333**

- ❍ **A.** Apply sterile gloves and untape the tube from the client's face
- ❍ **B.** Pull the tube out 2 inches, pause for 2 minutes, and repeat until the entire tube is removed
- ❍ **C.** Instill 30mL of normal saline before removing the tube
- ❍ **D.** Pull the tube out steadily and smoothly while keeping it pinched

Quick Check

132. The nurse is preparing a client with cirrhosis for a paracentesis. How will the nurse position the client for this procedure?

Quick Answers: 319
Detailed Answer: 333

- ❍ **A.** Trendelenburg
- ❍ **B.** Lying on the right side
- ❍ **C.** Lying on the left side
- ❍ **D.** Sitting position

133. A client has a vagal nerve stimulator in place to prevent seizures. Which would indicate that the device is working properly?

Quick Answers: 319
Detailed Answer: 333

- ❍ **A.** The client's voice changes when operating.
- ❍ **B.** Hiccups occur with each stimulation.
- ❍ **C.** The client can feel vibrations in the area of the vagal nerve stimulator when operational.
- ❍ **D.** The client's radial pulse obliterates when the stimulator is activated.

134. The nurse working on a surgical unit would identify which client as having the highest risk for pulmonary complications after surgery?

Quick Answers: 319
Detailed Answer: 333

- ❍ **A.** A 24-year-old with open reduction internal fixation of the ulnar
- ❍ **B.** A 45-year-old with an open cholecystectomy
- ❍ **C.** A 36-year-old after a hysterectomy
- ❍ **D.** A 50-year-old after a lumbar laminectomy

135. A client arrives after a house fire. What clinical manifestation is most indicative of possible carbon monoxide poisoning?

Quick Answers: 319
Detailed Answer: 333

- ❍ **A.** Pulse oximetry reading of 80%
- ❍ **B.** Expiratory stridor and nasal flaring
- ❍ **C.** Cherry-red color to the mucous membranes
- ❍ **D.** Presence of carbonaceous particles in the sputum

136. A client is admitted after a motor vehicle accident. The nurse suspects that the client is in the compensatory stage of shock due to which clinical manifestations?

Quick Answers: 319
Detailed Answer: 333

- ❍ **A.** Blood pressure 120/70, confusion, heart rate 120
- ❍ **B.** Crackles on chest auscultation, mottled skin, lethargy
- ❍ **C.** Skin color jaundice, urine output less than 30mL the past hour, heart rate 170
- ❍ **D.** Rapid, shallow respirations; unconscious; petechiae anterior chest

Quick Check

137. Which medication should the nurse have available in case a client has an anaphylactic reaction to penicillin G benzathine (Bicillin)?

Quick Answers: **319**
Detailed Answer: **333**

- ❍ **A.** Epinephrine
- ❍ **B.** Diazepam (Valium)
- ❍ **C.** Sodium bicarbonate
- ❍ **D.** Phentolamine mesylate (Regitine)

138. A client is admitted with benign prostatic hypertrophy. Which clinical manifestation should the nurse expect?

Quick Answers: **319**
Detailed Answer: **334**

- ❍ **A.** Frequent urge to void
- ❍ **B.** Foul-smelling urine
- ❍ **C.** Copious urine output
- ❍ **D.** Pain on urination

139. Which clinical manifestation during a bone marrow transplant alerts the nurse to the possibility of an adverse reaction?

Quick Answers: **319**
Detailed Answer: **334**

- ❍ **A.** Fever
- ❍ **B.** Red urine
- ❍ **C.** Hypertension
- ❍ **D.** Shortness of breath

140. Which area in dark-skinned individuals would be the most likely to show a skin cancerous lesion?

Quick Answers: **319**
Detailed Answer: **334**

- ❍ **A.** Chest
- ❍ **B.** Arms
- ❍ **C.** Face
- ❍ **D.** Palms

141. A client with a gastrointestinal bleed has an NG tube to low continuous wall suction. To assess bowel sounds, the nurse should perform which of the following procedures?

Quick Answers: **319**
Detailed Answer: **334**

- ❍ **A.** Insert 10mL of air in NG tube and listen over the abdomen with a stethoscope
- ❍ **B.** Clamp the tube while listening to the abdomen with a stethoscope
- ❍ **C.** Irrigate the tube with 30mL of NS while auscultating the abdomen
- ❍ **D.** Turn the suction on high and auscultate over the naval area

Quick Check

142. A burn client's care plan reveals an expected outcome of no localized or systemic infection. Which assessment by the nurse supports this outcome?

Quick Answers: **319**
Detailed Answer: **334**

❍ **A.** Wound culture results show minimal bacteria
❍ **B.** Cloudy, foul-smelling urine output
❍ **C.** White blood cell count of 14,000
❍ **D.** Temperature of 101°F

143. The nurse is preparing to administer promethazine hydrochloride (Phenergan). This drug should produce which therapeutic effect?

Quick Answers: **319**
Detailed Answer: **334**

❍ **A.** Marked diuresis
❍ **B.** Decreased nausea
❍ **C.** Constriction of the pupils
❍ **D.** Increased seizure threshold

144. Which antibiotic is safest to administer to a client who is allergic to penicillin?

Quick Answers: **319**
Detailed Answer: **334**

❍ **A.** Cefazolin (Ancef)
❍ **B.** Amoxicillin (Amoxil)
❍ **C.** Erythromycin (Erythrocin)
❍ **D.** Ceftriazone (Rocephin)

145. The nurse notes the following laboratory test results on a 24-hour post-burn client. Which abnormality should be of particular concern?

Quick Answers: **319**
Detailed Answer: **334**

❍ **A.** Potassium 7.5mEq/L
❍ **B.** Sodium 131mEq/L
❍ **C.** Arterial pH 7.34
❍ **D.** Hematocrit 52%

146. Which technique is correct for administration of ear drops to a 3-year-old?

Quick Answers: **319**
Detailed Answer: **334**

❍ **A.** Hold the child's head up and extended
❍ **B.** Place the head in chin tuck position
❍ **C.** Pull the pinna down and back
❍ **D.** Irrigate the ear before medication administration

Quick Check

147. The nurse is caring for a client with scalding burns across the face, neck, entire anterior chest, and entire right arm. Using the rule of nines, what is the estimated percentage of body burned?

Quick Answers: **319**
Detailed Answer: **335**

❍ **A.** 18%
❍ **B.** 23%
❍ **C.** 32%
❍ **D.** 36%

148. The nurse caring for a client in shock recognizes that the glomerular filtration rate of the kidneys will remain intact if the client's mean arterial pressure remains above which minimal value?

Quick Answers: **319**
Detailed Answer: **335**

❍ **A.** 80
❍ **B.** 70
❍ **C.** 60
❍ **D.** 50

149. Which assessment data on a child with hydrocephalus would be the most objective?

Quick Answers: **319**
Detailed Answer: **335**

❍ **A.** Anorexia
❍ **B.** Vomiting
❍ **C.** Head measurement
❍ **D.** Temperature

150. The nurse recognizes which of the following types of leukemia as being more common in an older adult?

Quick Answers: **319**
Detailed Answer: **335**

❍ **A.** Acute myelocytic leukemia
❍ **B.** Acute lymphocytic leukemia
❍ **C.** Chronic lymphocytic leukemia
❍ **D.** Chronic granulocytic leukemia

151. A client has pneumonia. Which assessment finding best indicates that the client's respiratory efforts are currently adequate?

Quick Answers: **319**
Detailed Answer: **335**

❍ **A.** The client is able to talk.
❍ **B.** The client is alert and oriented.
❍ **C.** The client's O_2 saturation is 97%.
❍ **D.** The client's chest movements are uninhibited.

Quick Check

152. The nurse is discussing with parents the recommended activities for children with asthma. Which sports activity would the nurse include in the discussion?

Quick Answers: **319**
Detailed Answer: **335**

❍ **A.** Soccer

❍ **B.** Swimming

❍ **C.** Football

❍ **D.** Track

153. Which of the following would the nurse perform when giving medication via an NG tube?

Quick Answers: **319**
Detailed Answer: **336**

❍ **A.** Ascertain tube patency and placement.

❍ **B.** Position the client dorsal recumbent.

❍ **C.** Reconnect the tube to suction immediately after administration of the drug.

❍ **D.** Administer the drug as rapidly as possible to prevent clogging the tube.

154. An infant in the nursery is 48 hours old and has not passed meconium. The nurse suspects which of the following?

Quick Answers: **319**
Detailed Answer: **336**

❍ **A.** Coarctation of the aorta

❍ **B.** Tetralogy of fallot

❍ **C.** Hyperbilirubinemia

❍ **D.** Cystic fibrosis

155. Which of the following laboratory results would cause the most concern in the immunosuppressed client?

Quick Answers: **319**
Detailed Answer: **336**

❍ **A.** A sodium level of 50mg/dL

❍ **B.** A blood glucose of 110mg/dL

❍ **C.** A platelet count of 100,000/cu mm

❍ **D.** A white cell count of 5,000/cu mm

156. The nurse has an order to administer meperidine (Demerol) 75 mg IM for pain. The drug available is Demerol 100mg in 2 mLs. How many mL(S) will the nurse administer?

Quick Answers: **319**
Detailed Answer: **336**

❍ **A.** 1.0 mL

❍ **B.** 1.3 mL

❍ **C.** 1.5 mL

❍ **D.** 1.7 mL

Quick Check

157. A client is diagnosed with left subclavian artery obstruction. What additional findings would the nurse expect?

Quick Answers: **319**
Detailed Answer: **336**

❍ **A.** Memory loss and disorientation

❍ **B.** Numbness in the face, mouth, and tongue

❍ **C.** Radial pulse differences over 10bpm

❍ **D.** Frontal headache with associated nausea or emesis

158. The nurse is giving information to a client at high risk for the development of skin cancer. Which instruction should be included?

Quick Answers: **319**
Detailed Answer: **336**

❍ **A.** "You should see the doctor every 6 months."

❍ **B.** "Sunbathing should be done between the hours of noon and 3 p.m."

❍ **C.** "If you have a mole, it should be removed and biopsied."

❍ **D.** "You should wear sunscreen when going outside."

159. A client who is complaining of nausea, has an order for hydroxyzine hydrochloride (Vistaril) 75mg every 3–4 hours IM p.r.n. for nausea. The vial contains 100mg per 2mL. How many milliliters will you give?

Quick Answers: **319**
Detailed Answer: **336**

❍ **A.** 0.8mL

❍ **B.** 1.5mL

❍ **C.** 2.0mL

❍ **D.** 2.5mL

160. The nurse is caring for a client who is experiencing pruritis. Which would be the most appropriate nursing intervention?

Quick Answers: **319**
Detailed Answer: **336**

❍ **A.** Suggest the client take warm showers B.I.D.

❍ **B.** Add baby oil to the client's bath water

❍ **C.** Apply powder to the client's skin

❍ **D.** Suggest a hot water rinse after bathing

161. What would the nurse expect to see included in the treatment plan of a 14-year-old with scoliosis and an 18° curvature of the spine?

Quick Answers: **319**
Detailed Answer: **336**

❍ **A.** Application of a Milwaukee brace

❍ **B.** Electrical stimulation to the outward side of the curve

❍ **C.** Re-evaluation with no treatment at this time

❍ **D.** Surgical realignment of the spine

Quick Check

162. The nurse is giving instructions on the removal of ticks at a Girl Scout meeting. Which information is proper procedure for tick removal?

Quick Answers: 319
Detailed Answer: 336

❍ A. "Use tweezers to remove the tick, disinfecting the area before and after removal."

❍ B. "Apply nail polish to the tick, then remove it with your gloved fingers."

❍ C. "Soak alcohol on a piece of cloth, smothering the tick, and pull it out with the cloth."

❍ D. "Apply a lighted match to the tick and wipe it off."

163. The nurse recognizes that which of the following protective equipment is most appropriate to wear when suctioning a client with a tracheostomy?

Quick Answers: 319
Detailed Answer: 336

❍ A. Gown, goggles, and gloves

❍ B. Gown only

❍ C. Gloves only

❍ D. Gown and shoe covers

164. Which statement made by a client's son signifies abnormal grieving by the client?

Quick Answers: 319
Detailed Answer: 336

❍ A. "Mother still has episodes of crying, and it's been 6 months since Daddy died."

❍ B. "Mother seems to have forgotten the bad things that Daddy did in his lifetime."

❍ C. "She really had a hard time after Daddy's funeral. She said that she had a sense of longing."

❍ D. "Mother has not been saddened at all by Daddy's death. She acts like nothing has happened."

165. Which statement made by the client would alert the nurse to a possible fluid and electrolyte imbalance in an 80-year-old client being admitted to a nursing home?

Quick Answers: 319
Detailed Answer: 336

❍ A. "My skin is always so dry."

❍ B. "I often use a laxative for constipation."

❍ C. "I have always liked to drink a lot of water."

❍ D. "I sometimes have a problem with dribbling urine."

Quick Check

166. The nurse is reviewing laboratory results. Serum sodium of 156mEq/L is noted. What changes would the nurse expect the client to exhibit?

Quick Answers: **319**
Detailed Answer: **337**

- ❍ **A.** Hyporeflexia
- ❍ **B.** Manic behavior
- ❍ **C.** Depression
- ❍ **D.** Muscle cramps

167. A nurse would expect a client admitted with congestive heart failure to be treated with which drug?

Quick Answers: **319**
Detailed Answer: **337**

- ❍ **A.** Furosemide (Lasix)
- ❍ **B.** Pentoxifyline (Trental)
- ❍ **C.** Warfarin (Coumadin)
- ❍ **D.** Metaxalone (Skelaxin)

168. The nurse is assessing the chart of a client admitted for surgery when an order is noted to administer Atropine 2mg IM as a pre-operative medication to a 40-year-old client. What initial nursing action is most appropriate?

Quick Answers: **319**
Detailed Answer: **337**

- ❍ **A.** Clarifying the order with the physician
- ❍ **B.** Administering the medication deep IM
- ❍ **C.** Checking the chart for client allergies
- ❍ **D.** Performing the mathematical calculation to determine dosage due

169. A client is admitted to the emergency room with a complaint of chest pain. The physician suspects a myocardial infarction and orders heparin and nitroglycerin. Which home medication, taken just before admission, would the nurse report to the ER physician immediately?

Quick Answers: **319**
Detailed Answer: **337**

- ❍ **A.** Acetaminophen (Tylenol)
- ❍ **B.** Sildenafil (Viagra)
- ❍ **C.** Chlordiazeproxide/clidnium (Librax)
- ❍ **D.** Escitalopram (Lexapro)

Quick Check

170. A client is to undergo a bone marrow aspiration. The nurse plans to include which statement in the client preparation?

Quick Answers: **319**
Detailed Answer: **337**

- ❍ **A.** "You will be sitting on the side of the bed during the procedure."
- ❍ **B.** "Portions of the procedure will cause pain or discomfort."
- ❍ **C.** "You will be given some medication to cause amnesia of the test."
- ❍ **D.** "You will not be able to drink fluids for 24 hours before the study."

171. A client is scheduled for surgical repair of an abdominal aortic aneurysm. Which assessment is most crucial during the preoperative period?

Quick Answers: **319**
Detailed Answer: **337**

- ❍ **A.** Assessment of the client's level of anxiety
- ❍ **B.** Evaluation of the client's exercise tolerance
- ❍ **C.** Identification of peripheral pulses
- ❍ **D.** Assessment of bowel sounds and activity

172. Which of the following dysrhythmias is most likely to occur during suctioning?

Quick Answers: **319**
Detailed Answer: **337**

- ❍ **A.** Bradycardia
- ❍ **B.** Tachycardia
- ❍ **C.** Ventricular ectopic beats
- ❍ **D.** Sick sinus syndrome

173. The nurse is providing discharge instructions for a client who requires oxygen therapy at home. The client asks the nurse, "Will Medicare and Medicaid services pay for the oxygen?" The nurse's response is based on the fact that the client's PO_2 must have been less than what level on room air for the client to receive financial reimbursement?

Quick Answers: **319**
Detailed Answer: **337**

- ❍ **A.** 40
- ❍ **B.** 50
- ❍ **C.** 55
- ❍ **D.** 65

Quick Check

174. The LPN/LVN is caring for a client with Clostidium difficile (C difficile). Which of the following observations indicates to the nurse that the client's condition is improving?

Quick Answers: **319**
Detailed Answer: **337**

- ❍ **A.** Increased watery stools
- ❍ **B.** Malaise
- ❍ **C.** Anorexia
- ❍ **D.** Moist mucous membranes

175. The LPN/LVN is describing a 24 hour urine collection to a client. Which of the following explanations is most accurate?

Quick Answers: **319**
Detailed Answer: **337**

- ❍ **A.** Void and save the urine at the start of the collection period to begin the process
- ❍ **B.** Wash the perineal area with soap and water before each void
- ❍ **C.** Collect the urine in a sterilized container or receptacle
- ❍ **D.** Empty the bladder at the end of the collection period and save this urine

176. A client who has had thoracic surgery has been instructed in arm and shoulder exercises. The nurse recognizes which of the following as the primary reason for these exercises?

Quick Answers: **319**
Detailed Answer: **338**

- ❍ **A.** Restore movement
- ❍ **B.** Prevent edema of the scapula
- ❍ **C.** Provide psychological stress relief
- ❍ **D.** Prevent respiratory complications

177. For the drugs Tamiflu and Relenza to be the most effective in eliminating the influenza virus, they should be administered within which time period?

Quick Answers: **319**
Detailed Answer: **338**

- ❍ **A.** 3 days of the client becoming ill
- ❍ **B.** 7 days of the client becoming ill
- ❍ **C.** 10 days of exposure to influenza
- ❍ **D.** 14 days of exposure to influenza

178. A 22-year-old female is being discharged after an admission for bipolar disorder. Discharge medications include valproate (Depakote). Which statement by the client would cause the nurse concern because of the prescription?

Quick Answers: **319**
Detailed Answer: **338**

- ❍ **A.** "I am trying to get pregnant."
- ❍ **B.** "My career as a secretary is just beginning."
- ❍ **C.** "I usually exercise 4 times a week."
- ❍ **D.** "I am on a well-balanced diet."

Quick Check

179. A tuberculin test has been administered to an elderly client in preparation for nursing home placement. Which of these skin reactions at the site of the test could indicate a positive result?

Quick Answers: **319**
Detailed Answer: **338**

❍ **A.** Induration
❍ **B.** Ulceration
❍ **C.** Rash
❍ **D.** Redness

180. The nurse is discussing discharge plans with a 30-year-old client who has sickle cell disease. Assessment findings include spleenomegaly. What information obtained in the discussion would cause the most concern? The client:

Quick Answers: **319**
Detailed Answer: **338**

❍ **A.** Eats fast food daily for lunch
❍ **B.** Drinks a beer occasionally
❍ **C.** Sometimes feels fatigued
❍ **D.** Works as a furniture mover

181. The influenza vaccine is contraindicated in clients with allergies to which of the following?

Quick Answers: **319**
Detailed Answer: **338**

❍ **A.** Eggs
❍ **B.** Shellfish
❍ **C.** Iodine
❍ **D.** Pork

182. The nurse is caring for a client who is of the Islam religious group. Which food selection would be inappropriate to offer to this client?

Quick Answers: **319**
Detailed Answer: **338**

❍ **A.** Jell-O
❍ **B.** Chicken
❍ **C.** Milk
❍ **D.** Broccoli

183. The nurse identifies which of the following as a side effect of the influenza vaccine?

Quick Answers: **319**
Detailed Answer: **338**

❍ **A.** Febrile reaction
❍ **B.** Hypothermia
❍ **C.** Dyspnea
❍ **D.** Generalized rash

Quick Check

184. Which breakfast selection by a client with osteopenia indicates that the client understands the dietary management of the disease?

Quick Answers: **320**
Detailed Answer: **338**

❍ **A.** Scrambled eggs, toast, and coffee

❍ **B.** Bran muffin with margarine

❍ **C.** Granola bar and half of a grapefruit

❍ **D.** Bagel with jam and skim milk

185. A client is admitted with cholethiasis and has obstructive jaundice. Which clinical manifestations does the LPN/LVN expect to observe?

Quick Answers: **320**
Detailed Answer: **338**

❍ **A.** Clear straw urine

❍ **B.** White sclera

❍ **C.** Clay colored stool

❍ **D.** Red nailbeds

186. The nurse is assessing a client with gastroenteritis for hypovolemia. Which laboratory result would help the nurse in confirming a volume deficit?

Quick Answers: **320**
Detailed Answer: **338**

❍ **A.** Hematocrit 55%

❍ **B.** Potassium 5.0mEq/L

❍ **C.** Urine specific gravity 1.016

❍ **D.** BUN 18mg/dL

187. A client has an order for Codeine 60 mg IM. An available vial contains Codeine 30 mg/mL. What volume of drug would the nurse administer?

Quick Answers: **320**
Detailed Answer: **339**

❍ **A.** 0.5mL

❍ **B.** 1.0mL

❍ **C.** 1.5mL

❍ **D.** 2.0mL

188. The nurse is assessing elderly clients at a nursing home. Which of the following findings would not be considered a normal part of the aging process?

Quick Answers: **320**
Detailed Answer: **339**

❍ **A.** Complaints of a dry mouth

❍ **B.** Loss of 1 inch of height in the last year

❍ **C.** Stiffened joints

❍ **D.** Rales bilaterally on chest auscultation

Quick Check

189. A client at the clinic reports to the nurse, "I have trouble seeing signs at a distance, but no trouble seeing things close up." The nurse identifies the correct term for this vision problem as:

Quick Answers: **320**
Detailed Answer: **339**

❍ **A.** Myopia

❍ **B.** Emmetropia

❍ **C.** Hyperopia

❍ **D.** Astigmatism

190. A client has signs of increased intracranial pressure. Which one of the following is an early indicator of increased intracranial pressure?

Quick Answers: **320**
Detailed Answer: **339**

❍ **A.** Widening pulse pressure

❍ **B.** Decrease in the pulse rate

❍ **C.** Dilated, fixed pupils

❍ **D.** Decrease in level of consciousness

191. Which statement by a client who is taking topiramate (Topamax) indicates that the client has understood the nurse's instruction?

Quick Answers: **320**
Detailed Answer: **339**

❍ **A.** "I will take the medicine before going to bed."

❍ **B.** "I will drink 8 to 10 ten-ounce glasses of water a day."

❍ **C.** "I will eat plenty of fresh fruits."

❍ **D.** "I must take the medicine with a meal or snack."

192. A client with AIDS is admitted to the unit. A family member asks the nurse, "How much longer will it be?" Which response by the nurse is most appropriate?

Quick Answers: **320**
Detailed Answer: **339**

❍ **A.** "This must be a terrible situation for you."

❍ **B.** "I don't know. I'll call the doctor."

❍ **C.** "I cannot say exactly. What are your concerns at this time?"

❍ **D.** "Don't worry, it will be very soon."

193. The LPN/LVN is working on a team that includes an RN and a nursing assistant. The LPN/LVN should be assigned which of the following clients?

Quick Answers: **320**
Detailed Answer: **339**

❍ **A.** A client with terminal pancreatic cancer in severe pain

❍ **B.** A client with peripheral vascular disease requiring a dressing change

❍ **C.** A client with alzheimers disease requiring ambulatory assistance

❍ **D.** A client with trauma who had a chest tube inserted 1 hour ago

Quick Check

194. The nurse is caring for a client with a basilar skull fracture. Fluid is assessed leaking from the ear. What is the nurse's first action?

Quick Answers: **320**
Detailed Answer: **339**

- ❍ **A.** Irrigate the ear canal gently
- ❍ **B.** Notify the physician
- ❍ **C.** Test the drainage for glucose
- ❍ **D.** Apply an occlusive dressing

195. The nurse has inserted an NG tube for enteral feedings. Which assessment result is the best indication that an NG tube is properly placed in the stomach?

Quick Answers: **320**
Detailed Answer: **339**

- ❍ **A.** Aspiration of tan-colored mucus
- ❍ **B.** Green aspirate with a pH of 3
- ❍ **C.** A swish auscultated with the injection of air
- ❍ **D.** Bubbling in a cup of NS when the end of the tube is placed in the cup

196. Which one of the following assessment findings is within normal expectations for a post-operative craniotomy client?

Quick Answers: **320**
Detailed Answer: **339**

- ❍ **A.** A decrease in responsiveness the third post-op day
- ❍ **B.** Sluggish pupil reaction the first 24–48 hours
- ❍ **C.** Dressing changes 3–4 times a day for the first 3 days
- ❍ **D.** Temperature range of 98.8°F–99.6°F the first 2–3 days

197. A client with alcoholism has been instructed to increase his intake of thiamine. Which food is highest in thiamine?

Quick Answers: **320**
Detailed Answer: **339**

- ❍ **A.** Roast beef
- ❍ **B.** Broiled fish
- ❍ **C.** Baked chicken
- ❍ **D.** Sliced pork

198. A client is immobile. Which nursing intervention would best improve tissue perfusion to prevent skin problems?

Quick Answers: **320**
Detailed Answer: **340**

- ❍ **A.** Assessing the skin daily
- ❍ **B.** Massaging any erythematous areas on the skin
- ❍ **C.** Changing incontinence pads as soon as they become soiled
- ❍ **D.** Performing range-of-motion exercises, and turning and repositioning the client

Quick Check

199. The nurse is discussing nutritional needs with the dietician at the nursing home. Which diet selection indicates a proper diet for healing of a decubitus ulcer?

Quick Answers: **320**
Detailed Answer: **340**

❍ **A.** Tossed salad, milk, and a slice of caramel cake

❍ **B.** Vegetable soup and crackers, and a glass of tea

❍ **C.** Baked chicken breast, broccoli, wheat roll, and an orange

❍ **D.** Hamburger, French fries, and corn on the cob

200. A client is admitted to the chemical dependency unit due to cocaine addiction. The client states, "I don't know why you are all so worried. I am in control. I don't have a problem." Which defense mechanism is being utilized?

Quick Answers: **320**
Detailed Answer: **340**

❍ **A.** Rationalization

❍ **B.** Projection

❍ **C.** Dissociation

❍ **D.** Denial

Quick Check Answer Key

1. A
2. C
3. A
4. A
5. D
6. B
7. A
8. C
9. D
10. A
11. A
12. C
13. B
14. C
15. C
16. C
17. C
18. B
19. B
20. D
21. C
22. C
23. B
24. C
25. A
26. A
27. B
28. D
29. A
30. B
31. D
32. C
33. D
34. D
35. C
36. B
37. D
38. D
39. C
40. A
41. B
42. D
43. C
44. A
45. D
46. D
47. D
48. A
49. B
50. D
51. B
52. C
53. D
54. B
55. C
56. B
57. A
58. C
59. A
60. D
61. B
62. B
63. A
64. A
65. B
66. C
67. A
68. B
69. A
70. D
71. A
72. C
73. C
74. D
75. C
76. A
77. A
78. C
79. C
80. D
81. C
82. A
83. D
84. D
85. A
86. A
87. C

88. C
89. A
90. C
91. C
92. A
93. A
94. B
95. C
96. C
97. C
98. C
99. C
100. B
101. D
102. A
103. D
104. C
105. B
106. A
107. A
108. C
109. A
110. B
111. A
112. C
113. A
114. D
115. B
116. B
117. B
118. D
119. D
120. B
121. A
122. B
123. B
124. B
125. A
126. C
127. C
128. C
129. A
130. B
131. D
132. D
133. A
134. B
135. C
136. A
137. A
138. A
139. D
140. D
141. B
142. A
143. B
144. C
145. A
146. C
147. C
148. A
149. C
150. C
151. C
152. B
153. A
154. D
155. A
156. C
157. C
158. D
159. B
160. B
161. C
162. A
163. A
164. D
165. B
166. B
167. A
168. A
169. B
170. B
171. C
172. A
173. C
174. D
175. D
176. A
177. A
178. A
179. A
180. D
181. A
182. A
183. A

184. D
185. C
186. A
187. D
188. D
189. A
190. D
191. B
192. C
193. B
194. C
195. B
196. D
197. D
198. D
199. C
200. D

Answers and Rationales

1. **Answer A is correct.** Administering Levofloxacin (Levaquin) and Mylanta at the same time will decrease the absorption of the fluoroquinolones. The drug combinations in answers B, C, and D are not contraindicated because the drugs in each combination do not affect one another.

2. **Answer C is correct.** A hyperactive thyroid causes hypermetabolism and increased sympathetic nervous system activity. Weight gain occurs with hypothyroidism, making answer A incorrect. Although tachycardia occurs with hyperthyroidism, diuresis and hypokalemia do not, so answer D is incorrect. Dyspnea can occur with this disorder, but clients exhibit increased libido, making answer B incorrect.

3. **Answer A is correct.** Tetany is caused by a decrease in calcium. Answers B, C, and D are not used in the treatment plan for clients with hypocalcemia.

4. **Answer A is correct.** Melena is blood in the stools, which would occur with bleeding in the gastrointestinal tract due to a peptic ulcer. Answers B, C, and D are not specific to the GI system so are incorrect. Hematuria (blood in the urine) is not indicative of a peptic ulcer, blood from the lungs can occur as hemoptysis but is not related to this problem, and ecchymosis indicates bruising.

5. **Answer D is correct.** When mixing insulins, air should be injected into both vials before drawing up the dose, and clear (Regular) insulin should be drawn up before cloudy (NPH). Answer A would require two injections, which is not necessary. Answers B and C are incorrect procedures because regular insulin, not NPH, should be drawn up first.

6. **Answer B is correct.** Pancreatic enzyme secretion is activated by food and fluid. Therefore, keeping the client NPO will prevent the pancreas from secreting, resulting in decreased pain and damage to the pancreas. Answers A and D would produce negative outcomes and would have no relationship to why food and fluids are withheld. Because pancreatic enzymes are decreased by withholding food and fluids, answer C is incorrect.

7. **Answer A is correct.** Digoxin (Lanoxin) increases the force of the contraction of the heart, thus increasing the cardiac output. Answer D is incorrect because Lanoxin increases cardiac output. Lanoxin slows the heart rate, making answer B incorrect. Answer C could result in a myocardial infarction and is not the effect of the drug.

8. **Answer C is correct.** A loss of gag reflex can occur due to the anesthetizing agent used for the tube insertion. It is most important to ensure an intact reflex before administering food or fluids because of the danger of aspiration. The position in answer A would be contraindicated because of possible increased secretions. Answer B would be instituted at a later time. Answer D would be necessary for clients with abdominal surgery.

9. **Answer D is correct.** Vital sign changes with hemorrhagic shock are decreasing blood pressure with an increased heart rate. Answer A is a normal BP and heart rate. Answers B and C are abnormal vital signs but do not correlate with hemorrhagic shock.

10. **Answer A is correct.** AIDS is transmitted by transfer of blood and bodily fluids, not by casual contact. Answers B, C, and D are incorrect statements about AIDS. Some states require sexual contact notification; otherwise, confidentially is maintained.

11. **Answer A is correct.** A tracheotomy set is placed at the bedside as a safety measure in case the client has severe edema or respiratory distress. The pieces of equipment in answers B, C, and D are not required or helpful after a thyroidectomy.

12. **Answer C is correct.** aPTTs should be monitored on clients receiving heparin. The goal is 1.5 to 2 times the control for prevention of deep vein thrombosis. Answer A is used for the monitoring of Coumadin therapy. Answer B is the antidote for too much Coumadin. Answer D is not a test used for heparin or Coumadin.

13. **Answer B is correct.** This is the American Cancer Society's recommendation for testicular examination. Answers A, C, and D are not the correct timing sequences for a testicular examination.

14. **Answer C is correct.** Remaining upright will decrease the chance of esophageal reflux. Clients should avoid fatty foods, coffee, tea, cola, chocolate, alcohol, and spicy and acidic foods, which makes answers B and D incorrect. Puréed diets, as in answer A, are not recommended.

15. **Answer C is correct.** With clients who are in end-stage cirrhosis, proteins are restricted because of the inability of the liver to convert the protein for excretion. This results in build-up of ammonia in the body. Answers A, B, and D are not restricted foods.

16. **Answer C is correct.** Cooling the burn stops the burn process, relieving pain and limiting edema. This is the initial action. Answers A and B are not initial actions to be performed in the field. Adherent clothing should remain in place after being cooled, so answer D is incorrect.

17. **Answer C is correct.** Clients with myasthenia gravis have a decrease in muscular strength because of a lack of acetylcholine. Tensilon administration halts the breakdown of acetylcholine, causing an increase in muscular strength that confirms the diagnosis. Answer A would indicate that the client does not have myasthenias gravis. Answers B and D are not an effect of the drug Tensilon.

18. **Answer B is correct.** These clients have a subnormal temperature and pulse rate, causing them to have a decreased tolerance of cold. Answers A, C, and D are symptoms of hyperthyroidism, so they are incorrect.

19. **Answer B is correct.** The nurse should give only one direction or step at a time when communicating to clients with Alzheimer's disease. Clients cannot comprehend when too much detailed information or too many instructions are given at one time, making answers A and D incorrect. Answer C forces the Alzheimer's client to make a choice and a decision, which is difficult for clients with this disorder.

20. **Answer D is correct.** The three main symptoms of diabetes are increased urination, increased thirst, and increased appetite. Answer A is incorrect because the client's appetite would be increased. Diabetics experience weight loss, which makes answer B incorrect. Answer C is not associated with diabetes.

21. **Answer C is correct.** Versed is used for conscious sedation and is an antianxiety agent. The antidote for this drug is Romazicon, a benzodiazepine. Answers A, B, and D

are not utilized as antagonists for Versed; however, answer B is the antagonist for narcotics.

22. **Answer C is correct.** Turning the client to the side will allow any vomit to drain from the mouth and decrease the risk for aspiration. Answers A, B, and D are all appropriate as nursing interventions, but a patent airway and prevention of aspiration is the priority.

23. **Answer B is correct.** When dehiscence and/or evisceration of a wound occurs, the nurse should apply a sterile saline dressing before notifying the physician. Answer A is not the appropriate position because the client should be placed in low Fowler's position. Answers C and D are not appropriate actions.

24. **Answer C is correct.** There is a risk of bleeding with this procedure; therefore, laboratory tests are done to determine any problems with coagulation before the test. Answers A, B, and D are incorrect statements. The client lies on the right side, not the left; no enemas are given; and the test is invasive and can cause some pain.

25. **Answer A is correct.** Obstruction of the tracheostomy can cause anxiety, increased respiratory rate, and a decrease in O_2 saturation. The nurse should first suction the client. If this doesn't work, she should notify the physician, as in answer C. Answer B would not help the client's breathing. Answer D would be done to assess for improvement after the suctioning was performed.

26. **Answer A is correct.** Clients who are taking INH should avoid tuna, red wine, soy sauce, and yeast extracts because of the side effects that can occur, such as headaches and hypotension. Answers B, C, and D are all allowed with this drug.

27. **Answer B is correct.** Any abnormal temperature should be reassessed in 30 minutes. A temperature above 101°F requires that the physician be notified, which makes answer D incorrect. Answer A would be done, but it would not be the only action. Answer C is incorrect because the nurse should wait 5 minutes after food or liquids to retake the temperature, for an accurate recording.

28. **Answer D is correct.** This cranial nerve deals with the function of the tongue and its movement. Clients can exhibit weakness and deviation with impairment of this cranial nerve. Answers A, B, and C are not tested by this procedure. Cranial nerve I is smell, cranial nerve II is visual, and cranial nerve X deals with the gag reflex.

29. **Answer A is correct.** Increased intracranial pressure vital sign changes include an elevated BP with a widening pulse pressure, decreased heart rate, and temperature elevation. Answer C could occur with shock or hypovolemia. Answer B does not correlate with increased ICP. Answer D shows increased intracranial pressure, but not as much as answer A.

30. **Answer B is correct.** The normal Dilantin level is 10–20mcg/mL. The 30 level exceeds the normal. The appropriate action would be to notify the physician for orders. Answer A would be inappropriate because of the high level. Answers C and D would require an order from the physician.

31. **Answer D is correct.** Hydration is needed to prevent slowing of blood flow and occlusion. It is important to perform assessments in answers A, B, and C, but answer D is the best intervention for preventing the crisis.

32. **Answer C is correct.** Vitamin B12 is an essential component for proper functioning of the peripheral nervous system. Clients without an adequate vitamin B12 level will have symptoms such as paresthesia due to the deficiency. Answers A and D don't occur with pernicious anemia. The client would have weight loss rather than weight gain, as in answer B.

33. **Answer D is correct.** Answers A, B, and C are all foods included on a low-purine diet. Spinach should be avoided on a low-purine diet. Other foods to avoid include poultry, liver, lobster, oysters, peas, fish, and oatmeal.

34. **Answer D is correct.** It is appropriate for the nursing assistant to perform activity orders for stable clients. It is beyond the role of the nurse's assistant to perform blood sugars and obtain vital signs on unstable clients, as in answers A and B. A client with a stroke might have dysphasia, which makes answer C inappropriate for the assistant, especially because the client is new and has not been evaluated.

35. **Answer C is correct.** Fat emboli occur more frequently with long bone or pelvic fractures and usually in young adults ages 20 to 30. The answers in A, B, and D are not high-risk groups for this complication.

36. **Answer B is correct.** This selection is the one with the highest iron content. Other foods high in iron include cream of wheat, oatmeal, liver, collard greens and mustard greens, clams, chili with beans, brown rice, and dried apricots. Answers A, C, and D are not high in iron.

37. **Answer D is correct.** Symptoms of a fractured right femoral neck include shortened, adducted, and external rotation. Answer A is incorrect because the patient usually is unable to move the leg because of pain. Answers B and C are incorrect because the fracture will cause adduction instead of abduction, and external rotation rather than internal rotation.

38. **Answer D is correct.** The 0.2mL of air that would be administered after the medication with an intramuscular injection would allow the medication to be dispersed into the muscle. In answer A, the muscle is too small. Answer C is an incorrect procedure, and answer B doesn't help prevent tracking.

39. **Answer C is correct.** The TENS unit is applied for pain relief. A TENS unit is a battery-operated unit applied to the skin that stimulates non–pain receptors in the same areas that transmit the pain. This is the only answer that actually does anything about the pain the client is experiencing. Answer A is a psychosocial acknowledgment. Answers B and D might help the pain, but answer C would help more.

40. **Answer A is correct.** In hemolytic anemia, destruction of red blood cells causes the release of bilirubin, leading to the yellow hue of the skin. Answers C and D occur with several anemias, but they are not specific to hemolytic. Answer B does not relate to anemia.

41. **Answer B is correct.** Neulasta is given to increase the white blood cell count in patients with leucopenia. This white blood cell count is within the normal range, showing an improvement. Answers A, C, and D are not specific to the drug's desired effect.

42. **Answer D is correct.** Clients with a diagnosis of polycythemia have an increased risk for thrombosis and must be aware of the symptoms. Answers A, B, and C do not relate to this disorder.

43. **Answer C is correct.** Ground pepper is an unprocessed food and will not be allowed because of the possible bacteria. The nurse would also ensure that this client receives no uncooked fruits and vegetables. Answers A, B, and D have all been through processing.

44. **Answer A is correct.** Alendronate (Fosamax) should be taken in the morning before food or other medications, with water as the only liquid. Answers B, C, and D are correct administrations. In answer B, remaining upright is important to prevent esophageal problems with Fosamax administration.

45. **Answer D is correct.** The dose of medication is too high, so the nurse should contact the physician. The infant weighs 5.45kg; the dose should be between 54.5 and 81.75. Answer A would be an incorrect dose. Answer B would require a new prescription. The action in answer C is not necessary and inappropriate to the situation.

46. **Answer D is correct.** This diet selection is the most balanced and best promotes healing. Answers A, B, and C are not as inclusive of food groups that promote healing as answer D.

47. **Answer D is correct.** Vomiting would be contraindicated with an acid, alkaline, or petroleum product. Answers A, B, and C do not contain any of the solutions mentioned in the previous statement.

48. **Answer A is correct.** Clients with ulcerative colitis experiencing diarrhea should avoid bowel irritants such as raw vegetables, nuts, and fatty and fried foods. Answers B, C, and D would not serve as irritants to the bowels.

49. **Answer B is correct.** The nurse should prioritize these clients and decide to see the client with the shortness of breath because this client is the least stable. Answer A has an abnormal PCO_2 (normal 35–45), but this would be expected in a client with COPD. Answer C can be corrected by pain medication and does not require the priority visit. Answer D is incorrect because a temperature elevation of this level would not be a reason for great concern with a client after gallbladder surgery.

50. **Answer D is correct.** A malignant mass is usually firm and hard, usually located in one breast, and not movable with an irregular shape. Answers A, B, and C are not characteristics of a malignancy.

51. **Answer B is correct.** The client has an open fracture. The priority would be to cover the wound and prevent further contamination. Swelling usually occurs with a fracture, making answer C incorrect. Manual traction, as in answer A, should not be attempted. In Answer D, the change in position would cause excessive movement and is an inappropriate action.

52. **Answer C is correct.** The child weighs 24kg and should receive 5 units/kg, or 120 units every 4 hours. This would be 720 units in 24 hours. The answers in A, B, and D are incorrect calculations.

53. **Answer D is correct.** This statement indicates that the client is retaining fluid and the condition is deteriorating. Answers A and B are normal and require no need for follow-up. Answer C indicates that the client is diuresing, which is a positive outcome of treatment.

54. **Answer B is correct.** Hypercalcemia is a common occurrence with cancer of the bone. Clinical manifestations of hypercalcemia include mental confusion and an elevated blood pressure. The potassium level in answer A is elevated but does not relate to the diagnosis. Answers C and D are both normal levels.

55. **Answer C is correct.** Clients with gallbladder (GB) disease complain of colicky pain usually after intake of fatty foods. The pain is located in the right upper quadrant of the abdomen or the right shoulder, so answer A is incorrect. Food intake causes more pain because of GB stimulation, so answer B is incorrect. Answer D is an incorrect statement because the gallbladder function is not associated with diarrhea or constipation.

56. **Answer B is correct.** A catheter will allow urine elimination without possible disruption of the implant. There is usually no restriction on TV or phone use, as in answer A. The client is placed on a low-residue diet, not a high-fiber diet, as in answer C. The client's radiation is not internal; therefore, there are no special precautions with excretions, as in answer D.

57. **Answer A is correct.** The liver fails to convert protein for excretion; therefore, protein converts to ammonia, which then builds up in the blood stream, causing mental changes and sometimes coma. An increased WBC and high blood sugar are not associated with liver cirrhosis, so answers C and D are incorrect. The protein levels are elevated, as evidenced by elevated ammonia in the serum, so answer B is incorrect.

58. **Answer C is correct.** The lung could be punctured inadvertently by the liver biopsy procedure, causing a pneumothorax. The nurse should also be alert for hemorrhage. Answers A, B, and D are not associated risks with a liver biopsy.

59. **Answer A is correct.** The client is at risk for a loss of fluid volume and shock, so obtaining the vital signs to assess for complications would be the priority. Answers B, C, and D can all be implemented, but they are not the priority so they are incorrect.

60. **Answer D is correct.** Platelets deal with the clotting of blood. Lack of platelets can cause bleeding. Answers A, B, and C do not directly relate to platelets.

61. **Answer B is correct.** Spasmodic eye winking could indicate a toxicity or overdose of the drug and should be reported to the physician. Other signs of toxicity include an involuntary twitching of muscles, facial grimaces, and severe tongue protrusion. Answers A, C, and D are side effects but do not indicate toxicity of the drug.

62. **Answer B is correct.** With neutropenia, the client is at risk for infection; therefore, the client must avoid crowds and people who are ill. Answer A would not be appropriate because there is no correlation between hypothermia and a WBC of 1000. Answers C and D would correlate with a risk for bleeding.

63. **Answer A is correct.** The nurse would monitor the client for hoarseness or a voice change, which could indicate damage to the laryngeal nerve during the surgical procedure. Although the nurse would monitor for edema, bleeding, and tetany, assessment of these problems would not be performed by asking the client to speak.

64. **Answer A is correct.** Vaginal bleeding or spotting is a common symptom of cervical cancer. Answers B and C, the nausea and vomiting and foul-smelling discharge, are not specific or common to cervical cancer. Hyperthermia, in answer D, does not relate to the diagnosis.

65. **Answer B is correct.** Heart failure can be life threatening and would be a priority for reporting. These clients are hyperactive and restless, making answers C and D incorrect. Urinary retention, as in answer A, is not a clinical manifestation of hyperthyroidism.

66. **Answer C is correct.** This procedure is usually done by the physician with specimens obtained from the sternum or the iliac crest. The high Fowler's position would be the best position of the ones listed to obtain a specimen from the client's sternum. Answers A, B, and D would be inappropriate positions for getting a biopsy from the sites indicated.

67. **Answer A is correct.** Hyperventilation is utilized to decrease the PCO_2 to 27–30, producing cerebral blood vessel constriction. Answers B, C, and D can decrease cerebral edema, but not by constricting cerebral blood vessels.

68. **Answer B is correct.** The client is experiencing autonomic hyperreflexia. This can be caused by a full bowel or bladder or a wrinkled sheet. Answer A is not the appropriate action before the assessment of the bladder. Answers C and D are not appropriate actions. There is no information to suggest a need for oxygen, and Procardia requires a doctor's order and would not be done prior to assessment.

69. **Answer A is correct.** Plavix is an antiplatelet. Bleeding could indicate a severe effect. Answers B, C, and D are not associated with Plavix.

70. **Answer D is correct.** Papilledema is a hallmark symptom of increased intracranial pressure. Answers A, B, and C are not as objective or specific to increased intracranial pressure as papilledema.

71. **Answer A is correct.** Imitrex results in cranial vasoconstriction to reduce pain, but it can also cause vasoconstrictive effects systemically. This drug is contraindicated in clients with angina, and the physician should be notified. Answers B and D are inappropriate actions from the information given. Answer C is appropriate, but answer A is most appropriate.

72. **Answer C is correct.** The pH is an accurate indicator of acute ventilatory failure and a need for mechanical ventilation. An elevated PCO_2, as in answer A, is not an adequate criterion for institution of ventilator support. Answer B, an oxygen saturation of 90, would not be very abnormal for a COPD client. Answer D is normal.

73. **Answer C is correct.** The absent breath sound and subcutaneous air, increased heart rate, dyspnea, and restlessness indicates a pneumothorax that would require immediate intervention. Answer A could occur with the pulmonary contusion and would be expected. Answer D, pain after breathing deeply, would be expected with fractured ribs. Answer B is not cause for great concern (the midline trachea is a normal finding).

74. **Answer D is correct.** Sitting or positioning the client in high Fowler's is best to assist the client in using respiratory muscles to breathe and lift the diaphragm from the abdominal area. Answer A would be contraindicated, and answers B and C would not help as much as answer D for breathing.

75. **Answer C is correct.** This client is exhibiting symptoms of heart failure. The client in answer A is being discharged, and a PO_2 of 85, as in answer D, would not be a cause for alarm in a COPD client. The client in answer B would not require immediate attention.

76. **Answer A is correct.** The occipital lobe is the visual lobe. If the client were having problems with the occipital lobe, it would mean that the edema, bleeding, and so on was increasing to that area. Answers B, C, and D do not relate to the occipital lobe.

77. **Answer A is correct.** The increase in venous pressure causes the jugular veins to distend. Other symptoms of right-sided heart failure include ascites, weakness, anorexia, dependent edema, and weight gain. The answers in B, C, and D result from the left ventricle's inability to pump blood out of the ventricle to the body and are specific for left-sided heart failure.

78. **Answer C is correct.** Lasix and Mannitol are given for their diuretic effects to decrease cerebral edema. Answers A, B, and D are not effects of the drugs in this stem.

79. **Answer C is correct.** Cyanosis and loss of consciousness will occur later as the obstruction worsens. Answers B and D are both earlier symptoms of obstruction. Answer A is not a definite clinical manifestation of obstruction.

80. **Answer D is correct.** Cigarette smoking directly affects the sweeping action of the cilia, which interferes with the ability to remove mucus and clear the airway. The answers in A and B are not specific to COPD. Answer C is not a direct effect of smoking.

81. **Answer C is correct.** An MRI uses a powerful magnetic force; therefore, any metal or jewelry should be removed before this test. Answers A, B, and D are not appropriate for this test.

82. **Answer A is correct.** Symptoms of diabetes insipidus include excretion of large amounts of dilute urine and extreme thirst. The clinical manifestations listed in options B, C, and D are not associated with diabetes insipidus so they are incorrect.

83. **Answer D is correct.** An acoustic neuroma tumor is one of the eighth cranial nerves. This cranial nerve deals with balance, hearing, and coordination, making the client at risk for injury from falls. Answers A, B, and C are not appropriate priorities with the information given in the stem.

84. **Answer D is correct.** The stem is describing subcutaneous emphysema (answer B), which is a symptom of air escaping. This can occur with a pneumothorax; therefore, the client should be further assessed for this problem. Answer A is another type of chest trauma, and answer C is not an appropriate assessment from the information given.

85. **Answer A is correct.** The flu vaccine has not been found to be safe in children younger than 6 months; therefore, is not recommended for them. It is especially important that the vaccine be given in the age groups in answers B and D because they are high-risk groups. The age group in C is not a high-risk group, but flu vaccine administration is not contraindicated.

86. **Answer A is correct.** Nimotop is a calcium channel blocker and is used to prevent the calcium influx. The etiology of vasospasm of the blood vessel has been thought to relate to this calcium influx; therefore, the drug is given to prevent this. Answers B, C, and D do not describe the action of this drug.

87. **Answer C is correct.** Simple partial seizures are characterized by the stated symptoms. Answers A and D are not characterized by these clinical manifestations. In answer B, a complex partial seizure, the client is not aware of the seizure.

88. **Answer C is correct.** The essential piece of equipment is the Ambu bag (manual resuscitator). Ventilator clients must always have another means of ventilation, in case of a problem with the ventilator, power, and so on. Answers A and B would be needed, but not as much as answer C. Answer D would be inappropriate for a client on the ventilator.

89. **Answer A is correct.** The suction source should not exceed 120mmHg when performing tracheal suctioning. The answers in B, C, and D exceed this amount and could cause damage to the trachea.

90. **Answer C is correct.** Contracting the abdominal muscles with each exhalation is the proper technique for pursed lip breathing. Answers A, B, and D are all incorrect techniques. The goal is to increase the exhalation phase.

91. **Answer C is correct.** A level of 15ug/mL is within the normal theophylline therapeutic range of 10-20ug/mL. Answers A, B, and D are not within the therapeutic range.

92. **Answer A is correct.** Zyban and Wellbutrin are classified as antidepressants and have been proven to increase long-term smoking abstinence. Answers B and C are bronchodilator drugs and are not used for smoking cessation. Answer D is a short-acting benzodiazepine that is not used for smoking cessation therapy.

93. **Answer A is correct.** Closed chest drainage is not usually used because it is helpful for serous fluid to accumulate in the space to prevent mediastinal shift. Answers B, C, and D are all parts of the care on a client with lung surgery.

94. **Answer B is correct.** Any posterior craniotomy requires the client to lie flat rather than with the head of the bed elevated, as in answer B. A posterior fossa procedure would be at the lower back of the head. Therefore, answer C would not be contraindicated and answer D would help to decrease intracranial pressure.

95. **Answer C is correct.** Raw or cooked vegetables are not allowed on a low-residue diet. Answers A, B, and D are all allowed foods.

96. **Answer C is correct.** A client with diverticulitis should avoid high-fiber foods containing seeds or nuts. Other foods to avoid include corn, popcorn, celery, figs, and strawberries. Answers A, B, and D are foods that do not contain nuts or seeds and would not need to be avoided.

97. **Answer C is correct.** Asking the client about his usual diet is the least helpful information in identifying the problem. Answer A would be important because the pain sometimes decreases as obstruction worsens. The distention in answer D indicates obstruction. Answer B is common because the vomiting can help differentiate the type of obstruction.

98. **Answer C is correct.** Tegretol can cause bone marrow depression, which is evident by the low WBC of 4,000 (normal 5,000–10,000). It can also cause problems with the liver that would raise the BUN (normal 5–25mg/dL). Answers A, B, and D are not related to the adverse effects of this drug.

99. **Answer C is correct.** The parietal lobe deals with sensation. Therefore, anyone with a problem in this area of the brain can have problems with sensation. Answers A, B, and D are not directly associated with this part of the brain.

100. **Answer B is correct.** The nurse must know military times, the Parkland formula, and how to calculate the amount of fluid. The Parkland formula is 4mL × weight in kilograms × percentage of body surface area burned = the amount to be given in 24 hours. The nurse is to give half this amount in the first 8 hours.

    4mL × 54kg × 40 BSA = 8640mL (amount to be given in 24 hours). Give half this amount in the first 8 hours:

    8640 ÷ 2 = 4320

    Answers A, C, and D are incorrect calculations.

101. **Answer D is correct.** A loss of pulses could indicate an occlusion in the graft, requiring surgical intervention. Answers A and C are expected post-operative occurrences with this surgical procedure, which makes them incorrect. Answer B is not classified as hyperthermia, so it is incorrect.

102. **Answer A is correct.** ECG changes associated with hypokalemia are peaked P waves, flat T waves, depressed ST segments, and prominent U waves. Answers B, C, and D are not associated with low potassium levels, so they are incorrect.

103. **Answer D is correct.** The Trendelenburg position is used for surgeries on the lower abdomen and pelvis. This position helps to displace intestines into the upper abdomen and out of the surgical area. Answer A is reserved for vaginal, perineal, and some rectal surgeries. Answer B is used for renal surgery, and answer C is used for back surgery and some rectal surgeries.

104. **Answer C is correct.** The left Sims position is the best position to use in this case because it follows the natural direction of the colon. Answer A places the client on the abdomen, and answers B and D position the client on the back, so they are all incorrect.

105. **Answer B is correct.** Trachea shift differentiates this clinical manifestation as a tension pneumothorax. When a person has a tension pneumothorax, air enters but cannot escape, causing a pressure build-up and a shifting of the great vessels, the heart, and the trachea to the unaffected side. Answer A correlates with a pulmonary contusion, so it is incorrect. Answers C and D are associated with a pneumothorax. This makes them nonspecific for tension pneumothorax and, thus, incorrect.

106. **Answer A is correct.** Abrupt withdrawal of steroids can lead to collapse of the cardiovascular system; therefore, the physician should be notified for drug coverage. The medications in answers B, C, and D would not be as important as the maintenance of the steroids. Answer B is an ace-inhibitor used as an antihypertensive. Answer C is a stool softener, and answer D is a calcium and vitamin agent; thus, all are incorrect.

107. **Answer A is correct.** Accolate should be taken 1 hour before or 2 hours after eating to prevent slow absorption of the drug caused by taking it with meals; therefore, this statement is incorrect and requires further teaching by the nurse. Answers B, C, and D are all true statements regarding this drug and are correct statements made by the client.

108. **Answer C is correct.** The assessment finding that causes the most concern is the finding that could indicate a possible stroke. The right-sided weakness would mean there is a loss of muscular functioning on the side opposite the surgical procedure. Answers A, B, and D might indicate a need for reassessments but not a cause for immediate concern or intervention, so they are incorrect.

109. **Answer A is correct.** Kubler Ross identified five stages of dying as the ways that people cope with death: denial, anger, bargaining, depression, and acceptance. Answer A is the first stage of denial that can be used as a buffer and a way to adapt. Other examples of statements made by the client in this stage are "This can't be true" and "I want another opinion." When dealing with these clients, the nurse needs to use open-ended statements, such as "Tell me more." Answers B, C, and D are a few of the other stages of dying and, thus, are incorrect.

110. **Answer B is correct.** The client with the stroke is the most stable client of the ones listed. The client in answer A would need extensive assessment. Answer C involves a client with a need for psychosocial support and nursing interventions. The client in answer D is a new admission with an infected diverticulum and would be less stable, with more unknowns.

111. **Answer A is correct.** Vitamin K would decrease the effects of Coumadin; therefore the client should be taught to restrict green, leafy vegetables, such as broccoli, cabbage, turnip greens, and lettuce. Answers B, C, and D are food choices that are low in vitamin K, so they are incorrect.

112. **Answer C is correct.** The clinical manifestation of clubbing of the fingers takes time. This indicates that the condition is chronic and not acute, making answer C the correct answer. Answers A, B, and D are all nonspecific for chronicity, so they are incorrect.

113. **Answer A is correct.** Ambulating the client should help to pass the air. The air is used during the surgical procedure to assist in performance of the surgery. Answers B and C would not help, so they are incorrect. Answer D is not necessary or appropriate at this time.

114. **Answer D is correct.** Assessment is not within the role of a nurse's assistant, which makes this the least appropriate of the tasks listed. Answers A, B, and C are all appropriate tasks for an assistant, so they are incorrect.

115. **Answer B is correct.** An NG is inserted to decrease the secretion of pancreatic juices and assist in pain relief. Answer A is incorrect because these clients are held NPO. Clients are placed in semi-Fowler's position, which makes answer C incorrect. Answer D is not appropriate because the wastes are not contaminated.

116. **Answer B is correct.** To test for vagus nerve problems, the nurse uses a tongue blade and depresses the back of the throat to elicit a gag reflex. Other ways to test for damage to the vagus nerve are by having the client say "Ah" while observing for uniform rising of the uvula and the soft palate. The absence of this reflex could indicate damage to the X cranial nerve. Answers A, C, and D are not tested in this manner, so they are incorrect.

117. **Answer B is correct.** The next step after calling for help is to begin chest compressions. Answers A and D are not performed until after answer B, so they are incorrect.

Answer C is not a correct procedure because this technique can be utilized only during a witnessed fibrillation.

118. **Answer D is correct.** Questran works by binding the bile acids in the GI tract and eliminating them, decreasing the itching associated with jaundice. Answers A, B, and C are not how Questran works to decrease itching.

119. **Answer D is correct.** Careful cleansing is necessary to prevent skin breakdown and skin irritation. Answer A is not an intervention used for illeostomies. Clients should avoid high fiber and gas-producing foods, as in answer B. Answer C is incorrect because these clients are not on fluid restriction.

120. **Answer B is correct.** Lomotil's desired effect is to decrease GI motility and the number of diarrhea stools. Answers A and D do not occur with the use of Lomotil. The drug should decrease cramping instead of increasing it, as in answer C.

121. **Answer A is correct.** This procedure prevents air entrance while the chest tube is being removed. Answer B is incorrect because it requires a lack of ventilation for too long of a period and exhalation is not allowed. Answers C and D allow air to enter the thoracic cavity during removal, so they are incorrect.

122. **Answer B is correct.** Tremors are an extrapyramidal side effect that can occur when taking Haldol. Answers A, C, and D are not side or adverse effects of Haldol.

123. **Answer B is correct.** Hemoptysis is a hallmark symptom of a pulmonary embolus. This client's fracture history and other clinical manifestation leads to this conclusion. The clinical manifestations as a group do not correlate with the diagnoses in answers A, C, and D.

124. **Answer B is correct.** A side effect of Aricept is dizziness; therefore, the client should be reminded to move slowly on rising from a lying or sitting position. Answer A is incorrect because it should be taken at bedtime, with no regard to food. Increasing the number of pills can increase the side effects, so answer C is incorrect. Another effect of the drug is bradycardia, making answer D incorrect.

125. **Answer A is correct.** Protein is a necessary component of wound healing. An inadequate amount of protein would correlate with the client's wound not healing properly. Answers B, C, and D do not directly relate to wound healing, so they are incorrect.

126. **Answer C is correct.** The client is exhibiting symptoms of hypoglycemia. The LPN needs to gather information related to the client's diagnosis. The questions in A, B, and D are appropriate. But the priority would be to find out the problem and treat it.

127. **Answer C is correct.** Although all of the tests listed can be used to diagnose an ulcer, an endoscopic exam is the only way to obtain accurate visual evidence. Answers A, B, and D are not as accurate or reliable, which makes them incorrect.

128. **Answer C is correct.** The parathyroid gland can be inadvertently removed or injured with thyroid removal. This can cause hypocalcemia and symptoms of tetany, which requires notifying the physician. Answers A and B are ineffective ways to treat or obtain treatment for hypocalcemia. Answer D would allow the condition to progress, so it is incorrect.

129. **Answer A is correct.** An esophageal gastric balloon tube is inserted for bleeding esophageal varices by placing direct pressure and stopping the bleeding. It cannot be used to prevent fluid build-up in the peritoneal cavity, as in answer B. The bleeding is a venous backup of blood, not an arterial one, so answer C is incorrect. Sclerotherapy is done by endoscopic procedure, so answer D is incorrect.

130. **Answer B is correct.** One of the questions on the CAGE assessment asks whether criticism of one's drinking is annoying. Other questions included in this assessment tool are "Have you ever felt you should cut down on your drinking?", "Have you felt guilty about your drinking?", and "Have you ever had a drink first thing in the morning to steady your nerves or get rid of a hangover?" The answers in A, C, and D are part of the Alcohol Use Disorders Identification Test (AUDIT), so they are incorrect.

131. **Answer D is correct.** The nurse should also ask the client to hold his breath to prevent aspiration, which is the correct procedure for discontinuing an NG tube. Clean gloves should be used for this procedure, making answer A incorrect. The tube should be removed continuously without pause, so answer B is incorrect. An amount of 30mL of air—not normal saline—can be inserted before removal, so answer C is incorrect.

132. **Answer D is correct.** Placing the client in the sitting position for a paracentesis is recommended. The side-lying and head-down positions in answers A, B, and C are not recommended for a paracentesis.

133. **Answer A is correct.** A vagal nerve stimulator is inserted surgically to treat seizure activity. If the device is working properly, the client will notice a voice change when the device is active. Answers B, C, and D don't occur with the operation of the device, which makes them incorrect.

134. **Answer B is correct.** The risk factors for pulmonary complications increase with abdominal surgery for clients over age 40, and for those with prolonged periods in bed. Answer B includes two risk factors, an age of more than 40 years and abdominal surgery in an area under the diaphragm. Answers A and C have one risk factor each, which makes them incorrect. Answer D involves a risk factor for deep vein thrombosis, so it is incorrect.

135. **Answer C is correct.** The hallmark symptom of carbon monoxide poisoning is the cherry-red color. The answers in A, B, and D are not specific to carbon monoxide poisoning.

136. **Answer A is correct.** When a person is in the compensatory stage of shock, the BP remains within normal limits. Increased heart rate occurs that allows cardiac output to be maintained. The client also exhibits confusion and cold and clammy skin. Answer B correlates with the progressive stage of shock, so it is incorrect. Answers C and D both indicate that the client is past compensation, so they are incorrect.

137. **Answer A is correct.** Epinephrine, antihistamines, and resuscitation equipment should be available in case of a reaction to penicillin. Epinephrine is used for allergic reactions. Answer B is an antianxiety agent, and answer D is used for high blood pressure. The anti-ulcer agent in answer C is not used for allergic reactions.

138. Answer A is correct. The person with benign prostatic hypertrophy (BPH) has clinical manifestations that are caused by the obstruction. Symptoms of BPH include frequency of urination, difficulty in starting the urine flow, and a frequent urge to void. If the client develops a urinary tract infection, the urine might smell, but it is not directly related to the BPH, so answer B is incorrect. Urinary retention also occurs, making answer C incorrect. Pain with urination is not a symptom of BPH, so answer D is incorrect.

139. Answer D is correct. Shortness of breath signifies an adverse reaction to the transplant procedure. Answers A and C can occur with the transplant process but do not signify an adverse reaction. Answer B is a normal finding with the bone marrow transplant.

140. Answer D is correct. The palms of the hands and soles of the feet are areas in dark-skinned clients where skin cancer is more likely to develop because of the decreased pigmentation found in these areas. Answers A, B, and C are areas where high pigmentation occurs and, therefore, are less likely to show signs of cancer.

141. Answer B is correct. It is important to clamp the tube while auscultating because the sound from the suction interferes with the auscultation process. Answer A is one measure used to determine whether NG is in the stomach, but not to assess bowel sounds. Answers C and D are not the correct procedure for assessment of bowel sounds, so they are incorrect.

142. Answer A is correct. A culture result that shows minimal bacteria is a favorable outcome. Answers B, C, and D are abnormal and negative outcomes, so they are incorrect.

143. Answer B is correct. Phenergan is used for prevention and treatment of nausea and vomiting, sedation, adjunct to pain and anesthesia medications, and allergic reactions. Answers A, C, and D are not desired effects of the drug Phenergan, which makes them incorrect.

144. Answer C is correct. Erythromycin is the only drug listed that is not penicillin based. Answers A, B, and D are in the same family as penicillin, so they are not as safe to administer, which makes them incorrect.

145. Answer A is correct. Normal potassium is 3.5–5.0. Severe life-threatening complications can occur with hyperkalemia, requiring the physician to be notified of any abnormality. Answers B, C, and D are normal results, which makes them incorrect.

146. Answer C is correct. Pulling the pinna down and back is correct for administering ear drops to a child because the child's ear canal is short and straight. The pinna is pulled up and back for adults. Answers A and B are improper technique and would make it harder for the drops to be administered. Answer D would be incorrect because this is not a necessary part of administering ear drops, even though irrigation might be done at times to cleanse the ear for assessment.

147. Answer C is correct. The rule of nines is a way to estimate the percentage of body surface area burned (see the following figure). The calculation would be 4.5% for the face and neck, 9% for the entire arm, and 18% for the entire anterior chest, which would be 31.5%, or approximately 32%. Answers A, B, and D are not correctly calculated sums of the burned areas.

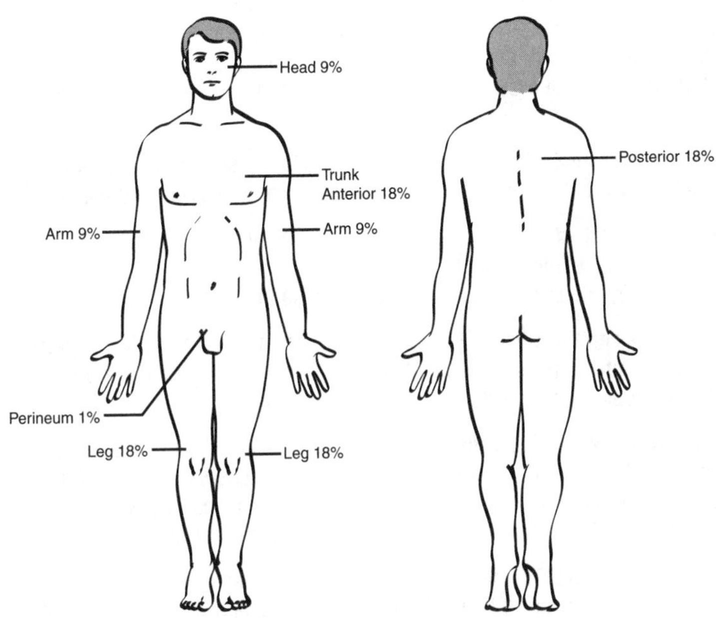

148. Answer A is correct. Acute renal failure can occur when the MAP drops below 80. The mean arterial pressures in answers B, C, and D are too low to allow proper functioning of the kidney, which makes these answers incorrect.

149. Answer C is correct. An increase in head growth is used as a diagnostic gauge for hydrocephalus. Answers A and B can also occur with hydrocephalus, but they are not as specific or diagnostic as head circumference, so they are incorrect. Answer D is not related to hydrocephalus, so it is incorrect.

150. Answer C is correct. Two-thirds of the clients with chronic lymphocytic leukemia are older than 60 years of age at diagnosis. Answers A, B, and D do not occur more often in the elderly, so they are incorrect.

151. Answer C is correct. The oxygen saturation is the best indicator of respiratory status because it is more objective. Answers A, B, and D are subjective and nonspecific, so they are incorrect.

152. Answer B is correct. Because of the moisturized air inhaled with swimming, it is an ideal sport for children with respiratory conditions, so this is correct. Answers A, C, and D could trigger an attack with asthma and would not be recommended.

153. **Answer A is correct.** Making sure that the tube is in the right location is an important first step. Clients should be positioned with the head elevated, the medication should be administered slowly, and the NG tube should be clamped for 20-30 minutes after medication administration; therefore, options B, C, and D are incorrect.

154. **Answer D is correct.** A newborn who has not passed meconium in the first 24 hours could have cystic fibrosis. This is due to the thick secretions preventing passage of the meconium, resulting in obstruction of the bowel. Answers A and B are both cardiovascular problems that are not associated with meconium passage, so these are incorrect. Answer C is not associated with meconium and is evidenced by a yellow skin tone and an elevated serum bilirubin level.

155. **Answer A is correct.** Normal sodium is 135–145mEq, so this is a low blood level that should be reported. Answers B, C, and D are normal or near-normal readings.

156. **Answer C is correct.** The correct calculation is 1.5 mL, which is calculated as follows:
75 mg?= 2mL/100mg= 150/100= 1.5 mL
Answers A, B, and D are incorrect calculations, so they are wrong.

157. **Answer C is correct.** Obstruction of the subclavian artery would show a decrease in radial heart rate on the side of the obstruction. Answers A, B, and D are related to neurological problems or deficits, which makes them incorrect.

158. **Answer D is correct.** Everyone should wear sunscreen when going outside, to protect them from the ultraviolet exposure. Answer A is not necessary. Answer C is incorrect because only moles that are suspicious require removal and biopsy. Answer B is the period of day when the sun rays are most detrimental to the skin.

159. **Answer B is correct.** The desired dose is 75mg. The dose on hand is 100mg in 2mL, making the correct dose 1.5mL. The answers in A, C, and D are incorrect calculations.

160. **Answer B is correct.** Adding baby oil to the client's bathwater could assist in soothing the itching. Answers A, C, and D would increase dryness and worsen the skin itching.

161. **Answer C is correct.** If a client has a curvature of less than 20°, it is considered mild, with no treatment required. If after reevaluation the curve is progressing, treatment might be necessary. Answer A and B are done with curvatures greater than 20°, so they are incorrect. Answer D might be required with curvatures greater than 40°, which makes it incorrect.

162. **Answer A is correct.** The recommended procedure is to use tweezers to remove the tick, using a slow steady force, and to disinfect the area before and after doing so. Answers B, C, and D are not the correct procedure to safely remove a tick.

163. **Answer A is correct.** Standard precautions require that goggles, a gown, and gloves be worn when there is a danger of contamination by splashing. Answers B and C are not adequate for the suctioning procedure. A gown is not an adequate precaution and shoe covers are not required, making answer D incorrect.

164. **Answer D is correct.** Abnormal grieving occurs when someone acts as if nothing has happened. Answers A, B, and C are normal parts of the grieving process, so they are incorrect.

165. **Answer B is correct.** The misuse and overuse of laxatives can cause serious fluid and electrolyte imbalances in the elderly, so this is the correct choice. Answers A and D

can be normal occurrences associated with the physiological changes of aging. Answer C is an incorrect response because the client states that increased fluid intake is not a new occurrence.

166. **Answer B is correct.** The normal sodium is 135–145mEq/L. When hypernatremia occurs, the client can exhibit manic and hyperactivity behaviors. Other symptoms of increased sodium include restlessness, twitching, seizures, and hyperreflexia. Answers A, and C are not symptoms of high sodium levels, so they are incorrect. Answer D is associated with low sodium levels.

167. **Answer A is correct.** Clients with congestive heart failure are usually treated with a diuretic, such as Lasix and Digoxin. Answer B is a hematologic, and answer C is an anticoagulant. Skelaxin, in answer D, is a muscle relaxer. These drugs are not used to decrease fluid or improve cardiac output necessary for the treatment of congestive heart failure, so they are incorrect.

168. **Answer A is correct.** The usual dosage of atropine as a preoperative medication is 0.4–0.6mg. The ordered dosage is too high, so the order requires clarification. Answer B is incorrect because of the ordered dosage. Answers C and D will be required, but not before getting a correct dosage order.

169. **Answer B is correct.** Nitroglycerin is contraindicated with the use of Viagra. The medications in B, C, and D have no adverse effects when administered with heparin or nitroglycerin, so they are incorrect.

170. **Answer B is correct.** There will be a sensation of pulling during the aspiration. This feeling is painful. Answer A is incorrect because the position is inappropriate for bone marrow aspiration. Answer D is not a required preprocedure diet change. Although the client might receive a local anesthetic and/or pain medication, amnesic medications such as Versed are not usually administered, so answer C is incorrect.

171. **Answer C is correct.** It is most important to identify the pulses preoperatively to have a baseline for post-operative evaluation. Answers A, B, and D are not priorities for the client preoperatively.

172. **Answer A is correct.** Excessive vagal stimulation causes bradycardia because of parasympathetic stimulation. Answers B, C, and D are not arrhythmias associated with suctioning, so they are incorrect.

173. **Answer C is correct.** This PO_2 level is required for the client to receive financial assistance from Medicare and Medicaid services. The answers in A, B, and D are either above or below the level of PO_2 requirement for reimbursement by Medicare and Medicaid services, so they are incorrect.

174. **Answer D is correct.** Dehydration is associated with C difficile due to the diarrhea and temperature elevation. Moist mucous membranes would indicate adequate hydration showing an improved patient outcome. Answers A, B, and D are manifestations of the condition and do not indicate an improvement, so they are incorrect.

175. **Answer D is correct.** Proper procedure is to empty the bladder and save the urine at the end of the collection period. Clients should void and discard the urine at the beginning of the collection period so answer A is incorrect. Answer B is utilized when collecting a mid stream (clean catch) specimen so it is incorrect. The urine doesn't have to be collected in a sterile container, therefore C is incorrect.

176. **Answer A is correct.** The reasons for these exercises are to restore movement, prevent stiffening of the shoulder area, and improve the client's muscle power. Answer B is not prevented by the exercises utilized. Although the answers in C and D might have a positive outcome from performing these exercises, they are not the primary reason the exercises are done.

177. **Answer A is correct.** The best effect of the medications occurs if given within 2–3 days of illness with the influenza virus. Answers B, C, and D are not within the allotted time period for the drugs to be effective in eliminating the influenza virus.

178. **Answer A is correct.** Depakote can cause neural tube defects in pregnant women, so the client should be on birth control or should not take this drug. A client's career, exercise level, and diet will not affect the dose or prescription for this drug, so answers B, C, and D are incorrect.

179. **Answer A is correct.** The hardening or induration could indicate a positive test result. A reaction of 0–4mm is not significant. A larger-size induration could indicate exposure to tuberculosis. Answers B, C, and D without induration are nonsignificant, so they are incorrect.

180. **Answer D is correct.** A client with an enlarged spleen has an increased risk for rupture; therefore, heavy lifting would be contraindicated. Answers A, B, and C would not be a cause for a concern because of the enlarged spleen.

181. **Answer A is correct.** The vaccine is made from eggs, so clients with allergies to eggs should not receive the vaccine. Shellfish and iodine are associated with the dye used for intravenous pyelograms, so answers B and C are incorrect. An allergy to pork, as in answer D, does not indicate a need to avoid the influenza virus.

182. **Answer A is correct.** People of the Islam religion are prohibited from eating foods with gelatin. They also must avoid pork, alcohol products and beverages, and animal shortening. Answers B, C, and D would all be appropriate because they can be included in the diet of people of the Islam religion.

183. **Answer A is correct.** The client, especially a child, could experience a febrile reaction. This makes hypothermia or a decreased temperature, as in answer B, incorrect. Another side effect is soreness at the injection site. A generalized rash and difficulty breathing are not side effects of the vaccine; therefore, answers C and D are incorrect.

184. **Answer D is correct.** The highest amount of calcium is in this answer. The client also needs to know that calcium in combination with high fiber and caffeine decreases the absorption; therefore, answers A, B, and C are incorrect.

185. **Answer C is correct.** The obstruction decreases the elimination of bile causing the collection of bilirubin in the blood instead of it being removed by the urinary and Gastrointestinal system. This leads to a lack of normal color of the stool and urine. Answers A, B, and D do not occur with obstructive jaundice so they are incorrect.

186. **Answer A is correct.** Hematocrit levels can be elevated with hypovolemia caused by fluid loss. Answers B, C, and D are all normal levels. Potassium (normal 3.5–5.3mEq/L) levels would be decreased with hypovolemia; BUN (normal 5–20mg/dL) and specific gravity (1.016–1.022) levels would be elevated with hypovolemia.

187. **Answer D is correct.** The dose to administer is 2mL, which is calculated as follows: 60 mg?= 1 mL/30 mg=60/30 = 2.0 mL
Answers A, B, and C are incorrect calculations.

188. **Answer D is correct.** Rales would indicate lung congestion and the need for follow-up. Answers A, B, and C are normal health-related changes with aging.

189. **Answer A is correct.** Myopia is nearsightedness due to the cornea being too steep or the eye being too long. This causes light to come into focus in front of the retina, resulting in blurred distant vision. Answer B is normal vision. Farsightedness is blurred near and often distant vision, as in answer C. Astigmatism occurs when light rays focus in multiple points, causing blurred vision not related to near or far vision; thus, answer D is incorrect.

190. **Answer D is correct.** The nurse observes sluggishness and lethargy as early indications of increased ICP in a client. A change in vital signs and papillary changes, as in answers A, B, and C, are late signs of increased ICP.

191. **Answer B is correct.** There is an increased risk for kidney stones with topiramate (Topamax) use, so fluids are an important part of problem prevention. The drug is not required to be taken with meals or at bedtime, so answers A and D are incorrect. Answer C is not required with the use of this medication.

192. **Answer C is correct.** The nurse responds appropriately by answering the question honestly and attempting to assess for more information that will allow the person to ventilate feelings. Answer A is an appropriate response but is not as appropriate as C. Answers B and D are nontherapeutic communication techniques.

193. **Answer B is correct.** The LPN should be assigned the client requiring a dressing change. This client is the one most correlated to the LPN's scope of practice. The clients described in answer options A and D are more appropriate to the RN. The nursing assistant should care for the client needing ambulatory assistance as described in answer C because this relates to the nurses assistants standards and practices.

194. **Answer C is correct.** Testing the drainage for glucose could indicate the presence of cerebrospinal fluid, making this the best initial action. The next action would be to notify the physician, as in answer B. Answers A and D would be contraindicated, so they are incorrect.

195. **Answer B is correct.** The aspirate of gastric content should be green, brown, clear, or colorless, with a gastric pH between 1 and 5. Answer A would most likely be from the lungs, so it is incorrect. Answers C and D are not as accurate as color and pH for confirming gastric location, so they are incorrect.

196. **Answer D is correct.** A slight elevation in temperature would be expected from surgical intervention and would not be a cause for concern. Answers A, B, and C could indicate a progressing complication, so they are incorrect.

197. **Answer D is correct.** Pork has more thiamine than beef, fish, or chicken, which makes answers A, B, and C incorrect.

198. **Answer D is correct.** Activity, exercise, and repositioning the client will increase circulation and improve tissue perfusion. Answer A will help to identify problem areas but will not improve the perfusion of the tissue. Answer B should be avoided because it could increase the damage if trauma was present. Answer C should be done to prevent irritation of the skin, but this action does not improve perfusion.

199. **Answer C is correct.** These clients need a balanced nutritional diet with protein and vitamin C, making it the most balanced meal plan. Answers A and B both lack protein, which is very important in maintaining a positive nitrogen balance. Answer D has protein but is lacking in vitamins.

200. **Answer D is correct.** The statement reflects the use of denial as a means of coping with the illness. Answers A, B, and C are defense mechanisms not reflected by the statement.

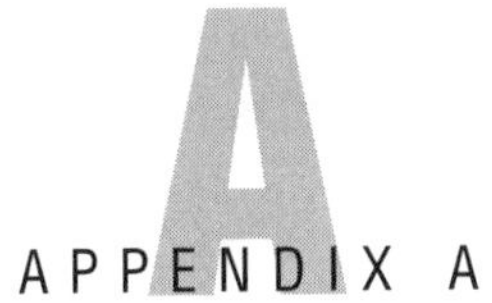

APPENDIX A

Things You Forgot

Throughout this book, we have tried to simplify your preparation for the NCLEX® exam. This appendix includes information you have learned during nursing school but might have forgotten.

Therapeutic Drug Levels

Therapeutic drug levels that are important for the nurse to remember when taking the NCLEX® exam include:

- Digoxin: 0.5–2.0 ng/mL
- Lithium: 0.8-1.2 mEq/L* (NIH value)
- Dilantin: 10–20 mcg/mL
- Theophylline: 10–20 mcg/mL

NOTE

*The therapeutic range for lithium may vary slightly according to laboratory methods used. Lithium toxicity occurs at levels greater than 1.5 mEq/L.

Vital Signs

Normal ranges for the vital signs of the adult and the newborn:

- Adult heart rate: 80–100 beats per minute
- Newborn heart rate: 100–180 beats per minute
- Adult respiratory rate: 12–20 respirations per minute
- Newborn respiratory rate: 30–60 respirations per minute
- Adult blood pressure: systolic pressure = 110–120 mm Hg; diastolic pressure = 60–90 mm Hg

- Newborn blood pressure: systolic pressure = 65 mm Hg; diastolic pressure = 41 mm Hg
- Temperature: 98.6° F plus or minus one degree

Intrapartal Normal Values

Here are some of the normal ranges to remember when caring for the client during the intrapartal period:

- Fetal heart rate: 120–160 beats per minute
- Variability: 6–10 beats per minute
- Contractions:
  - Frequency of contractions: every 2–5 minutes
  - Duration of contractions: less than 90 seconds
  - Intensity of contractions: less than 100 mmHg

Anticoagulant Therapy

The nurse should be familiar with the tests ordered for the client receiving anticoagulant therapy and for the control levels. Remember that the therapeutic range is 1.5–2 times the control:

- Coumadin (sodium warfarin) PT/Protime: 12–20 seconds.
- International normalizing ratio (INR): 2–3.
- The antidote for sodium warfarin is vitamin K.

NOTE

Lab values may vary according to methods used.

- Heparin and heparin derivatives partial thromboplastin time (PTT): 30–60 seconds.
- The antidote for heparin is protamine sulfate.

TABLE A.1 *Continued*

Diseases Being Treated	Foods to Include	Foods to Avoid
Renal transplantation	Meats, dairy products, breads and starches, vegetables, and sweets.	Eggs, organ meats, fried or fattyfood, foods containing salt, driedfoods, salt substitutes, and fruits.

Immunization Schedule

It is important for the nurse to be aware of the recommended immunization schedule for various age groups. Figure A.1 is a recommended schedule for childhood and adolescent immunizations. Figure A.2 is a recommended schedule for adult immunizations.

Recommended Childhood and Adolescent Immunization Schedule

CDC

UNITED STATES • 2006

Vaccine ▼ / Age ▶	Birth	1 month	2 months	4 months	6 months	12 months	15 months	18 months	24 months	4–6 years	11–12 years	13–14 years	15 years	16–18 years
Hepatitis B	HepB	HepB		*HepB*[1]		HepB					HepB Series			
Diphtheria, Tetanus, Pertussis			DTaP	DTaP	DTaP		DTaP			DTaP	Tdap		Tdap	
Haemophilus influenzae type b			Hib	Hib	*Hib*[3]	Hib								
Inactivated Poliovirus			IPV	IPV		IPV				IPV				
Measles, Mumps, Rubella						MMR				MMR		MMR		
Varicella							Varicella				Varicella			
Meningococcal							Vaccines within broken line are for selected populations		MPSV4		MCV4		MCV4 MCV4	
Pneumococcal			PCV	PCV	PCV	PCV			PCV		PPV			
Influenza						Influenza (Yearly)					Influenza (Yearly)			
Hepatitis A										HepA Series				

This schedule indicates the recommended ages for routine administration of currently licensed childhood vaccines, as of December 1, 2005, for children through age 18 years. Any dose not administered at the recommended age should be administered at any subsequent visit when indicated and feasible. ▇ Indicates age groups that warrant special effort to administer those vaccines not previously administered. Additional vaccines may be licensed and recommended during the year. Licensed combination vaccines may be used whenever any components of the combination are indicated and other components of the vaccine are not contraindicated and if approved by the Food and Drug Administration for that dose of the series. Providers should consult the respective ACIP statement for detailed recommendations. Clinically significant adverse events that follow immunization should be reported to the Vaccine Adverse Event Reporting System (VAERS). Guidance about how to obtain and complete a VAERS form is available at www.vaers.hhs.gov or by telephone, 800-822-7967.

Range of recommended ages | Catch-up immunization | 11–12 year old assessment

FIGURE A.1 Recommended childhood and adolescent immunization schedule.

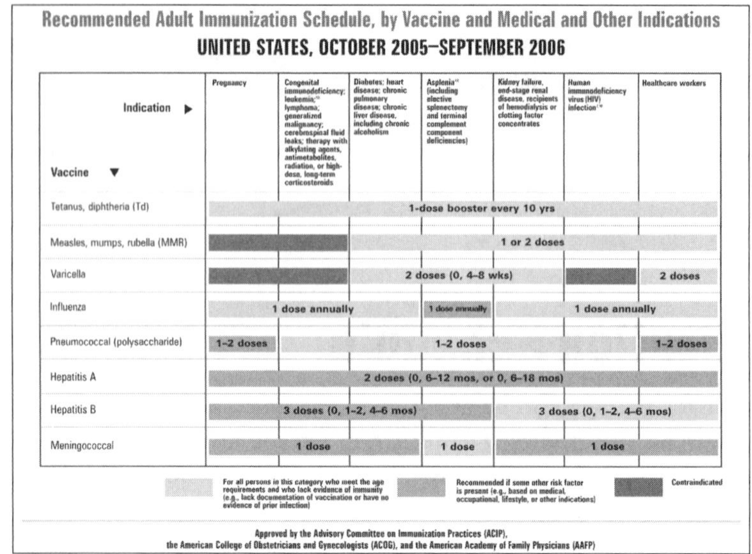

Recommended Adult Immunization Schedule, by Vaccine and Medical and Other Indications
UNITED STATES, OCTOBER 2005–SEPTEMBER 2006

Indication ▶ / Vaccine ▼	Pregnancy	Congenital immunodeficiency; leukemia; lymphoma; generalized malignancy; cerebrospinal fluid leaks; therapy with alkylating agents, antimetabolites, radiation, or high-dose, long-term corticosteroids	Diabetes; heart disease; chronic pulmonary disease; chronic liver disease, including chronic alcoholism	Asplenia (including elective splenectomy and terminal complement component deficiencies)	Kidney failure, end-stage renal disease, recipients of hemodialysis or clotting factor concentrates	Human immunodeficiency virus (HIV) infection	Healthcare workers
Tetanus, diphtheria (Td)	1-dose booster every 10 yrs						
Measles, mumps, rubella (MMR)			1 or 2 doses				
Varicella			2 doses (0, 4–8 wks)				2 doses
Influenza	1 dose annually			1 dose annually	1 dose annually		
Pneumococcal (polysaccharide)	1–2 doses	1–2 doses					1–2 doses
Hepatitis A	2 doses (0, 6–12 mos, or 0, 6–18 mos)						
Hepatitis B	3 doses (0, 1–2, 4–6 mos)				3 doses (0, 1–2, 4–6 mos)		
Meningococcal	1 dose			1 dose	1 dose		

For all persons in this category who meet the age requirements and who lack evidence of immunity (e.g., lack documentation of vaccination or have no evidence of prior infection)

Recommended if some other risk factor is present (e.g., based on medical, occupational, lifestyle, or other indications)

Contraindicated

Approved by the Advisory Committee on Immunization Practices (ACIP), the American College of Obstetricians and Gynecologists (ACOG), and the American Academy of Family Physicians (AAFP)

FIGURE A.2 Recommended adult immunization schedule.

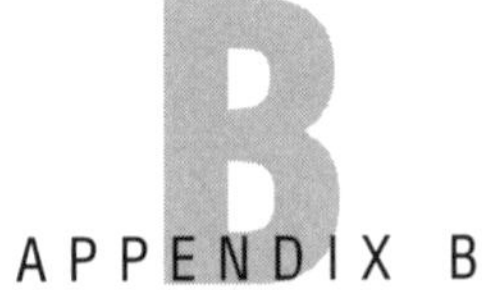

APPENDIX B

Need to Know More?

Pharmacology

http://www.druginfonet.com

http://www.fda.gov/search/databases.html

http://www.globalrph.com

http://www.mosbysdrugconsult.com

http://www.needymeds.com

http://www.nlm.nih.gov/medlineplus

http://www.nursespdr.com

http://www.nursespdr.com

Deglin, J., and Vallerand, A., *Davis Drug Guide for Nurses*. Philadelphia: F.A. Davis, 2009.

Care of the Client with Respiratory Disorders

http://www.aaaai.org—The website for the American Academy of Allergy, Asthma, and Immunology

http://www.cdc.gov—The website for the Centers for Disease Control and Prevention

http://www.lungusa.org—The website for the American Lung Association

Ignatavicius, D., and Workman, S. *Medical Surgical Nursing: Critical Thinking for Collaborative Care.* 5th ed. Philadelphia: Elsevier, 2007.

Brunner, L., and Suddarth, D. *Textbook of Medical Surgical Nursing*. 12th ed. Philadelphia: Lippincott Williams & Wilkins, 2009.

LeMone, P., and Burke, K. in *Medical Surgical Nursing: Critical Thinking in Client Care.* 4th ed. Upper Saddle River, NJ: Pearson Prentice Hall, 2008.

Lewis, S., Heitkemper, M., Dirksen, S., Obrien, P., and Bucher, L. *Medical Surgical Nursing: Assessment and Management of Clinical Problems.* 7th ed. Philadelphia: Elsevier, 2007.

Lehne, R. *Pharmacology for Nursing Care.* 7th ed. Philadelphia: Elsevier, 2009.

Care of the Client with Genitourinary Disorders

http://www.kidney.org—The website for the National Kidney Foundation

http://www.pkd.cure.org—The website for the Polycystic Kidney Disease Foundation

Ignatavicius, D., and Workman, S. *Medical Surgical Nursing: Critical Thinking for Collaborative Care.* 5th ed. Philadelphia: Elsevier, 2007.

Brunner, L., and Suddarth, D. *Textbook of Medical Surgical Nursing.* 12th ed. Philadelphia: Lippincott Williams & Wilkins, 2009.

LeMone, P., and Burke, K. in *Medical Surgical Nursing: Critical Thinking in Client Care.* 4th ed. Upper Saddle River, NJ: Pearson Prentice Hall, 2008.

Lewis, S., Heitkemper, M., Dirksen, S., Obrien, P., and Bucher, L. *Medical Surgical Nursing: Assessment and Management of Clinical Problems.* 7th ed. Philadelphia: Elsevier, 2007.

Lehne, R. *Pharmacology for Nursing Care.* 7th ed. Philadelphia: Elsevier, 2009.

Care of the Client with Hematological Disorders

http://www.americanhs.org—The website for the American Hemochromatosis Society

http://www.aplastic.org—The website for the Aplastic Anemia and MDS International Foundation

http://www.emedicine.com/med/topic3387.htm

http://www.hemophilia.org—The website for the National Hemophilia Foundation

http://www.marrow.org

http://www.nci.nih.gov—The website for the National Cancer Institute Information Center

http://www.ons.org—The website for the Oncology Nursing Society

http://www.sicklecelldisease.org—The website for the Sickle Cell Disease Association of America, Inc.

Brunner, L., and Suddarth, D. *Textbook of Medical Surgical Nursing*. 12th ed. Philadelphia: Lippincott Williams & Wilkins, 2009.

Lewis, S., Heitkemper, M., Dirksen, S., O'Brien, P., and Bucher, L. *Medical Surgical Nursing: Assessment and Management of Clinical Problems.* 7th ed. Philadelphia: Elsevier, 2007.

Care of the Client with Fluid and Electrolytes and Acid/Base Balance

http://www.enursescribe.com

http://www.umed.utah.edu/ms2/renal

Ignatavicius, D., and Workman, S. *Medical Surgical Nursing: Critical Thinking for Collaborative Care.* 5th ed. Philadelphia: Elsevier, 2007.

Brunner, L., and Suddarth, D. *Textbook of Medical Surgical Nursing*. 12th ed. Philadelphia: Lippincott Williams & Wilkins, 2009.

Care of the Client with Burns

Ignatavicius, D., and Workman, S. *Medical Surgical Nursing: Critical Thinking for Collaborative Care.* 5th ed. Philadelphia: Elsevier, 2007.

Brunner, L., and Suddarth, D. *Textbook of Medical Surgical Nursing*. 12th ed. Philadelphia: Lippincott Williams & Wilkins, 2009.

LeMone, P., and Burke, K. in *Medical Surgical Nursing: Critical Thinking in Client Care.* 4th ed. Upper Saddle River, NJ: Pearson Prentice Hall, 2008.

Lewis, S., Heitkemper, M., Dirksen, S., Obrien, P., and Bucher, L. *Medical Surgical Nursing: Assessment and Management of Clinical Problems.* 7th ed. Philadelphia: Elsevier, 2007.

Lehne, R. *Pharmacology for Nursing Care.* 7th ed. Philadelphia: Elsevier, 2009.

Care of the Client with Sensory Disorders

http://www.afb.org—The website for the American Foundation for the Blind

http://www.loc.gov.nis—The website for the National Library Services for the Blind and Physically Handicapped

Ignatavicius, D., and Workman, S. *Medical Surgical Nursing: Critical Thinking for Collaborative Care.* 5th ed. Philadelphia: Elsevier, 2007.

Brunner, L., and Suddarth, D. *Textbook of Medical Surgical Nursing.* 12th ed. Philadelphia: Lippincott Williams & Wilkins, 2009.

LeMone, P., and Burke, K. in *Medical Surgical Nursing: Critical Thinking in Client Care.* 4th ed. Upper Saddle River, NJ: Pearson Prentice Hall, 2008.

Lewis, S., Heitkemper, M., Dirksen, S., Obrien, P., and Bucher, L. *Medical Surgical Nursing: Assessment and Management of Clinical Problems.* 7th ed. Philadelphia: Elsevier, 2007.

Lehne, R. *Pharmacology for Nursing Care.* 7th ed. Philadelphia: Elsevier, 2009.

Care of the Client with Neoplastic Disorders

http://www.abta.org—The website for the American Brain Tumor Association

http://www.cancer.gov—The website for the National Cancer Institute

http://www.komen.org—The website for the Susan G. Komen Breast Cancer Foundation

http://www.leukemia.org

http://www.leukemia-research.org

http://www.ons.org—The website for the Oncology Nursing Society

http://www.skincancer.org—The website for the Skin Cancer Foundation

Ignatavicius, D., and Workman, S. *Medical Surgical Nursing: Critical Thinking for Collaborative Care.* 5th ed. Philadelphia: Elsevier, 2007.

Brunner, L., and Suddarth, D. *Textbook of Medical Surgical Nursing.* 12th ed. Philadelphia: Lippincott Williams & Wilkins, 2009.

Care of the Client with Gastrointestinal Disorders

http://www.asge.org—The website for the American Society for Gastrointestinal Endoscopy

http://www.ccfa.org—The website for the Crohn's and Colitis Foundation

http://www.cdc.gov—The website for the Centers for Disease Control and Prevention

http://www.uoaa.org—The website for the United Ostomy Association

Brunner, L., and Suddarth, D. *Textbook of Medical Surgical Nursing.* 12th ed. Philadelphia: Lippincott Williams & Wilkins, 2009.

Ignatavicius, D., and Workman, S. *Medical Surgical Nursing: Critical Thinking for Collaborative Care.* 5th ed. Philadelphia: Elsevier, 2007.

Lewis, S., Heitkemper, M., Dirksen, S., O'Brien, P., and Bucher, L. *Medical Surgical Nursing: Assessment and Management of Clinical Problems.* 7th ed. Philadelphia: Elsevier, 2007.

Lemone, P., and Burke, K. *Medical-Surgical Nursing Critical Thinking in Client Care.* 4th ed. Upper Saddle River, NJ: Pearson Prentice Hall, 2008.

Care of the Client with Musculoskeletal and Connective Tissue Disorder

http://www.amputee-coalition.org—The website for the Amputee Coalition of America

http://www.niams.nih.gov—The website for the National Institute of Arthritis and Musculoskeletal and Skin Diseases

http://www.nof.org—The website for the National Osteoporosis Foundation

http://www.orthonurse.org—The website for the National Association of Orthopaedic Nurses

Ignatavicius, D., and Workman, S. *Medical Surgical Nursing: Critical Thinking for Collaborative Care.* 5th ed. Philadelphia: Elsevier, 2007.

Lewis, S., Heitkemper, M., Dirksen, S., O'Brien, P., and Bucher, L. *Medical Surgical Nursing: Assessment and Management of Clinical Problems.* 7th ed. Philadelphia: Elsevier, 2007.

Lemone, P., Burke, K. *Medical-Surgical Nursing Critical Thinking in Client Care*. 4th ed. Upper Saddle River, NJ: Pearson Prentice Hall, 2008.

Care of the Client with Endocrine Disorders

http://www.cdc.gov/diabetes—The website for the Centers for Disease Control and Prevention

http://www.diabetes.org—The website for the American Diabetes Association

http://www.diabetesnet.com—The website for the American Association of Diabetes Educators

http://www.eatright.org—The website for the American Dietetic Association

http://www.endo-society.org—The website for the National Endocrine Society

http://www.medhelp.org/nadf—The website for the National Adrenal Disease Foundation

http://www.niddk.nih.gov—The website for the National Diabetes Clearing House

http://www.pancreasfoundation.org—The website for the National Pancreas Foundation

http://www.thyroid.org—The website for the American Thyroid Association

Ignatavicius, D., and Workman, S. *Medical Surgical Nursing: Critical Thinking for Collaborative Care*. 5th ed. Philadelphia: Elsevier, 2007.

Brunner, L., and Suddarth, D. *Textbook of Medical Surgical Nursing*. 12th ed. Philadelphia: Lippincott Williams & Wilkins, 2009.

Care of the Client with Cardiac Disorders

http://www.americanheart.org—The website for the American Heart Association

http://www.nursebeat.com—The website for the *Nurse Beat: Cardiac Nursing Electronic Journal*

Ignatavicius, D., and Workman, S. *Medical Surgical Nursing: Critical Thinking for Collaborative Care*. 5th ed. Philadelphia: Elsevier, 2007.

Brunner, L., and Suddarth, D. *Textbook of Medical Surgical Nursing*. 12th ed. Philadelphia: Lippincott Williams & Wilkins, 2009.

Woods, A. "An ACE Up Your Sleeve and an ARB in Your Back Pocket," *Nursing Made Incredibly Easy*, Sept.–Oct. 2003, 36–42.

Care of the Client with Neurological Disorders

http://www.apdaparkinson.com—The website for the American Parkinson's Disease Association

http://www.biausa.org—The website for the Brain Injury Association

http://www.epilepsyfoundation.org—The website for the Epilepsy Foundation

http://www.gbs-cidp.org—The website for the Guillain-Barré Syndrome Foundation

http://www.nmss.org—The website for the National Multiple Sclerosis Society

http://www.parkinson.org—The website for the National Parkinson's Foundation

http://www.stroke.org—The website for the American Stroke Association

Ignatavicius, D., and Workman, S. *Medical Surgical Nursing: Critical Thinking for Collaborative Care.* 5th ed. Philadelphia: Elsevier, 2007.

Lewis, S., Heitkemper, M., Dirksen, S., O'Brien, P., and Bucher, L. *Medical Surgical Nursing: Assessment and Management of Clinical Problems.* 7th ed. Philadelphia: Elsevier, 2007.

Lemone, P., Burke, K. *Medical-Surgical Nursing Critical Thinking in Client Care.* 4th ed. Upper Saddle River, NJ: Pearson Prentice Hall, 2008.

Brunner, L., and Suddarth, D. *Textbook of Medical Surgical Nursing.* 12th ed. Philadelphia: Lippincott Williams & Wilkins, 2009.

Care of the Client with Psychiatric Disorders

http://www.nami.org—The website for the National Alliance on Mental Illness

Kneisl, C., and Trigoboff, E. *Contemporary Psychiatric Mental Health Nursing.* 2nd ed. Upper Saddle River, NJ: Pearson Prentice Hall, 2009.

Townsend, M. *Essentials of Psychiatric Mental Health Nursing.* 4th ed. Philadelphia: F.A. Davis, 2008.

Lehne, R. *Pharmacology for Nursing Care.* 7th ed. Philadelphia: Elsevier, 2009.

Ball, J., and Bindler, R. *Pediatric Nursing: Caring for Children.* 4th ed. Upper Saddle River, NJ: Pearson Prentice Hall, 2008.

Care of the Client with Maternal-Newborn Care

Lowdermilk, D., et al. (eds.). *Maternity and Women's Health Care. 8th ed.* St. Louis: C.V. Mosby, 2000.

McKinney, E. et al. (eds.). *Maternal-Child Nursing. 2nd ed.* St. Louis: W.B. Saunders, 2005.

Wong, D. et al. (eds.). *Maternal-Child Nursing Care. 3rd ed.* St. Louis: C.V. Mosby, 2002.

Care of the Pediatric Client

Hockenberry, M., and Wilson, D. *Wong's Essentials of Pediatric Nursing.* 8th ed. St. Louis: Elsevier, 2009.

Ball, J., and Bindler, R. *Pediatric Nursing: Caring for Children.* 4th ed. Upper Saddle River, NJ: Pearson Prentice Hall, 2008.

www.aaai.org—American Academy of Allergy, Asthma, and Immunology

www.cdc.gov—Centers for Disease Control

www.lungusa.org—The American Lung Association

www.aafp.org—The American Academy of Family Practice

www.pathguy.com—Dr. Ed Friedlander, pathologist

www.cff.org—Cystic Fibrosis Foundation

www.candlelighters.org—Candlelighters Childhood Cancer Foundation

Cultural Practices Influencing Nursing Care

Brunner, L., and Suddarth, D. *Textbook of Medical Surgical Nursing.* 12th ed. Philadelphia: Lippincott Williams & Wilkins, 2009.

Ignatavicius, D., and Workman, S. *Medical Surgical Nursing: Critical Thinking for Collaborative Care.* 5th ed. Philadelphia: Elsevier, 2007.

Potter, P., and Perry, A. *Fundamentals of Nursing. 6th ed.* St. Louis: C.V. Mosby, 2005.

Legal Issues in Nursing Practice

Tappen, R. *Nursing Leadership and Management: Concepts and Practice. 5th ed.* Philadelphia: F.A. Davis, 2004.

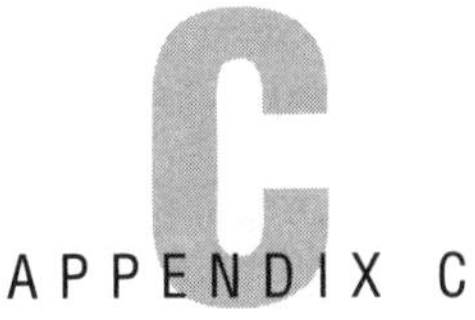

APPENDIX C

Alphabetical Listing of Nursing Boards in the United States and Protectorates

This appendix contains contact information for nursing boards found throughout the United States. The information found here is current as of this writing, but be aware that names, phone numbers, and websites do change. If the information found here is not completely current, most likely some of the information will be useful enough for you to still make contact with the organization. If all the information is incorrect, a helpful hint is to use an Internet search engine, such as Yahoo! or Google, and enter the name of the nursing board you are trying to contact. In addition, the following website keeps an up to date register of the different boards of nursing in the U.S. and its territories: https://www.ncsbn.org/515.htm. Most likely, you'll find some contact information. Also, if you don't have access to the Internet, contact your state government because they should be able to help you find the information you need.

Alabama Board of Nursing
Mailing Address:

P O Box 303900
Montgomery, AL 36130-3900

Physical Address:

770 Washington Avenue
RSA Plaza, Suite 250
Montgomery, AL 36104

Phone: 800.656.5318
Fax: 334.293.5201

Contact person: N. Genell Lee, MSN, JD, RN, Executive Officer
Website: http://www.abn.alabama.gov

Alaska Board of Nursing
550 West Seventh Avenue, Suite 1500
Anchorage, AK 99501-3567

Phone: 907-269-8161
Fax: 907-269-8196

Contact person: Nancy Sanders, PhD, RN, Executive Administrator
Website: http://www.dced.state.ak.us/occ/pnur.htm

American Samoa Health Services
Regulatory Board
LBJ Tropical Medical Center
Pago Pago, AS 96799

Phone: 684-633-1222
Fax: 684-633-1869

Contact person: Toaga Atuatasi Seumalo, MS, RN, Executive Secretary

Arizona State Board of Nursing
4747 North 7th Street, Suite 200
Phoenix, AZ 85014-3655

Phone: 602-771-7800
Fax: 602-771-7888

Contact person: Joey Ridenour, MN, RN, FANN, Executive Director
Website: http://www.azbn.gov/

Arkansas State Board of Nursing
University Tower Building
1123 S. University, Suite 800
Little Rock, AR 72204-1619

Phone: 501-686-2700
Fax: 501-686-2714

Contact person: Sue Tedford, MSNc, RN, Executive Director
Website: http://www.arsbn.org/

California Board of Registered Nursing
1625 North Market Boulevard, Suite N-217, Sacramento, CA 95834-1924

Phone: 916-322-3350
Fax: 916-574-8637

Contact person: Louise Bailey, MEd, RN, Executive Officer
Website: http://www.rn.ca.gov/

California Board of Vocational Nurses and Psychiatric Technicians
2535 Capitol Oaks Drive, Suite 205
Sacramento, CA 95833

Phone: 916-263-7800
Fax: 916-263-7859

Contact person: Teresa Bello-Jones, JD, MSN, RN, Executive Officer
Website: http://www.bvnpt.ca.gov/

Colorado Board of Nursing
1560 Broadway, Suite 880
Denver, CO 80202

Phone: 303-894-2430
Fax: 303-894-2821

Contact person: Kenneth Julien, JD, Program Director
Website: http://www.dora.state.co.us/nursing/

Connecticut Board of Examiners for Nursing
Dept. of Public Health
410 Capitol Avenue, MS# 13PHO
P.O. Box 340308
Hartford, CT 06134-0328

Phone: 860-509-7624
Fax: 860-509-7553

Contact person: Jennifer L. Filippone, Chief, Practitioner Licensing and Investigations Section
Website: http://www.ct.gov/dph/cwp/view.asp?a=3143&q=388910

Delaware Board of Nursing
861 Silver Lake Boulevard
Cannon Building, Suite 203
Dover, DE 19904

Phone: 302-744-4500
Fax: 302-739-2711

Contact person: Pamela Zickafoose, Ed.D, RN, CNA-BC, CNE, Executive Director
Website: http://dpr.delaware.gov/boards/nursing/

District of Columbia Board of Nursing
Department of Health
Health Professional Licensing Administration
899 North Capitol Street, NE
Washington, DC 20002

Phone: 877-672-2174
Fax: 202-727-8471

Contact person: Karen Scipio-Skinner, MSN, RNC, Executive Director
Website: http://hpla.doh.dc.gov/hpla/cwp/view,A,1195,Q,488526,hplaNav,|30661|,.asp

Florida Board of Nursing
Mailing address:
4052 Bald Cypress Way, BIN C02
Tallahassee, FL 32399-3252

Street address:
4042 Bald Cypress Way, Room 120
Tallahassee, FL 32399

Phone: 850-245-4125
Fax: 850-245-4172

Contact person: Joe Baker, Jr., Executive Director
Website: http://www.doh.state.fl.us/mqa/nursing/index.html

Georgia Board of Nursing
237 Coliseum Drive
Macon, GA 31217-3858

Phone: 478-207-2440
Fax: 877.571.3712

Contact person: Jim Cleghorn, Executive Director
Website: http://sos.georgia.gov/plb/rn/

Georgia Board of Examiners and Licensed Practical Nurses
237 Coliseum Drive
Macon, GA 31217-3858

Phone: 478-207-2440
Fax: 877.571.3712

Contact person: Sylvia Bond, RN, MSN, MBA, Executive Director
Website: http://sos.georgia.gov/plb/lpn/

Guam Board of Nurse Examiners
#123 Chalan Kareta
Mangilao, Guam 96913-6304

Phone: 671-735-7407
Fax: 671-735-7413

Contact person: Margarita Bautista-Gay, RN, BSN, MN, Interim Executive Officer
Website: http://www.dphss.guam.gov/

Hawaii Board of Nursing
Mailing Address:
PVLD/DCCA
Attn: Board of Nursing
P.O. Box 3469
Honolulu, HI 96801

Physical Address:
King Kalakaua Building
335 Merchant Street, 3rd Floor
Honolulu, HI 96813

Phone: 808-586-3000
Fax: 808-586-2689

Contact person: Lee Ann Teshima, Executive Officer
Website: www.hawaii.gov/dcca/areas/pvl/boards/nursing

Idaho Board of Nursing
280 N. 8th Street, Suite 210
P.O. Box 83720
Boise, ID 83720

Phone: 208-334-3110
Fax: 208-334-3262

Contact person: Sandra Evans, MA.Ed, RN, Executive Director
Website: www2.state.id.us/ibn

Illinois Board of Nursing
James R. Thompson Center
100 West Randolph, Suite 9-300
Chicago, IL 60601

Phone: 312-814-2715
Fax: 312-814-3145

Contact person: Michele Bromberg, MSN, APN, BC, Nursing Act Coordinator
Website: http://www.idfpr.com/dpr/WHO/nurs.asp

Indiana State Board of Nursing
Professional Licensing Agency
402 W. Washington Street, Room W072
Indianapolis, IN 46204
Phone: 317-234-2043
Fax: 317-233-4236
Contact person Elizabeth Kiefner Crawford, Board Director
Website: http://www.in.gov/pla/nursing.htm

Iowa Board of Nursing
RiverPoint Business Park
400 S.W. 8th Street, Suite B
Des Moines, IA 50309-4685
Phone: 515-281-3255
Fax: 515-281-4825
Contact person: Lorinda Inman, MSN, RN, Executive Director
Website: http://nursing.iowa.gov/

Kansas State Board of Nursing
Landon State Office Building
900 S.W. Jackson, Suite 1051
Topeka, KS 66612
Phone: 785-296-4929
Fax: 785-296-3929
Contact person: Mary Blubaugh, MSN, RN, Executive Administrator
Website: http://www.ksbn.org/

Kentucky Board of Nursing
312 Whittington Parkway, Suite 300
Louisville, KY 40222
Phone: 502-429-3300
Fax: 502-429-3311
Contact person: Charlotte F. Beason, Ed.D, RN, NEA, Executive Director
Website: http://www.kbn.ky.gov/

Louisiana State Board of Nursing
17373 Perkins Road
Baton Rouge, Louisiana 70810
Phone: 225-755-7500
Fax: 225-755-7585
Contact person: Barbara Morvant, MN, RN, Executive Director
Website: http://www.lsbn.state.la.us/

Louisiana State Board of Practical Nurse Examiners
3421 N. Causeway Boulevard, Suite 505
Metairie, LA 70002
Phone: 504-838-5791
Fax: 504-838-5279
Contact person: Claire Doody Glaviano, BSN, MN, RN, Executive Director
Website: http://www.lsbpne.com/

Maine State Board of Nursing
Regular mailing address:
158 State House Station
Augusta, ME 04333
Street address (for FedEx & UPS):
161 Capitol Street
Augusta, ME 04333
Phone: 207-287-1133
Fax: 207-287-1149
Contact person: Myra Broadway, JD, MS, RN, Executive Director
Website: http://www.maine.gov/boardofnursing/

Maryland Board of Nursing
4140 Patterson Avenue
Baltimore, MD 21215
Phone: 410-585-1900
Fax: 410-358-3530
Contact person: Patricia Ann Noble, MSN, RN Executive Director
Website: http://www.mbon.org/

Massachusetts Board of Registration in Nursing
Commonwealth of Massachusetts
239 Causeway Street, Suite 500, 5th Floor
Boston, MA 02114

Phone: 617-973-0900 / 800-414-0168
Fax: 617-973-0984

Contact person: Rula Faris Harb, MS, RN, Executive Director
Website: http://www.mass.gov/dpl/boards/rn/

Michigan/DCH/Bureau of Health Professions
Ottawa Towers North
611 W. Ottawa, 1st Floor
Lansing, MI 48933

Phone: 517-335-0918
Fax: 517-373-2179

Contact person: Vacant
Website: http://www.michigan.gov/healthlicense

Minnesota Board of Nursing
2829 University Avenue SE
Suite 200
Minneapolis, MN 55414

Phone: 612-617-2270
Fax: 612-617-2190

Contact person: Shirley Brekken, MS, RN, Executive Director
Website: http://www.nursingboard.state.mn.us/

Mississippi Board of Nursing
1080 River Oaks Drive
Flowood, MS 39232

Phone: 601-664-9303
Fax: 601-664-9304

Contact person: Melinda E. Rush, DSN, FNP, Executive Director
Website: http://www.msbn.state.ms.us/

Missouri State Board of Nursing
3605 Missouri Boulevard
P.O. Box 656
Jefferson City, MO 65102-0656

Phone: 573-751-0681
Fax: 573-751-0075

Contact person: Lori Scheidt, BS, Executive Director
Website: http://pr.mo.gov/nursing.asp

Montana State Board of Nursing
301 South Park
Suite 401
P.O. Box 200513
Helena, MT 59620-0513

Phone: 406-841-2340
Fax: 406-841-2305

Contact person: Cynthia Gustafson, PhD, RN, Executive Director
Website: http://bsd.dli.mt.gov/license/bsd_boards/nur_board/board_page.asp

Nebraska Board of Nursing
301 Centennial Mall South
Lincoln, NE 68509-4986

Phone: 402-471-4376
Fax: 402-471-1066

Contact person: Diana Baker, MSN, RN, Executive Director
Website: www.hhs.state.ne.us/crl/nursing/nursingindex.htm

Nevada State Board of Nursing
5011 Meadowood Mall, Suite 300
Reno, NV 89502

Phone: 775-687-7700
Fax: 775-687-7707

Contact person: Debra Scott, MS, RN, FRE, Executive Director
Website: http://www.nursingboard.state.nv.us/

New Hampshire Board of Nursing
21 South Fruit Street, Suite 16
Concord, NH 03301-2341

Phone: 603-271-2323
Fax: 603-271-6605

Contact person: Margaret Walker, MBA, BSN, RN, Executive Director
Website: http://www.state.nh.us/nursing/

New Jersey Board of Nursing
P.O. Box 45010
124 Halsey Street, 6th Floor
Newark, NJ 07101

Phone: 973-504-6430
Fax: 973-648-3481

Contact person: George Hebert, Executive Director
Website: http://www.state.nj.us/lps/ca/medical/nursing.htm

New Mexico Board of Nursing
6301 Indian School Road, NE
Suite 710
Albuquerque, NM 87110

Phone: 505-841-8340
Fax: 505-841-8347

Contact person: Nancy Darbro, PhD, APRN, CNS, LPCC, LADAC, Interim Executive Director
Website: http://www.bon.state.nm.us/

New York State Board of Nursing
Education Bldg.
89 Washington Avenue
2nd Floor West Wing
Albany, NY 12234

Phone: 518-474-3817, extension 120
Fax: 518-474-3706

Contact person: Barbara Zittel, PhD, RN, Executive Secretary
Website: www.op.nysed.gov/prof/nurse/

North Carolina Board of Nursing
4516 Lake Boone Trail
Raleigh, NC 27607

Phone: 919-782-3211
Fax: 919-781-9461

Contact person: Julia L. George, RN, MSN, FRE, Executive Director
Website: http://www.ncbon.com/

North Dakota Board of Nursing
919 South 7th Street, Suite 504
Bismarck, ND 58504

Phone: 701-328-9777
Fax: 701-328-9785

Contact person: Constance Kalanek, PhD, RN, Executive Director
Website: http://www.ndbon.org/

Northern Mariana Islands
Regular Mailing Address
P.O. Box 501458
Saipan, MP 96950

Street Address (for FedEx and UPS)
Commonwealth Health Center,
New Administration Bldg.
Navy Hill
Saipan, MP 96950

Phone: 670-234-8950, ext. 3587
Fax: 670-664-4813

Contact person: Aurelia G. Long, RNC, FNP, Board Chairperson

Ohio Board of Nursing
17 South High Street, Suite 400
Columbus, OH 43215-3413

Phone: 614-466-3947
Fax: 614-466-0388

Contact person: Betsy J. Houchen, RN, MS, JD, Executive Director
Website: http://www.nursing.ohio.gov/

Oklahoma Board of Nursing
2915 N. Classen Boulevard, Suite 524
Oklahoma City, OK 73106

Phone: 405-962-1800
Fax: 405-962-1821

Contact person: Kimberly Glazier, M.Ed., RN, Executive Director
Website: http://www.ok.gov/nursing/

Oregon State Board of Nursing
17938 SW Upper Boones Ferry Rd
Portland, OR 97224

Phone: 971-673-0865
Fax: 971-673-0684

Contact person: Holly Mercer, JD, RN, Executive Director
Website: http://www.osbn.state.or.us/

Pennsylvania State Board of Nursing
P.O. Box 2649
Harrisburg, PA 17105-2649

Phone: 717-783-7142
Fax: 717-783-0822

Contact person: Laurette D. Keiser, RN, MSN, Executive Secretary/Section Chief
Website: http://www.portal.state.pa.us/portal/server.pt/community/state_board_of_nursing/12515

Rhode Island Board of Nurse Registration and Nursing Education
105 Cannon Building
Three Capitol Hill
Providence, RI 02908

Phone: 401-222-5700
Fax: 401-222-3352

Contact person: Pamela McCue, MS, RN, Executive Officer
Website: http://www.health.ri.gov/

South Carolina State Board of Nursing
Mailing Address:
P.O. Box 12367
Columbia, SC 29211

Physical Address:
Synergy Business Park, Kingstree Building
110 Centerview Drive, Suite 202
Columbia, SC 29210

Phone: 803-896-4550
Fax: 803-896-4525

Contact person: Joan K. Bainer, MN, RN, NE, BC, Administrator
Website: http://www.llr.state.sc.us/pol/nursing

South Dakota Board of Nursing
4305 South Louise Avenue, Suite 201
Sioux Falls, SD 57106-3115

Phone: 605-362-2760
Fax: 605-362-2768

Contact person: Gloria Damgaard, RN, MS, Executive Secretary
Website: http://www.state.sd.us/doh/nursing/

Tennessee State Board of Nursing
227 French Landing, Suite 300
Heritage Place MetroCenter
Nashville, TN 37243

Phone: 615-532-5166
Fax: 615-741-7899

Contact person: Elizabeth Lund, MSN, RN, Executive Director
Website: http://health.state.tn.us/Boards/Nursing/index.htm

Texas Board of Nurse Examiners
333 Guadalupe, Suite 3-460
Austin, TX 78701

Phone: 512-305-7400
Fax: 512-305-7401

Contact person: Katherine Thomas, MN, RN, Executive Director
Website: http://www.bon.state.tx.us/

Utah State Board of Nursing
Heber M. Wells Bldg., 4th Floor
160 East 300 South
Salt Lake City, UT 84111

Phone: 801-530-6628
Fax: 801-530-6511

Contact person: Laura Poe, MS, RN, Executive Administrator
Website: http://www.dopl.utah.gov/licensing/nursing.html

Vermont State Board of Nursing
Office of Professional Regulation
National Life Building North F1.2
Montpelier, Vermont 05620-3402

Phone: 802-828-2396
Fax: 802-828-2484

Contact person: Linda Davidson, APRN, Executive Director
Website: http://www.vtprofessionals.org/opr1/nurses/

Virgin Islands Board of Nurse Licensure
Mailing Address:
P.O. Box 304247, Veterans Drive Station
St. Thomas, Virgin Islands 00803

Physical Address (For FedEx and UPS):
Virgin Island Board of Nurse Licensure
#3 Kongens Gade (Government Hill)
St. Thomas, Virgin Islands 00802

Phone: 340-776-7131
Fax: 340-777-4003

Contact person: Diane Ruan-Viville, MA, BSN, RN, Executive Director
Website: http://www.vibnl.org/

Virginia Board of Nursing
Department of Health Professions
Perimeter Center
9960 Mayland Drive, Suite 300
Henrico, Virginia 23233

Phone: 804-367-4515
Fax: 804-527-4455

Contact person: Jay Douglas, RN, MSM, CSAC, Executive Director
Website: www.dhp.virginia.gov/nursing

Washington State Nursing Care Quality Assurance Commission
Department of Health
HPQA #6
310 Israel Rd. SE
Tumwater, WA 98501-7864

Phone: 360.236.4700
Fax: 360.236.4738
Contact Person: Paula Meyer, MSN, RN, Executive Director
Website: www.doh.wa.gov/hsqa/professions/nursing/default.htm

West Virginia Board of Examiners for Registered Professional Nurses
101 Dee Drive
Charleston, WV 25311

Phone: 304-558-3596
Fax: 304-558-3666

Contact person: Laura Rhodes, MSN, RN, Executive Director
Website: http://www.wvrnboard.com/

West Virginia State Board of Examiners for Licensed Practical Nurses
101 Dee Drive
Charleston, WV 25311

Phone: 304-558-3572
Fax: 304-558-4367

Contact person: Lanette Anderson, RN, BSN, JD, Executive Director
Website: http://www.lpnboard.state.wv.us/

Wisconsin Department of Regulation and Licensing
Mailing Address:
P.O. Box 8935
Madison, WI 53708-8935

Physical Address:
1400 E. Washington Avenue
Madison, WI 53703

Phone: 608-266-2112
Fax: 608-261-7083

Contact person: Dan Williams, Bureau Director – Division of Board Services
Website: http://drl..wi.gov/

Wyoming State Board of Nursing
1810 Pioneer Avenue
Cheyenne, WY 82001

Phone: 307-777-7601
Fax: 307-777-3519

Contact person: Mary Kay Goetter, Executive Officer
Website: http://nursing.state.wy.us/